ATTACHMENT IN MIDDLE CHILDHOOD

ATTACHMENT
IN MIDDLE CHILDHOOD

◆ ◆ ◆

edited by
Kathryn A. Kerns
Rhonda A. Richardson

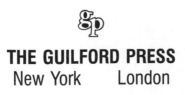

THE GUILFORD PRESS
New York   London

© 2005 The Guilford Press
A Division of Guilford Publications, Inc.
72 Spring Street, New York, NY 10012
www.guilford.com

Printed in the United States of America

This book is printed on acid-free paper.

Last digit is print number: 9 8 7 6 5 4 3 2 1

Library of Congress Cataloging-in-Publication Data

Attachment in middle childhood / edited by Kathryn A. Kerns and Rhonda A.
Richardson.
   p. cm.
  Includes bibliographical references and index.
  ISBN 1-59385-121-9 (hardcover)
  1. Attachment behavior in children. I. Kerns, Kathryn A., 1961–
II. Richardson, Rhonda A.
  BF723.A75A86 2005
  155.42′48—dc22

                                2004016929

About the Editors

Kathryn A. Kerns, PhD, is Professor in the Department of Psychology at Kent State University. Dr. Kerns's current research focuses on parent–child attachment in middle childhood, including assessment issues and how attachment is related to children's social and emotional development. She has over 30 publications, including the edited book *Family and Peers: Linking Two Social Worlds* (2000, Praeger). Dr. Kerns's research has been funded by the National Institute of Child Health and Human Development and the National Institute of Mental Health.

Rhonda A. Richardson, PhD, is Associate Professor in the School of Family and Consumer Studies at Kent State University. Her research interests relate to understanding and strengthening the family as a context for adolescent development, with a particular focus on parent–child communication in early adolescence, and parenting education for parents of middle school students. Dr. Richardson holds the Certified Family Life Educator credential, awarded by the National Council on Family Relations.

Contributors

Michelle M. Abraham, BA, Department of Psychology, Kent State University, Kent, Ohio

Massimo Ammaniti, PhD, Department of Clinical Psychology, University of Rome, Rome, Italy

Cathryn Booth-LaForce, PhD, Department of Family and Child Nursing, University of Washington, Seattle, Washington

Kim B. Burgess, PhD, Center for Children, Relationships, and Culture, Department of Human Development, University of Maryland, College Park, Maryland

Brooke C. Corby, MA, Department of Psychology, Florida Atlantic University, Boca Raton, Florida

Chantal Cyr, MA, Department of Psychology, University of Quebec at Montreal, Montreal, Quebec, Canada

Karine Dubois-Comtois, MPs, Department of Psychology, University of Quebec at Montreal, Montreal, Quebec, Canada

Silvia Fedele, PhD, Department of Clinical Psychology, University of Rome, Rome, Italy

Kathryn A. Kerns, PhD, Department of Psychology, Kent State University, Kent, Ohio

Roger Kobak, PhD, Department of Psychology, University of Delaware, Newark, Delaware

Alfons Marcoen, PhD, Department of Psychology, Catholic University of Leuven, Leuven, Belgium

Ofra Mayseless, PhD, Faculty of Education, University of Haifa, Haifa, Israel

Theresa A. Morgan, BA, Department of Psychology, Kent State University, Kent, Ohio

Ellen Moss, PhD, Department of Psychology, University of Quebec at Montreal, Montreal, Quebec, Canada

David G. Perry, PhD, Department of Psychology, Florida Atlantic University, Boca Raton, Florida

H. Abigail Raikes, MA, MPH, Department of Psychology, University of Nebraska, Lincoln, Nebraska

Rhonda A. Richardson, PhD, School of Family and Consumer Studies, Kent State University, Kent, Ohio

Linda Rose-Krasnor, PhD, Department of Psychology, Brock University, St. Catharines, Ontario, Canada

Natalie Rosenthal, BA, Department of Psychology, University of Delaware, Newark, Delaware

Kenneth H. Rubin, PhD, Center for Children, Relationships, and Culture, Department of Human Development, University of Maryland, College Park, Maryland

Andrew Schlegelmilch, MA, Department of Psychology, Kent State University, Kent, Ohio

Asia Serwik, BA, Department of Psychology, University of Delaware, Newark, Delaware

Anna Maria Speranza, PhD, Department of Clinical Psychology, University of Rome, Rome, Italy

Diane St-Laurent, PhD, Department of Psychology, University of Quebec at Trois-Rivières, Trois-Rivières, Quebec, Canada

Howard Steele, PhD, Graduate Faculty of Political and Social Science, New School University, New York, New York

Miriam Steele, PhD, Graduate Faculty of Political and Social Science, New School University, New York, New York

Ross A. Thompson, PhD, Department of Psychology, University of California, Davis, California

Karine Verschueren, PhD, Center for School Psychology, University of Leuven, Leuven, Belgium

Jennifer L. Yunger, MA, Department of Psychology, Florida Atlantic University, Boca Raton, Florida

Laura T. Zionts, PhD, Department of Educational Foundations and Special Services, Kent State University, Kent, Ohio

Preface

This book grew out of a small conference sponsored by Kent State University on the topic of attachment in middle childhood (roughly 6–12 years of age). The goal of the conference and the book is to advance theory and research on attachment in this understudied period. middle childhood (roughly 6–12 years of age). We already know a great deal about the operation, measurement, and correlates of parent–child attachment in infancy, early childhood, and adolescence. By contrast, although research exists on other aspects of parent–child relationships, very little research has been done on parent–child attachment in middle childhood. For example, the *Handbook of Attachment* (Cassidy & Shaver, 1999), which provides a very comprehensive survey of the field, has no chapters devoted to attachment in middle childhood. In fact, the topic is addressed in only one chapter (a one-page discussion on developmental changes in attachment; see Marvin & Britner, 1999). The present volume is intended to help fill that gap.

It is important to study attachment in middle childhood for several reasons. Middle childhood is an important time because many of the problems that emerge in adolescence (e.g., school dropout, delinquency, drug use) have antecedents in middle childhood. In addition, parents continue to be important sources of support to children in the middle childhood years. Despite a decline in the frequency and intensity of attachment behavior, parents continue to function as children's primary attachment figures and providers of social support during this age period. Furthermore, in order to address issues regarding continuity and change in attachment, we need conceptual approaches and assessment tools for all periods of childhood.

The authors in this volume have begun to develop a research agenda for work on attachment in middle childhood. In their issue-oriented chapters, they identify key conceptual and methodological questions, and several themes emerge from their work. First, it is clear that we need to understand attachment in relation to the normative developmental processes that occur in middle childhood. Two chapters explicitly address this challenge. Ofra Mayseless (Chapter 1) discusses several ways that the attachment behavioral system may change across the middle childhood years, and also considers how these changes may lay the groundwork for a reorienting and refocusing of the attachment system away from parents and toward others in adolescence. Rhonda A. Richardson (Chapter 2) embeds the study of attachment within a larger social context by describing individual characteristics of and changes in both parent and child that occur in later middle childhood, and asking how these changes might then affect the nature of parent–child attachment.

A second set of chapters focus on questions regarding the assessment of attachment. One reason for the lack of work on attachment in middle childhood has been the lack of well-validated methods. Investigators have started to make some progress in this area. In Chapter 3, Kathryn A. Kerns, Andrew Schlegelmilch, Theresa A. Morgan, and Michelle M. Abraham review available measures of attachment, and also discuss several questions regarding assessment that still need to be addressed. Two other chapters focus on specific approaches to measuring attachment. Roger Kobak, Natalie Rosenthal, and Asia Serwik (Chapter 4) discuss criteria for identifying attachment relationships in middle childhood and the importance of the attachment hierarchy, and also present a technique to assess whom children identify as attachment figures. Jennifer L. Yunger, Brooke C. Corby, and David G. Perry (Chapter 5) discuss their work examining avoidant and preoccupied styles for coping with attachment insecurity, which they argue are two organized styles in which there is a failure to use a parent as a secure base, considering especially how styles of insecurity are related to parenting.

A third set of chapters address issues of continuity and change in attachment from infancy to the later middle childhood years. Both chapters ask how attachment in middle childhood, as assessed in an interview, is related to child attachment and parent state of mind in regard to attachment as assessed in earlier developmental periods. The studies include parent–child attachment measures that have been well validated at younger ages. In Chapter 6, Massimo Ammaniti, Anna Maria Speranza, and Silvia Fedele assess child attachment at ages 1, 5, and 10 years, and consider factors that may explain change over time in attachment. Howard Steele and Miriam Steele (Chapter 7) assess child attachment at ages 1 and 11 years, and they investigate how parent state of mind and early attachment forecast children's later capacity to provide a coherent narrative of attachment experiences.

A fourth set of chapters examine how attachment is related to children's social and emotional adjustment. Cathryn Booth-LaForce, Kenneth H. Rubin, Linda Rose-Krasnor, and Kim B. Burgess (Chapter 8) examine in two samples how attachment is related to psychosocial functioning, with a consideration of what other variables might mediate these associations. In a similar vein, Karine Verschueren and Alfons Marcoen (Chapter 10) investigate how mother–child and father–child attachment are related to peer relationships at two points in middle childhood, while further testing whether self-worth mediates these links. Ellen Moss, Diane St-Laurent, Karine Dubois-Comtois, and Chantal Cyr (Chapter 9) examine how attachment and parent–child relationships predict children's social-emotional and academic development, with special attention to the developmental trajectories of children who form disorganized attachments to mothers. Laura T. Zionts (Chapter 11) considers how attachments to teachers may be an important factor in understanding the school adjustment of disorganized children. In addition, she considers how culture may affect the development and interpretation of attachment patterns.

In their commentary in Chapter 12, H. Abigail Raikes and Ross A. Thompson amplify and extend these themes. They identify several changes in children's cognitive, social, and emotional competencies in middle childhood, as well as changes in the larger social context, and then consider how these changes might affect the operation of the attachment system. In addition, they discuss how the developmental transitions of middle childhood have implications for assessing attachment during this age period.

We wish to thank many people for their contributions to this project. We extend our thanks to the Applied Psychology Center at Kent State University for providing funding for the conference and administrative help with organizing the conference and preparing the book. We especially owe our gratitude to Kathy Floody, who handled all of these tasks with both skill and good cheer and in the process made this project go smoothly. We also thank the participating authors for their lively and thoughtful contributions at the conference, their thought-provoking chapters, and their cooperative spirit.

KATHRYN A. KERNS
RHONDA A. RICHARDSON

REFERENCES

Cassidy, J., & Shaver, P. R. (Eds.). (1999). *Handbook of attachment: Theory, research, and clinical applications*. New York: Guilford Press.

Marvin, R. S., & Britner, P. A. (1999). Normative development: The ontogeny of attachment. In J. Cassidy & P. R. Shaver (Eds.), *Handbook of attachment: Theory, research, and clinical applications* (pp. 44–67). New York: Guilford Press.

Contents

CHAPTER 1

◆ ◆ ◆

Ontogeny of Attachment in Middle Childhood

Conceptualization of Normative Changes

OFRA MAYSELESS

Until quite recently middle childhood has been a relatively neglected period in attachment research. For example, though infancy, the preschool years, adolescence, and adulthood are all largely covered by several chapters in the recent *Handbook of Attachment* (Cassidy & Shaver, 1999), this handbook does not include any chapter that specifically refers to middle childhood. Even Marvin and Britner (1999), in their elaboration on the ontogeny of attachment theory, devote most of the chapter to infancy and the preschool years and only two pages to changes in attachment behavior beyond the preschool years. As Waters and Cummings (2000) have pointed out, this lacuna may be related to Bowlby's focus on the four developmental phases of the attachment behavioral system, which end at the goal-corrected partnership phase at age 3 or 4. Bowlby (1977, 1988) suggested that at this age the intensity of attachment behavior is much reduced, but he did not specify what happens next and only briefly elaborated on the changes expected during adolescence and young adulthood. In the words of Waters and Cummings (2000, p. 166):

1

Traditionally, attachment theory has been a theory of infancy and of adult relationships, with a great deal of what lies in between left to the imagination. Completing this picture is essential to understanding the effects of early experience, the mechanisms underlying stability and change, and the relevance of ordinary socialization processes in attachment development.

Nevertheless, in recent years quite a large number of researchers (as evident in this volume) have become interested in the interplay of attachment in middle childhood and have examined, in particular, the sequelae of attachment security and insecurity in middle childhood. Most of these stimulating approaches have looked at individual differences in middle childhood and examined their longitudinal stability or various outcomes associated with them. In this chapter I pursue a different direction. In following some of the ideas set forth by Bowlby regarding the ontogeny of the attachment behavioral system and suggestions and insights by others (Crittenden, 1992; Main, 1990, 1991; Marvin & Britner, 1999; Thompson & Raikes, 2003; Waters & Cummings, 2000), I draw attention to several ontogenetic processes that might be expected to occur in middle childhood. The following analysis is not intended as a conservative approach to theory building but as a somewhat exploratory and hopefully challenging proposal that includes various suggestions for empirical testing.

In doing so I rely on close reading of Bowlby's original works and on conceptualizations offered by Ainsworth (e.g., 1989, 1991) and others (e.g., Cassidy, 1999; Kobak, 1999; Thompson & Raikes, 2003; Waters & Cummings, 2000). In line with these conceptualizations, the attachment behavioral system is seen as a "safety regulating system." Namely, its main function is conceptualized as promoting safety, both physically and psychologically, in the context of close relationships (Crittenden, 2000). In general, two major classes of events will activate it: the presence of potential danger or stress (internal or external) and threat to the accessibility and or availability of the attachment figure. Termination of its activity will result when the situation is experienced as resulting in feeling comforted (not stressed) and secure by the actions or the presence of an attachment figure. These are considered the set goals of the system.

In this sense affect regulation of felt security may be described as a set goal. However, this similarity is based on the assumption of close correspondence between actual protection and safety and felt security. If a mismatch occurs, the person may be at evolutionary risk to be injured or to lose his or her life. Furthermore, as outlined by Kobak (1999) and by Waters and Cummings (2000), because people may derive a sense of security from various sources (e.g., good health, religious values) the set goal of the attachment behavioral system cannot be conceived as felt security in general but should probably be conceived as *felt security in the context of availability of protection in a relationship*. Thus, when the fear system becomes activated in times of perceived threat or danger, gaining access to others may be conceived as the set goal of attachment (the safe-haven function). In addition, attachment processes may be manifested when individuals are faced with challenges that only moderately activate their fear system. In such situations children and adults would use their relationships with other people who provide them with a sense of availability of support and protection as a secure base from which to explore the environment.

The operation of these attachment processes (the safe-haven and the secure-base functions) should not be equated with the existence of an attachment *relationship*. Safe-haven and secure-base behavior may be manifested even within relationships that do not qualify as attachment bonds (i.e., they are not enduring emotional ties). For example, children may feel safer and better able to explore the academic and social challenges at school because their favorite teacher or friend is there, even though these people do not serve as their attachment figures. Finally, in line with the depiction of these motivational processes as based on a behavioral system (Sroufe & Waters, 1977), the specific actions utilized to achieve the set goals are not central, and they may vary considerably depending on age, experience, culture, context, and so forth.

According to Bowlby (1969/1982), the ontogeny of instinctive behavior follows three major principles: (1) restriction of range of effective stimuli (e.g., turning to mother for comfort rather than to every adult); (2) elaboration of primitive behavioral systems and their supersession by sophisticated systems; and (3) integration of behavioral systems into functional wholes. Bowlby articulated four stages in the progression of attachment relationships whereby these principles are revealed. For example, the last phase, *formation of goal-corrected partnership*, which characterizes children mostly around the age of 3, involves the child's capacity to conceive of the attachment figure as having her own goals and interests and to take them into account (Bowlby, 1969/1982), thus demonstrating a high level of sophistication and integration. Though Bowlby himself did not suggest specific further developmental phases, several researchers discussed some of the subsequent characteristic changes in attachment organization. For example, Waters and Cummings (2000, p. 166) suggested that middle childhood is marked by "formulating and consolidating representations of secure-base experience, expectations, and skills." Similarly, Marvin and Britner (1999, p. 62) suggested that attachment at that age becomes "more sophisticated, more abstract, and less dependent on proximity and contact." In the following analysis, five different developmental processes are noted and discussed in an attempt to articulate some of the expected normative, ontogenetic changes of the attachment behavioral system in middle childhood.

THE ATTACHMENT BEHAVIORAL SYSTEM BECOMES MORE SOPHISTICATED AND GOVERNED BY COGNITIVE–AFFECTIVE INTERNALIZATIONS

Although goal-corrected partnership that includes the capacity to take into account the partners' plans and preferences evolves in the preschool years, the limited cognitive capacity at that age precludes the child from forming elaborate and sophisticated plans or symbolic internalizations. However, in middle childhood children evince growing ability (1) to reason in terms of abstract representations of objects and events, (2) to employ planned behavior that includes "adopting goals for their activities, subordinating knowledge and actions in the service of a superordinate plan, and monitoring one's activities and mental processes" (Collins, Madsen, & Susman-Stillman, 2002, p. 75), and (3) to acquire new information and use it in reasoning and problem solving. These capacities are employed also in the service of attachment processes. Thus children in middle childhood are better able than younger ones to understand their own point of view, as well as that of their caregiver; are better able to regulate their emotions and communicate about them; are more sophisticated in the plans they employ; and can better articulate and organize these plans (Thompson & Raikes, 2003). Consequently, their behavioral systems operate more smoothly as goal-corrected systems and become highly regulated by cognitive-affective internalizations, conscious as well as unconscious. Specifically, behavior becomes organized in terms of set goals and plans and includes subordinate plans and alternative ways to achieve a desired set goal, including the capacity to change the set goal. The child develops elaborate plan hierarchies and becomes increasingly aware of the set goals he or she has adopted.

This capacity for top-down processing is manifested in a more proactive approach in the child's negotiations with the caregiver and in a better capability to mesh his or her plans with those of the caregiver. These plans and the cognitive-affective internalizations are also more elaborate and flexible. Children in middle childhood find it easier to change their plans when required and are better able to implement different behaviors with different people in different circumstances, depending among other things on contextual expectations (i.e., crying or misbehaving at home but not in school). Part of this sophistication is also apparent in the verbal fluency with which children in middle childhood are able to articulate their wishes and plans regarding themselves and their attachment figures. Finally, as part of this process of sophistication in middle childhood, semantic memory becomes more multifaceted and differentiated from episodic and procedural memory. It is therefore also more susceptible to defensive manipulation.

One of the consequences of this new elaborate level of organization and operation is that individual differences in attachment security or insecurity may be construed, even more than in earlier periods, as differences in strategies whose goal is the attainment of protection from another person (e.g., Crittenden, 1992; Waters & Cummings, 2000). This position is similar to yet distinct from the statement that individual differences reflect strategies of affect regulation (e.g., Cassidy, 1994). Affect regulation (e.g., minimizing affective display) is only one of the actions that could be employed in the service of each strategy. These strategies could include different classes of behaviors, such as physical distancing, reasoning, not communicating, crying, withdrawing, clinging, and so forth. In terms of individual differences, it is not the specific behaviors that matter but which strategy they serve: The same behavior may serve different strategies. For example, withdrawal may serve a distancing strategy whose main purpose is an effort not to overtax an attachment figure with demands that she may not be able to meet in an attempt to preserve her limited protection instead of alienating her completely. Alternatively, withdrawal may serve as an elicitor of pursuit by the attachment figure. In this case it serves a coercive strategy in which different actions are employed to coerce an unresponsive attachment figure to remain available (Crittenden, 1992, 2000). Though such elaborate strategies are already displayed in the preschool years, they become more organized, sophisticated, and smoothly activated in middle childhood. Thus, when examining individual differences in middle childhood, the meaning of behavior and the purpose it serves should be the main focus rather than the overt action itself (e.g., Granot & Mayseless, 2001).

THE ATTACHMENT BEHAVIORAL SYSTEM
BECOMES MORE INTEGRATED AND GENERALIZED

One of the most intriguing processes in the ontogeny of attachment is the process of integration. As the child matures, attachment behaviors become integrated first into a strategy that encompasses various moments and experiences with one caregiver. Later attachment behaviors also become integrated into a general strategy that reflects contributions from relationships with various figures. In adolescence and adulthood, most assessment methods of individual differences identify one major attachment style, pattern, or state of mind (Crowell, Fraley, & Shaver, 1999). Thompson and Raikes (2003) discuss this presumed process and point out that as children mature attachment security or insecurity becomes increasingly an attribute of the person rather than of a specific relationship. However, they also point out that this effect may be also related to the specific measures employed in adolescence and adulthood to examine individual differences in attachment strategies or organization (i.e., the Adult Attachment Interview [AAI] and the attachment style questionnaires). Indeed, it was demonstrated (Mayseless, Sharabany, & Sagi, 1997; Ross & Spinner, 2001; Trinke & Bartholomew, 1997) that when researchers employ measures that do not require the respondent to choose one overarching attachment style, a diversity of styles with different figures can be identified. Nevertheless, a large body of research in adulthood has demonstrated that a person's generalized attachment style is associated in predictable ways with a host of relevant outcomes assessed using self-reports, reports by others, observations, and even physiological indicators (see a recent review by Shaver & Mikulincer, 2002). Thus clearly some form of integration and generalization across different attachment relationships occurs (Bretherton & Munholland, 1999).

As discussed in detail by Thompson and Raikes (2003) and by Kobak, Rosenthal, and Serwik (Chapter 4, this volume), several important questions remain unanswered. For example, how does this integration take place? What determines the relative importance of the different relationships? Do relationships with one dominant figure become the prototype, or is there a tendency to prefer secure relationships? Is there a weighing of input by each relationship depending on its significance? Are generalized models later organized in some sort of hierarchy, as suggested by Collins and Read (1994), in which there is an overarching style but also different modules depending on the type of the relationship (with parents, friends, romantic partners)? Are these modules activated as a function of key triggers depending on the context or the personality of the other person? When does this integration happen?

Preliminary findings (Kerns, Schlegelmilch, Morgan, & Abraham, Chapter 3, this volume) suggest that middle childhood may be the period in which such a process begins. However, very little is currently known about it. Thus middle childhood may be an especially fertile period in which to examine this process, preferably with the employment of a longitudinal design and assessments of attachment relationships with different figures at each point in time, along with concurrent observations of the relationships with these figures. (See Kobak, Rosenthal, & Serwick, Chapter 4, and Steele and Steele, Chapter 7, in this volume.) The significance of this process is discussed later.

THE ATTACHMENT BEHAVIORAL SYSTEM
BECOMES MORE DIFFERENTIATED AND DIVERSIFIED

Several researchers noted that during middle childhood several processes of differentiation and diversification can be identified. First, as noted by Ainsworth (1989, 1991), Weiss (1982, 1991) and others (e.g., Cassidy, 1999; Collins et al., 2002) children at that age form close affectional bonds with several additional figures besides their primary caregivers. These may include other adults, such as teachers, coaches, or members of the extended family, as well as peers and siblings. One of the intriguing lines of research facing attachment researchers is related to the questions: Are these other people attachment figures? Are these relationships attachment relationships? Can we apply attachment notions to relationships that only partially fulfill these functions? Several researchers—in particular Weiss (1991) and Ainsworth (1989, 1991; see also Cassidy, 1999)—suggested definitions of an attachment relationship as contrasted with the larger category of affectional bonds. Attachment relationships are viewed as involving a relatively long-enduring tie, in which the partner is not interchangeable with another person and in which there is a desire to maintain closeness and to reestablish proximity if it is threatened, thus regulating a sense of security. This is a relationship in which inexplicable separation tends to cause distress and permanent loss causes grief. In particular, the safe-haven and the secure-base functions are conceived as the hallmark of attachment relationships (e.g., Waters & Cummings, 2000).

In some of the relationships formed in middle childhood with other people besides the primary caregivers, attachment-related dynamics might be apparent. For example, children may derive a sense of security from being in proximity to these people (secure-base function) and may turn to them for comfort and reassurance (safe-haven function) when distressed or alarmed. For example, children in middle childhood may feel more secure and bold in their exploration if a close friend or a favorite teacher is nearby (the secure-base function). Similarly they may choose to confide in their friends regarding various upsetting situations and derive comfort and a sense of security from the friend's support (the safe-haven function). They may even become distressed if a threat of separation is perceived and protest if they become separated, for example, when a close friend moves to a different city. Though in most of these relationships only some of these elements are apparent, and though they may not be construed as attachment relationships, they are clearly relationships in which *attachment-related dynamics* operate.

In fact, as suggested by Bowlby (1969/1982) and discussed by others (e.g., Ainsworth, 1991; Waters & Cummings, 2000), even social groups may become sources of security and protection, and some attachment-related dynamics may apply even to them (see also Smith, Murphy, & Coats, 1999). In the words of Bowlby (1969/1982, p. 207):

> During adolescence and adult life a measure of attachment behavior is commonly directed not only towards persons outside the family but also towards groups and institutions other than the family. A school or college, a work group, a religious group or a political group can come to constitute for many people a subordinate attachment-"figure," and for some people a principal attachment-"figure."

Thus attachment-related processes seem to become applied and to generalize to other relationships besides those with the primary caregivers. Several important questions are related to these processes. For example, how do these relationships interact with each other? Which relationship will become a full-blown attachment relationship and which will not, and why? When do these relationships become attachment relationships? What is the impact of the relationships that do not become full-blown attachment relationships but that still provide some attachment-related functions? Are attachment figures just added, or do they replace parents in that capacity? Or do they only exchange places in a hierarchy? Because middle childhood marks the first period in which children highly invest in other relationships besides those with their primary caregivers, these questions become salient at this period. Consequently, the investigation of these relationships could shed light on these highly important normative developmental processes.

In general it seems that this process of forming affectional bonds with several additional figures takes the form of diversification: namely, a child may rely on one of the figures (e.g., a friend) to help her with one type of distress (e.g., a problem at school) and yet rely on another figure (e.g., an older sibling) for a different type of distress (e.g., problems with her dad). Whereas in infancy and probably also in the preschool years children tend to turn to one dominant figure in most of the conditions that activate the attachment behavioral system (termed "monotropy" by Bowlby), in middle childhood we may witness a diversification of "investment" in that different eliciting or activating conditions may lead the child to look for reassurance and help from different figures. Thus diversification is observed (1) with regard to the existence of a diverse group of individuals who serve attachment-related functions and (2) the tendency to regulate the request for protection and support depending on a diverse set of conditions that differentially affect who will be called. The sophistication of the cognitive–affective internalizations of middle childhood may aid in this process.

A third way in which diversification in the attachment behavioral system might be manifested involves changes in the range of possible attachment strategies. In infancy and the preschool years, four major attachment patterns have been identified. Though subtypes exist, very few researchers have ever employed this subclassification for research purposes, and in most cases researchers would collapse the subtypes into one major category. However, as noted by Crittenden (1992, 2000), close observations of preschool children, especially in non-normative samples, can expose a larger pool of individual differences. In addition, the identification of the disorganized group and the observation that these children exhibit two very different patterns as 4- and 6-year-olds (Cicchetti, Cummings, Greenberg, & Marvin, 1990; Lyons-Ruth, Bronfman, & Atwood, 1999) opened the way to the consideration of more alternatives to the usual three- or four-style classification system identified in infancy (for an observation of the sequelae of disorganization in middle childhood, see Moss, St-Laurent, Dubois-Comtois, & Cyr, Chapter 9, this volume). Similarly, in adulthood, researchers have noted the richness and diversity of styles identified in the Adult Attachment Interview (AAI), in particular with less normative samples (e.g., Turton, McGauley, Marin, & Hughes, 2001).

As underscored by Thompson and Raikes (2003), we might expect developmental changes in middle childhood to be manifested in a "broadening array of behavioral strategies reflecting more differentiated variations in security and insecurity." Taking this suggestion seriously, attachment researchers in middle childhood may need to retain open minds in terms of identification of patterns and strategies during this period and to try to refrain from imposing the three- or four-pattern format on their observations. In fact, given the expanded experience of middle childhood, the larger array of figures with whom attachment-related dynamics are activated, and the growing cognitive capacities, it might be quite naive to assume that the same three- or four-style categorization that was identified in infancy will be documented. One of the realms in which diversification in terms of strategies may occur is related to gender differences.

Although in infancy no gender differences were found in the Strange Situation classifications, several reports regarding attachment security and, in particular, patterns of insecurity in middle childhood and adolescence underscore that beginning in middle childhood we might witness some gender differences. For example, girls were found to be more secure than boys, and boys tended to show higher avoidance than girls (Granot & Mayseless, 2001; Kerns, Tomich, Aspelmeier, & Contreras, 2000). Not surprisingly, these differences start emerging following the internalization of stable gender identity and the enhanced operation of gender role socialization by the end of the preschool years. Do these differences reflect cultural norms or "true" differences? For example, are girls "really" more secure and boys "really" more avoidant? Or are these differences reflective of a behavioral style and not internal dynamics and attachment strategy? Do these differences reflect different cultural expectations for boys and girls? Or are these differences an issue of different ontogenetic normative routes for boys and girls? I believe that these questions need to be examined carefully with an open eye to the possibility of "real" gender differences. Currently, in following infancy research and the results of the Strange Situation procedure as a gold standard, researchers who find gender differences tend to minimize this finding or to refer to it as a possible caveat in their research. A careful delineation of normative changes in activating and terminating conditions in middle childhood, keeping an open mind to the possibility of observing deviations from expectations that are based on infancy research or cultural biases, is needed.

The idea that the attachment behavioral system becomes more differentiated over time looks, at first glance, contrary to the claim discussed previously that it becomes more integrated. On the one hand, middle childhood is seen as involving the beginning of a consolidation of representational models into a general one (Kerns, Schlegelmilch, Morgan, & Abraham, Chapter 3, this volume; Steele & Steele, Chapter 7, this volume; Waters & Cummings, 2000), and yet on the other hand it is assumed to involve diversification in terms of people or social groups to whom one can turn (Waters & Cummings, 2000), in terms of types of distress (e.g., pain, fear, hurt feelings) and in terms of strategies. These seeming contradictions are discussed later.

SHIFT IN RESPONSIBILITY BETWEEN CHILD AND PARENT FOR MONITORING AND MAINTAINING THE AVAILABILITY AND ACCESSIBILITY OF THE CAREGIVER

Though in the preschool years parents keep a close eye on children's whereabouts and often may feel utterly exhausted at the end of the day (Edwards & Liu, 2002), parents of children in middle childhood let them play in the park unsupervised, go to friends' houses without being escorted, and even stay home without the supervision of an adult for long hours (Collins et al., 2002). Thus at this stage parents do not have to constantly monitor the children, who are able to call the caregivers when in need or to tackle by themselves many of the challenges inherent in what previously constituted alarming situations. As Bowlby (1969/1982, p. 243) suggested: "During the course of infancy and childhood in all higher primate species responsibility for maintaining proximity between mother and young shifts progressively from the mother to the young." This shift relies on the children's better knowledge of the world and alarming situations, their better capacity to represent time and space, their better employment of various alternative plans of actions, including plans of communication, and their better capacity to take care of themselves by themselves.

The negotiation of this shift may take place smoothly or abruptly, depending on the quality of the relationship and on circumstances (e.g., the parents suddenly need to work long hours and leave the child unattended after school). In the more gradual case, the parents adjust their monitoring as they observe the child's growing capacities to correctly identify dangers and threats and to act sensibly in these situations, either by tackling them on his or her own or by summoning help. In this process the parent is seen as reacting to the child's growing capacities, and it is the child who is leading the change. Alternatively, the parent may be the one to purposefully teach the child to assume responsibility for his or her well-being; namely, the parent may be seen as leading this process of shifting responsibility. Of course, both processes may be operating in different degrees. In other, less gradual situations, the child may be pulling strongly for more responsibility, which the parent is unwilling to give, or the parent may be giving the child more freedom and responsibility than warranted by his or her capacities. Empirical examinations of this normative shift and deviations from it, as well as of the way parents and children negotiate this process, are called for. This shift in responsibility is closely tied to one of the most noted characteristics of middle childhood—the decrease in the intensity of attachment behavior, which is discussed in the next section.

DECREASE IN INTENSITY OF ATTACHMENT BEHAVIOR

Compared with earlier periods, in middle childhood attachment behaviors are displayed less urgently and less frequently. In the words of Bowlby (1969/1982, p. 179): "Until about the time a child reaches his third birthday the systems continue to be very readily activated. Thenceforward in most children they become less readily activated and they also undergo other changes that make proximity to mother less urgent." Bowlby even termed this process "waning of attachment behavior." Interestingly, Freud deemed this a latency period—namely, a period in which drives are quiescent and few libidinal processes occur; he too noted the less urgent nature of motivational forces in middle childhood.

In general, as the child grows older we might expect changes in two major domains (Bowlby, 1969/1982, p. 373): (1) the conditions that elicit/activate the system—namely, what constitutes potential danger or stress and what constitutes threat to the accessibility (availability) of the attachment figure; (2) the conditions that terminate the operation of the behavioral system.

With regard to activating conditions, we might expect two interrelated and opposing processes. On the one hand, many conditions that tended to arouse fear and a sense of threat in infancy and the preschool years may no longer pose a threat to children in middle childhood—in particular, strange people and strange places, as well as moderate levels of pain or hunger. Similarly, changes occur in what constitutes a threat to a caregiver's availability or accessibility. With the growing cognitive and executive capacities of middle childhood, long duration of separations and large distances may no longer be perceived as a threat to the accessibility of the attachment figure. This might be related to the restriction in the range of stimuli noted by Bowlby as characterizing the ontogenetic progression of behavioral systems (see the preceding discussion). On the other hand, new conditions that elicit fear or distress in older children, but not in younger ones, emerge. Many of these conditions involve self-related threats, such as hurt pride, shame, guilt, inability to measure up to expectations, and being rejected by peers. Thus it is not clear that in the final count we should expect a decrease in the number and prevalence of cases or conditions that could potentially activate the attachment behavioral system. Similarly, these changes do not imply that the intensity of the distress (and hence the intensity of the attachment behavior) should decrease. A rejection by peers may cause as much distress as a hurt knee.

A related change in the conditions that terminate the operation of the behavioral system occurs. In general, in middle childhood a larger range of conditions is available (not just touch and proximity). These new conditions are in most cases less intense (a reassuring glance instead of picking up the child), and some are even symbolic (letters, e-mail messages). Yet, again, in and of themselves these changes do not necessitate the decrease in intensity. For example, a child using phone calls instead of visibility or actual touch to assure accessibility may still engage in this behavior many times a day. Thus, though the decrease in intensity and frequency of activation of attachment behavior was clearly noted by Bowlby and others (Marvin & Britner, 1999; Thompson & Raikes, 2003), the changes described in activating and terminating conditions do not automatically imply such a drop, which still remains unexplained.

Interestingly, there has been little attempt to note and describe this normative process. Observational studies in naturalistic settings and survey studies (asking children and caregivers to report on their experience) are needed to help elucidate what constitutes normative activation of attachment behavior during this period. For example, would we consider it ontogenetically normative if a 10-year-old cried upon hurting her knee after falling and from that time on wanted to stay close to her mom? Would we consider it ontogenetically normative if a 12-year-old missed his dad so much after several days in a camp that he terminated the stay in the camp and came home a week earlier than planned? This question is highly important for descriptive purposes and for policy making. For example, should we observe that at this age separations longer than a week are perceived by most children as stressing and as a threat to the accessibility of their attachment figures, we might want to caution institutions and parents against devising a 4-week summer camp with no visitation.

Research on attachment in infancy needed several studies and films by the Robertson couple (Robertson & Robertson, 1972, 1989) and careful natural observations by researchers such as Mary Ainsworth (1967) in naturalistic settings in order to present descriptions of normative activation of attachment behavior—observations that refuted some of the strongly held beliefs of that time. Nothing like that has been done in research on middle childhood. This is not a trivial task. Similar arguments regarding the need to examine normative manifestations of attachment in different age groups have been raised by Fonagy (2001). The lacunae in descriptions of normative changes in activating and terminating conditions have been especially apparent during the construction of assessment tools of individual differences in attachment security in middle childhood. Most researchers who have attempted to develop measures to assess individual differences in attachment in middle childhood had to struggle with this question. For example, when employing a narrative approach, should we have a departure story stem with one night separation, two nights, or a whole week (e.g., Granot & Mayseless, 2001)? Should a child who says he does not need his mom to stay with him in the mall be considered avoidant or secure (see Yunger, Corby, & Perry, Chapter 5, this volume)? In addition, what is normative may also differ across cultures.

As indicated by Bowlby and others (e.g., Thompson & Raikes, 2003), the changes in the intensity of attachment behaviors are a direct result of experience (e.g., much of what was strange is now familiar), learned capacities (e.g., major advances in children's capacity to take care of themselves in many daily yet possibly dangerous situations), cognitive changes that allow a better grasp of time and place and representations of various situations, and last but not least biological changes in the central nervous system and its related endocrine system. It is my contention that the presumed drop in arousal of the attachment behavioral system cannot be ascribed only to learning processes that are gradual and ongoing. Thus the current point of view assumes a central role for maturational processes that are biological in their nature. This is also related to the fact that, despite marked individual differences in attachment relationships and experiences, the very large majority of children in middle childhood are able to tolerate much longer separations than toddlers are, and this ability is not related only to changes in their cognitive capacity in representing time, space, and the caregiver. For example, cognitive capacity cannot easily account for the fact that most 10-year-olds will probably find 1 week of separation tolerable but 3 weeks too much to bear (Bowlby, 1973). Thus attachment research might need to consider biological changes and try to incorporate these aspects as well into research designs. The works by Insel (1997) and others regarding the neurobiological basis of attachment behavior could be illuminating in this respect.

EVOLUTIONARY ANALYSIS: MIDDLE CHILDHOOD AS A PHASE OF "LAYING THE GROUNDWORK FOR REFOCUSING AND REORIENTING ATTACHMENT INVESTMENT FROM PRIMARY CAREGIVERS TO OTHERS"

Besides the need to describe the normative drop in the intensity of display of attachment behavior, one of the exciting challenges is an attempt to explain *why* all this occurs. Interestingly, though Bowlby (1969/1982) noted this process and briefly described some of the other normative changes elucidated previously (e.g., diversification), he did not explain why, in his opinion, these changes take place or what is *the evolutionary significance of this presumably universal process*. Nevertheless, he suggested several proximal causes: mother's rebuff of attachment behavior, child's growing curiosity and exploration, growing cognitive capacity and hormonal changes. Yet the ultimate cause was not fully explicated. In general I suggest that this decrease in the intensity of attachment behavior, which characterizes the move to middle childhood, marks the phase in which *preparations for refocusing and reorienting the investment in affectional attachment bond between children and their parents or primary caregivers* occurs.

For most of human evolutionary history, children during middle childhood were already considered little adults in terms of responsibilities and expectations. In a chapter addressing parenting in middle childhood, Collins, Madsen, and Susman-Stillman summarize this as follows (2002, p. 74):

> In diverse cultures, early-middle childhood historically has marked a major shift in children's relationships with adults. The age of 6 or 7 years was the time at which children were absorbed into the world of adults, helping to shoulder family responsibilities and working alongside their elders. Well into the 18th century in Western nations, many children left home by the age of 6 or 7 years to work as servants in other households (Aries, 1965). If children remained at home, their parents became more like supervisors or overseers.

Though in today's industrialized nations most children are no longer "absorbed into the world of adults," they nevertheless leave their parents for long hours to start their compulsory schooling and to play and socialize with peers, preparing for eventual responsibilities. The noted decline in intensity of attachment behavior, which probably rests on evolutionary origin, might therefore be the basis enabling this normative change toward greater investment in exploration and learning.

Applying an evolutionary rationale, it might be expected that once children secure a moderate level of protection and safety, they need: (1) to learn to be *self-sustaining and autonomous*—to fend for themselves and eventually to protect themselves and their progeny (Caporael, 2001); (2) to learn to live in a group and *get along with peers their own age* so that they will be better able to protect themselves, find food, and survive (Ainsworth, 1989; Smith, Coats & Murphy, 2001); and eventually (3) to *find a mate who does not share their gene pool* (Caporael, 2001; Simpson, 1999; Smith et al., 2001). To be better able to accomplish most of these tasks, children need eventually to partially withdraw behaviorally and emotionally from their investment in the close relationships with their parents or primary caregivers. Freud referred to this process as *decathexis* of primary objects (Rycroft, 1995). "Cathexis" represents the conscious or unconscious attachment or binding of emotional feeling and significance (psychic energy) to an idea or a person. The withdrawal of cathexis, or "decathexis," refers to detachment of interest, attention, emotional involvement, or energy (libido) from one person or problem so that it can be reinvested in oneself or in another area. Though Freud's terminology is based on a different model of human motivation and human development than the model adopted by attachment theory, I suggest that a process reminiscent of decathexis starts to occur in middle childhood. This process involves some form of preliminary withdrawal of investment, which includes change in focus and reorientation of the affectional attachment bond between children and their parents or primary caregivers toward peers or non–family members.

Current research clearly demonstrates (e.g., Zarit & Eggebeen, 2002) that the withdrawal of investment is only partial and that, in most human societies, some form of affectional bond, sometimes quite strong, continues to be present between children and their parents throughout adulthood. Yet the affectional focus changes, and in adulthood individuals primarily focus on peers and romantic partners (Hazan & Zeifman, 1994; Trinke & Bartholomew, 1997). This process of partial withdrawal of investment is evolutionary expected because children who do not develop relationships with a group of agemates but instead continue to rely on their parents for protection may eventually find themselves unprotected when their parents age, lose their capacity to help their children, and eventually die. Similarly, in our evolutionary history, if children did not transfer their emotional investment from parents to a sexual mate and then to their own children, they had lower chances of ever finding a mate and much lower chances of ever having their own children grow up to be adults themselves. Hence their genes may have not survived human evolutionary history.

Employing an evolutionary adaptability rationale, this phase is considered highly important as a preparatory phase for adolescence. By early adolescence, when puberty begins, children's rising sexual motivation should be directed outside their gene pool—namely, not toward the family or toward primary caregivers. Indeed, most researchers of adolescence noted the drop in quality of relationships with parents around puberty (see a summary in Steinberg & Silk, 2002), and psychoanalytically oriented researchers (e.g., Blos, 1979) suggested that this drop serves to distance the young adolescent from the possibility of directing sexual desires toward primary caregivers. Combining these psychoanalytic and evolutionary points of view with tenets of attachment theory (e.g., Allen & Land, 1999), it seems that to be able to feel secure and protected even during this phase (puberty) adolescents may need to have *already* secured other sources of attachment security besides their relationships with their primary caregivers.

In other words, it is here suggested that humans have an evolutionary-based developmental tendency to partially withdraw from their investment in close relationships with their parents or primary caregivers (to refocus and reorient their investment) and to invest instead in (1) building their autonomous capacities, (2) getting along with their peer group and securing their cooperation and protection, and (3) finding a sexual mate and raising their own progeny. It is further proposed that this process starts to be evident during middle childhood, when children start laying the foundation for the possibility of partial transfer later on.

The various normative developmental processes of attachment in middle childhood described here may be viewed as reflecting the general evolutionary process that prepares the child for this partial transfer in investment. This is reflected in four different ways. First, the intensity of attachment behavior decreases and the behavioral system is activated less often, thus allowing more time and energy to be invested in other domains. Second, the shift in responsibility between child and parent for monitoring and maintaining the availability and accessibility of the caregiver may also be seen as serving the same function. Namely, by allowing the child more autonomy in the decision of when to summon the attachment figure and by reducing the frequency of such calls, this change leaves the child more freedom to explore the inanimate world, as well as other relationships. Much of the knowledge about the world that humans need to acquire to become autonomous, to reach adulthood unharmed, and to raise their own progeny is not prewired but is learned by engaging in explorations and negotiations with the inanimate world, as well as with the peer group. A strong internal (evolutionary-based) motivation to learn these capacities in these contexts (e.g., the sociable or affiliative behavioral system, Cassidy, 1999; the exploratory behavioral system or effectance motivation, White, 1959) might be one of the main driving forces in middle childhood and might be more of a concern at this age than protection and safety, which are the most apparent concerns in infancy and even the preschool years.

Third, the process by which the attachment behavioral system becomes more sophisticated and governed by cognitive–affective internalizations opens the door for the consolidation of attachment representations from different figures to an overarching generalized internal model, though the unique contributions of the different figures may still exert their influence. This process leads eventually to a situation in which attachment security becomes more an attribute of the person, part of the individual's personality, than a characteristic of a specific relationship. This allows some independence from the actual relationship with the specific figure and the possibility of transfer of emotional investment to other figures.

Fourth, while holding on to the attachment relationship with the primary caregiver (in which attachment behaviors are nevertheless activated less intensely), children in middle childhood are able to explore close relationships with others. Primary caregivers still remain the main anchor, and if a serious threat arises children are most likely to use their primary caregivers as a safe haven and a secure base. Nevertheless, the partial withdrawal of investment and its refocusing is reflected in the tendency to turn also to others in times of distress or when upset. Furthermore, in some situations children may even *prefer* to rely on peers for support rather than on primary caregivers (e.g., disclosing a secret about wrongdoing).

Bowlby coined the term "monotropy" to refer to the tendency of infants to prefer a principal attachment figure. Some researchers contend that even in adulthood an individual tends to prefer a principal attachment figure (e.g., Hazan & Zeifman, 1999). Nevertheless, preliminary results (e.g., Trinke & Bartholomew, 1997) highlight that in many cases adults form several close relationships in which attachment-related dynamics are evident, and, in addition, for different activating conditions they may have a different preferred figure. As described previously, similar tendencies are evident in middle childhood. Though at that age primary caregivers still constitute the principal attachment figures, children tend to invest in several close relationships in which attachment-related dynamics can be manifested and show a somewhat lower tendency to fo-

cus on one principal substitute figure. These new close relationships
evince only components of the attachment-related dynamics, and in any
event the investment is diversified (different people may be relied on for
different functions or in different activating conditions). This process of
differentiation and diversification serves well the evolutionary-based developmental process of refocusing as the child gradually and cautiously
examines the possibility of transfer and does not take the risk of being unprotected either by performing a quick transfer or by relying on only one
substitute figure.

These analyses may mistakenly be taken to imply that by middle childhood children no longer have attachment relationships with their parents.
As indicated herein, this is clearly not the case. Children in middle childhood continue to use their parents as attachment figures even if they display attachment behaviors less often and less intensely and even when
they explore other relationships as potential attachment-related sources.
In the words of Bowlby (1969/1982, pp. 206–207):

> Thus, although most children after their third birthday show attachment
> behavior less urgently and frequently than before, it nonetheless still consti-
> tutes a major part of behavior. Furthermore, though becoming attenuated,
> attachment behavior of a kind not very different from that seen in four-year-
> olds persists throughout the early school years. . . . Thus, throughout the la-
> tency of an ordinary child, attachment behavior continues as a dominant
> strand in his life.

It is only in adolescence, Bowlby assumes, that the attachment relationships with the parents, not just their manifestations, actually change
(Bowlby (1969/1982, p. 207): "During adolescence a child's attachment to
his parents changes. Other adults may come to assume an importance
equal to or greater than that of the parents, and sexual attraction to agemates begins to extend the picture."

SUMMARY AND CONCLUSION

Together, these processes—(1) the decrease in intensity of attachment
behavior, (2) the shift in responsibility between child and parent, (3) the
regulation of attachment behaviors by cognitive–affective internalizations
and their consolidation and integration, and (4) the processes of differentiation and diversification—are viewed as serving the general evolutionary
process of partial withdrawal from the strong emotional and instrumental
investment in primary caregivers and of refocusing and reorienting these

investments to allow the development of autonomous capacities, the formation of close relations with peers, finding a sexual mate, and raising children.

Following Ainsworth (1989, 1991) and Hinde (1979), Cassidy (1999, p. 13) discusses this process by employing the concept of "penetration." She suggests that, as the child matures, the bond with primary caregivers does not become weaker; however, the relationships may "penetrate fewer aspects of the growing child's life as he or she comes to spend more time away from the parents and to develop new relationships." Similarly Ammaniti, van IJzendoorn, Speranza, and Tambelli (2000) discuss the possibility that by early adolescence children partly withdraw from their relationships with their parents and distance themselves from them by evincing more dismissive tendencies. Thus attachment theorists acknowledge that some form of withdrawal or distancing occurs, yet they are unclear about the whole process—how it starts, what drives it, and for what purpose. The approach presented in this chapter is more radical. In some respects it echoes the psychoanalytic literature, which refers to the need of the maturing child to relinquish dependency needs and libidinal investments in primary caregivers, and the term employed by Freud and others to describe the process of disengagement from parental internalized objects—"decathexis." As discussed, unlike earlier psychoanalytic writers, I do not at all contend that a renunciation of parental relationships occurs. However, middle childhood is seen as involving the preparatory phase for refocusing and reorienting the investment in primary caregivers by laying the groundwork for nonsexual and sexual peer relationships that involve attachment-related dynamics and that develop more fully in adolescence. Still, it seems that in the efforts of attachment theory to counter psychoanalytic notions regarding the need of adolescents to sever their emotional ties with their parents (e.g., Blos, 1979), attachment theory has played down the importance of the normative (evolutionary-based) process of withdrawal of emotional and behavioral investment in primary caregivers.

Recently several researchers within the attachment paradigm (e.g., Fonagy, 2001; Steele & Steele, 1998) called for an attempt at a conceptual "reunion" between the two paradigms—attachment and psychoanalysis. In fact, several such attempts were recently published (e.g., Diamond, Blatt, & Lichtenberg, 2003; Sandler, 2003). However, these attempts mostly looked at infancy or the therapeutic relationships (but see Ammaniti & Sergi, 2003). The current approach, which is heavily based on an evolutionary approach and involves an attempt to apply insights from psychoanalytic conceptualizations to attachment processes in middle childhood, follows suit.

REFERENCES

Ainsworth, M. D. S. (1967). *Infancy in Uganda: Infant care and the growth of love.* Baltimore: Johns Hopkins Press.

Ainsworth, M. D. S. (1989). Attachment beyond infancy. *American Psychologist, 44,* 709–716.

Ainsworth, M. D. S. (1991). Attachment and other affectional bonds across the life cycle. In C. M. Parkes, J. Stevenson-Hinde, & P. Marris (Eds.), *Attachment across the life cycle* (pp. 33–51). New York: Routledge.

Allen, J. P., & Land, D. (1999). Attachment in adolescence. In J. Cassidy & P. R. Shaver (Eds.), *Handbook of attachment: Theory, research, and clinical applications* (pp. 319–335). New York: Guilford Press.

Ammaniti, M., & Sergi, G. (2003). Clinical dynamics during adolescence: Psychoanalytic and attachment perspectives. *Psychoanalytic Inquiry, 23*(1), 54–80.

Ammaniti, M., van IJzendoorn, M. H., Speranza, A. M., & Tambelli, R. (2000). Internal working models of attachment during late childhood and early adolescence: An exploration of stability and change. *Attachment and Human Development, 2*(3), 328–346.

Aries, P. (1965). *Centuries of childhood: A social history of family life.* Oxford, UK: Vintage Books. (Original work published 1960)

Blos, P. (1979). Modifications in the classical psychoanalytical model of adolescence. *Adolescent-Psychiatry, 7,* 6–25.

Bowlby, J. (1973). *Attachment and loss: Vol 2. Separation, anxiety, and anger.* New York: Basic Books.

Bowlby, J. (1977). The making and breaking of affectional bonds. *British Journal of Psychiatry, 130,* 201–210.

Bowlby, J. (1982). *Attachment and loss: Vol. 1. Attachment.* New York: Basic Books. (Original work published 1969)

Bowlby, J. (1988). *A secure base: Clinical applications of attachment theory.* London: Routledge.

Bretherton, I., & Munholland, K. A. (1999). Internal working models in attachment relationships: A construct revisited. In J. Cassidy & P. R. Shaver (Eds.), *Handbook of attachment: Theory, research, and clinical applications* (pp. 89–111). New York: Guilford Press.

Caporael, L. R. (2001). Parts and wholes: The evolutionary importance of groups. In C. Sedikides & M. B. Brewer (Eds.), *Individual self, relational self, collective self* (pp. 241–258). Philadelphia: Psychology Press.

Cassidy, J. (1994). Emotion regulation: Influences of attachment relationships. In N. A. Fox (Ed.), The development of emotion regulation: Biological and behavioral considerations. *Monographs of the Society for Research in Child Development, 59*(2–3, Serial No. 240), 228–249.

Cassidy, J. (1999). The nature of the child's ties. In J. Cassidy & P. R. Shaver (Eds.), *Handbook of attachment: Theory, research, and clinical applications* (pp. 3–20). New York: Guilford Press.

Cassidy, J., & Shaver, P. R. (Eds.). (1999). *Handbook of attachment: Theory, research, and clinical applications.* New York: Guilford Press.

Cicchetti, D., Cummings, E. M., Greenberg, M. T., & Marvin, R. S. (1990). An organizational perspective on attachment beyond infancy: Implications for theory, measurement, and research. In M. T. Greenberg & D. Cicchetti (Eds.), *Attachment in the preschool years: Theory, research, and intervention* (pp. 3–49). Chicago: University of Chicago Press.

Collins, N. L., & Read, S. J. (1994). Cognitive representations of attachment: The structure and function of working models. In K. Bartholomew & D. Perlman (Eds.), *Advances in personal relationships: Vol. 5. Attachment processes in adulthood* (pp. 53–90). Greenwich, CT: JAI Press.

Collins, W. A., Madsen, S. D., & Susman-Stillman, A. (2002). Parenting during middle childhood. In M. H. Bornstein (Ed.), *Handbook of parenting* (Vol. 1, pp. 73–101). Mahwah, NJ: Erlbaum.

Crittenden, P. M. (1992). Quality of attachment in the preschool years. *Development and Psychopathology, 4*(2), 209–241.

Crittenden, P. M. (2000). A dynamic maturational exploration of the meaning of security and adaptation: Empirical, cultural and theoretical considerations. In P. M. Crittenden & A. H. Claussen (Ed.), *The organization of attachment relationships: Maturation, culture and context* (pp. 358–383). New York: Cambridge University Press.

Crowell, J. A., Fraley, R. C., & Shaver, P. R. (1999). Measurement of individual differences in adolescent and adult attachment. In J. Cassidy & P. R. Shaver (Eds.), *Handbook of attachment: Theory, research, and clinical applications* (pp. 434–465). New York: Guilford Press.

Diamond, D., Blatt, S. J., & Lichtenberg, J. (2003). Epilogue. *Psychoanalytic Inquiry, 23*(1), 207–209.

Edwards, C. P., & Liu, W. L. (2002). Parenting toddlers. In M. H. Bornstein (Ed.), *Handbook of parenting* (Vol. 1, pp. 45–71). Mahwah, NJ: Erlbaum.

Fonagy, P. (2001). *Attachment theory and psychoanalysis*. New York: Other Press.

Granot, D., & Mayseless, O. (2001). Attachment security and adjustment to school in middle childhood. *International Journal of Behavioral Development, 25*, 530–541.

Hazan, C., & Zeifman, D. (1994). Sex and the psychological tether. In K. Bartholomew & D. Perlman (Eds.), *Advances in personal relationships: Vol. 5. Attachment processes in adulthood* (pp. 151–178). Greenwich, CT: JAI Press.

Hazan, C., & Zeifman, D. (1999). Pair bonds as attachments: Evaluating the evidence. In J. Cassidy & P. R. Shaver (Eds.), *Handbook of attachment: Theory, research, and clinical applications* (pp. 336–354). New York: Guilford Press.

Hinde, R. A. (1979). *Towards understanding relationships*. London: Academic Press.

Insel, T. R. (1997). A neurobiological basis of social attachment. *American Journal of Psychiatry, 154*(6), 726–735.

Kerns, K. A., Tomich, P. L., Aspelmeier, J. E., & Contreras, J. M. (2000). Attachment-based assessments of parent–child relationships in middle childhood. *Developmental Psychology, 36*, 614–626.

Kobak, R. (1999). The emotional dynamics of disruptions in attachment relationships: Implications for theory, research, and clinical intervention. In J. Cassidy & P. R. Shaver (Eds.), *Handbook of attachment: Theory, research, and clinical applications* (pp. 21–43). New York: Guilford Press.

Lyons-Ruth, K., Bronfman, E., & Atwood, G. (1999). A relational diathesis model of hostile–helpless states of mind: Expressions in mother–infant interaction. In J. Solomon & C. George (Eds.), *Attachment disorganization* (pp. 33–70). New York: Guilford Press.

Main, M. (1990). Cross-cultural studies of attachment organization: Recent studies, changing methodologies, and the concept of conditional strategies. *Human Development, 33*, 48–61.

Main, M. (1991). Metacognitive knowledge, metacognitive monitoring, and singular (coherent) vs. multiple (incoherent) model of attachment: Findings and directions for future research. In C. M. Parkes & H. J. Stevenson (Eds.), *Attachment across the life cycle* (pp. 127–159). New York: Tavistock/Routledge.

Marvin, R. S., & Britner, P. A. (1999). Normative development: The ontogeny of attachment. In J. Cassidy & P. R. Shaver (Eds.), *Handbook of attachment: Theory, research, and clinical applications* (pp. 44–67). New York: Guilford Press.

Mayseless, O., Sharabany, R., & Sagi, A. (1997). Attachment concerns of others as manifested in parental, spousal and friendship relationships. *Personal Relationships, 4*, 255–269.

Robertson, J., & Robertson, J. (1972). Quality of substitute care as an influence on separation responses. *Journal of Psychosomatic Research, 16*, 261–265.

Robertson, J., & Robertson, J. (1989). *Separation and the very young.* Oxford, UK: Free Association Books.

Ross, L. R., & Spinner, B. (2001). General and specific attachment representations in adulthood: Is there a relationship? *Journal of Social and Personal Relationships, 18*, 747–766.

Rycroft, C. (1995). *A critical dictionary of psychoanalysis* (2nd ed.). London: Penguin Books.

Sandler, J. (2003). On attachment to internal objects. *Psychoanalytic Inquiry, 23*(1), 12–26.

Shaver, P. R., & Mikulincer, M. (2002). Attachment-related psychodynamics. *Attachment and Human Development, 4*, 133–161.

Simpson, J. A. (1999). Attachment theory in modern evolutionary perspective. In J. Cassidy & P. R. Shaver (Eds.), *Handbook of attachment: Theory, research, and clinical applications* (pp. 115–140). New York: Guilford Press.

Smith, E. R., Coats, S., & Murphy, J. (2001). The self and attachment to relationship partners and groups: Theoretical parallels and new insights. In C. Sedikides & M. B. Brewer (Eds.), *Individual self, relational self, collective self* (pp. 109–122). Philadelphia: Psychology Press.

Smith, E. R., Murphy, J., & Coats, S. (1999). Attachment to groups: Theory and measurement. *Journal of Personality and Social Psychology, 77*, 94–110.

Sroufe, L. A., & Waters, E. (1977). Attachment as an organizational construct. *Child Development, 48*, 1184–1199.

Steele, H., & Steele, M. (1998). Attachment and psychoanalysis: Time for a reunion. *Social development, 7*(1), 92–119.

Steinberg, L., & Silk, J. S. (2002). Parenting adolescents. In M. H. Bornstein (Ed.), *Handbook of parenting: Vol. 1. Children and parenting* (2nd ed., pp. 103–133). Mahwah, NJ: Erlbaum.

Thompson, R. A., & Raikes, H. A. (2003). Toward the next quarter-century: Conceptual and methodological challenges for attachment theory. *Development and Psychopathology, 15,* 691–718.

Trinke, S. J., & Bartholomew, K. (1997). Hierarchies of attachment relationships in young adulthood. *Journal of Social and Personal Relationships, 14,* 603–625.

Turton, P., McGauley, G., Marin, A. L., & Hughes, P. (2001). The Adult Attachment Interview: Rating and classification problems posed by non-normative samples. *Attachment and Human Development, 3,* 284–303.

Waters, E., & Cummings, E. M. (2000). A secure base from which to explore close relationships. *Child Development, 71*(1), 164–172.

Weiss, R. S. (1982). Attachment in adult life. In C. M. Parkes & J. Stevenson-Hinde (Eds.), *The place of attachment in human behavior* (pp. 171–184). New York: Basic Books.

Weiss, R. S. (1991). The attachment bond in childhood and adulthood. In C. M. Parkes, J. Stevenson-Hinde, & P. Marris (Eds.), *Attachment across the life cycle* (pp. 66–76). New York: Routledge.

White, R. W. (1959). Motivation reconsidered: The concept of competence. *Psychological Review, 66,* 297–333.

Zarit, S. H., & Eggebeen, D. J. (2002). Parent–child relationships in adulthood and later years. In M. H. Bornstein (Ed.), *Handbook of parenting: Vol. 1. Children and parenting* (2nd ed., pp. 135–161). Mahwah, NJ: Erlbaum.

CHAPTER 2

◆ ◆ ◆

Developmental Contextual Considerations of Parent–Child Attachment in the Later Middle Childhood Years

RHONDA A. RICHARDSON

The later middle childhood years, from ages 10 to 12, coincide with the beginning of early adolescence, a period of great transition as youngsters undergo multiple physical, cognitive, and social changes (Hill, 1983). Little research has examined issues of attachment in middle childhood, and even less has focused specifically on these particular transitional years. Yet there are a number of ways in which the contexts of early adolescence may be important for a complete understanding of the parent–child relationship. The purpose of this chapter is to describe early adolescence from a developmental contextual perspective and to discuss implications for attachment-related behaviors within the parent–child relationship.

Developmental contextualism is a perspective that views the essential process of human development as being composed of changing, reciprocal relations between individuals and the multiple contexts within which they live. From this perspective three key themes arise for the study of human development:

1. Children are active producers of their own development.
2. Development is a lifespan phenomenon.
3. Human development is embedded within social contexts (Lerner, 1995).

Each of these suggests implications for examining the parent–child relationship during the later middle childhood years.

First is the notion that children are active producers of their own development. According to this perspective, the relationship between child and parent is bidirectional, or reciprocal, such that not only does parental behavior influence child development but parent behavior and characteristics are also influenced by characteristics of the child. Child effects emerge largely as a consequence of a child's individual distinctiveness (Lerner, 1995). This distinctiveness includes not only genetic inheritance and temperament but also intraindividual change. That is, some characteristics of individuality are altered over time. The later years of middle childhood are a period of particularly notable transformation as children experience numerous and rapid physical changes associated with puberty. According to a developmental contextual perspective, the attachment relationship between parent and child would be expected to respond to these intraindividual changes.

A second theme of developmental contextualism is the principle that development is a lifespan phenomenon. This implies that parents, as well as children, develop as distinct individuals across life. Parents are as individually distinct as are their children. Based on their own unique individuality, parents will differentially react to the stimulation provided by the child. For example, the influence of a child on his or her parents will depend in part on prior experience the adult has had with the parental role and on the other roles in which the parent is engaged (Lerner, 1995). In this way, parent characteristics will affect the parent–child attachment relationship. Demands are placed on the child by virtue of the social and physical components of the setting, such as attitudes, values, or stereotypes that are held by others in the context regarding the child's attributes (Lerner, 1995). During the later middle childhood years, when children are transitioning into early adolescence, parents' attitudes, values, and/or stereotypes about adolescence may partially define the context of parent–child attachment. Those children whose characteristics best fit with the demands of the setting will have the most adaptive development (Lerner, 1995). In other words, those children who best fit their parents' expectations about the way a child moves into early adolescence may have the most optimal attachment relationship during this time. Thus it is important to include consideration of parental expectations and beliefs about adolescence when examining the parent–child relationship in later middle childhood.

The third important theme emerging from developmental contextualism is that human development is embedded within social contexts.
The parent–child relationship does not exist in isolation; both parent and
child are encircled by a broader social network. The parent–child relationship cannot be understood independent of the various social contexts that
surround it. Bronfenbrenner (1979) has identified multiple layers of this
broader context. Specifically, the microsystem is composed of the immediate settings in which a child is involved. In the later middle childhood
years, these typically include the family, the peer group, and the middle
school. This chapter considers these microsystem contexts in relation to
parent–child attachment. Bronfenbrenner also has defined the meso-
system (interrelations between microsystems), exosystems (systems in
which the child has no direct role but which nevertheless indirectly influence what goes on in the microsystem), the macrosystem (broader cultural values and beliefs and historical events), and the chronosystem
(movement of the entire ecological system through time). Although all of
these latter system levels have potential importance for understanding attachment-related behaviors in the parent–child relationship, they will not
be discussed in this chapter due to space limitations.

Collectively, the three key themes of the developmental contextual
perspective are reflected in this chapter in several ways. One is recognition of reciprocity in the parent–child relationship. In examining attachment during middle childhood, this chapter considers not just the child's
attachment to the parent but also the parent's caregiving behaviors toward the child. This is not a new idea, as Bowlby (1982) also described attachment as bidirectional. Attachment research has, however, tended to
focus primarily on the child's side of the relationship (Bradley, Whiteside-
Mansell, Birsby, & Caldwell, 1997). Second, the parent–child relationship
is viewed as a dynamic construct influenced by the individual characteristics and development of each party and also by contexts and changes in
contexts. This chapter considers individual characteristics and changes of
both parent and child that are particularly salient during the beginning of
early adolescence, such as physical and behavioral changes associated
with puberty and parental expectations and beliefs about adolescence. It
also considers microsystem contexts that are particularly salient because
of the changes they undergo during the beginning of early adolescence.
Specifically, family, middle school, and peer group contexts are examined
in relation to attachment in the parent–child relationship.

In this chapter, attachment is viewed in terms of behaviors and attitudes that make up the attachment behavioral system of parent or child
and reflect the attachment relationship between parent and child. These
are attitudes and behaviors that relate to the parent serving as a safe haven for the child in times of distress and as a secure base from which the

child can face new challenges (see Kobak, Rosenthal, & Serwik, Chapter 4, this volume, and Mayseless, Chapter 1, this volume). As stated previously, the focus of most attachment research and measures has been on the child's side of the relationship (Bradley et al., 1997). Child attachment to parent can include such constructs as perceptions of security (Kerns, Tomich, Aspelmeier, & Contreras, 2000); preoccupied versus avoidant coping strategies (Finnegan, Hodges & Perry, 1996); thoughts and feelings regarding attachment (Resnick, 1993, cited in Kerns et al., 2000); parental communication, trust, and alienation (Woodward, Fergusson, & Belsky, 2000); and use of the parent as a safe haven and secure base (Mayseless, Chapter 1, this volume). As operationalized in measures of these constructs, specific attachment-related behaviors and attitudes of a child in the later middle childhood years would include such things as believing the parent is responsive and available, relying on the parent for comfort and support in times of stress, ease and interest in communicating with the parent, emotional openness with and expression of vulnerable feelings to the parent, feelings of closeness to the parent, dismissing or devaluing of attachment relationships, preoccupying anger, and pessimism or optimism regarding the outcome of separation from the parent. This chapter considers ways in which these behaviors and attitudes may influence or respond to developmental changes and microsystem contexts of early adolescence.

Although less frequently studied, parent attachment-related caregiving toward a child is reflected in a variety of parenting behaviors and attitudes related to serving as a safe haven and secure base. Most extensively studied has been maternal sensitivity (see DeWolff & van IJzendoorn, 1997, for a review). Bradley and colleagues (1997) refer more broadly to parents' socioemotional investment in their child as an indicator of attachment-related behaviors and attitudes. As defined by these researchers, components of socioemotional investment include not only sensitivity (knowledge of child's needs and responsiveness to these needs) but also delight or joy, acceptance of the parenting role, and separation anxiety (worry and concern about the child's well-being). The latter has been the focus of recent work identifying anxiety about adolescent distancing and comfort with serving in a secure-base role as dimensions of parent attachment (Bartle-Haring, Brucker, & Hock, 2002; Hock, Eberly, Bartle-Haring, Ellwanger, & Widaman, 2001). For this chapter the following behaviors and attitudes have been gleaned from these and other studies as expressions of parental attachment-related caregiving toward a child in early adolescence: shared activities or spending time together; parental monitoring or knowledge of the whereabouts and activities of the child; provision of emotional or social support to the child; expressions of affection (physical and/or verbal) toward the child; open, nonconflictual communication between parent and child; acceptance of the child; sensitive responsiveness to the child; allowing decision-making input from the child; willingness to serve as a secure base for the child; and enjoying or liking the child.

INTRAINDIVIDUAL CHANGES OF EARLY ADOLESCENCE

As stated previously, a developmental contextual perspective includes recognition of the fact that characteristics of the child influence the parent–child relationship. This becomes particularly important when considering issues of parent–child attachment in the later middle childhood years, because the transition into early adolescence is marked by rapid and dramatic physical changes that make up the process of puberty. These changes in physical features of the child may yield alterations in the parent–child relationship, as reflected in attachment-related behaviors. Although a thorough discussion of all physical changes of early adolescence is not practical here, several aspects of growth are briefly reviewed because of their potential for influencing parent–child attachment.

Increases in height often begin between 10 and 12 years of age, particularly for girls. Although there is considerable variability in the timing and tempo of this growth spurt, on average girls grow 3.5 inches per year between the ages of 10 and 12 (Tanner & Davies, 1985). Boys may not reach their peak height velocity until a few years later, but when they do they average 4.5 inches of growth per year (Tanner & Davies, 1985). For both boys and girls, the later middle childhood years also mark the beginning of the emergence of secondary sex characteristics. In girls, this includes breast growth and pubic hair growth. Although the latter may not be noticeable to parents, the emergence of breast buds is more obvious and often signals to parents, as well as to the girl herself, that she is moving into adolescence. The parallel change for boys is growth of the testes and pubic hair, both of which are more private. The timing of the emergence of secondary sex characteristics in boys and girls varies somewhat by race. Recent data on girls indicate that at age 8, 48% of African Americans and 15% of European Americans show signs of either breast development or pubic hair (Herman-Giddens et al., 1997). At age 9, the corresponding percentages are 77% and 38%, and at age 10, 95% of African American girls and 68% of European American girls exhibit breast and/or pubic hair growth. By the time they reach 12 years of age, nearly all girls of both races have developed these secondary sex characteristics. Data for boys show a similar racial difference. At age 8, 38% of African American boys and 28% of European American and Mexican American boys have started genital development; at age 9, the corresponding percentages are 58% and 33% (Herman-Giddens, Wang, & Koch, 2001). By age 13, nearly all boys have begun puberty.

In addition to increase in physical stature and the emergence of secondary sex characteristics, there is a third intraindividual change at the beginning of early adolescence that may have implications for parent–child attachment-related behaviors and/or attitudes. This is an increase in moodiness. There is evidence that during the later middle childhood years when the hormone system is being activitated there are often rapid increases in hormones such as testosterone, estrogen, and adrenal androgens. These rapid increases and fluctuations in hormone levels have been found to be associated with increased aggression in boys, depression in girls, and irritability and impulsivity in both boys and girls (Brooks-Gunn & Warren, 1989; Buchanan, Eccles, & Becker, 1992; Flannery, Torquati, & Lindemeier, 1994). Additionally, research on neurological change at the beginning of early adolescence has found changes in levels of the neurotransmitters dopamine and serotonin in the limbic system. These changes make young adolescents more emotional and more responsive to stress (Spear, 2000).

There has been minimal research exploring the relation between these physical changes of early adolescence and the parent–child relationship. The research that has been done has utilized broad measures of physical change such as menarcheal status in girls or a composite measure of pubertal status (Petersen, Crockett, Richards, & Boxer, 1988), which makes it difficult to delineate effects of particular aspects of physical development. Furthermore, parent–child attachment has not been included among the examined outcomes, although many of the parent–child relationship dimensions studied could be considered attachment-related behaviors. Although this body of research is small and does not suggest specific effects of intraindividual change on attachment, it does offer evidence that this is an area worthy of future investigation.

It is plausible that how parents perceive their child's changing body may influence their expectations and interactions with them (Dorn, Susman, Nottelmann, Inoff-Germain, & Chrousos, 1990). For example, research using samples of European American children has found that as youngsters experience the physical changes of puberty, feelings of distance between them and their parents increase and conflict intensifies, especially between the adolescent and his or her mother (Laursen, Coy, & Collins, 1998). Specifically, there tends to be an increase in expressions of negative affect (e.g., conflict, anger, complaints) and a decrease in expressions of positive affect (e.g., support, smiles, laughter; Flannery et al., 1994; Holmbeck & Hill, 1991). In a study of fathers and sons between the ages of 7 and 12, Salt (1991) found that when boys reached early adolescence, both fathers and sons were less accepting of paternal touch to boys, and the amount of touch between fathers and sons decreased. More recent research has documented a similar pattern of decrease in levels of physical affection between fathers and sons following pubertal development, although other measures of paternal involvement, such as general support and spending time, remain stable (Ogletree, Jones, & Coyl, 2002). This stability of paternal involvement is less likely for girls, however. In a cross-sectional study of 9- to 11-year-olds and 12- to 14-year-olds, Lieberman, Doyle and Markiewicz (1999) found that older girls, but not boys, perceived their fathers as less available than younger girls. The distancing effect of puberty on the parent–child relationship is not as consistently observed in ethnic minority families (Molina & Chassin, 1996; Sagrestano, McCormick, Paikoff, & Holmbeck, 1999).

Extrapolating from this research, one can offer speculative suggestions about ways in which some of the specific physical changes of later middle childhood may influence a parent's caregiving behaviors toward his or her child, as well as the child's attachment to the parent. For example, moody children may be harder for parents to like and enjoy, leading to fewer shared activities and less time spent together and ultimately decreasing children's feelings of closeness to parents. Children's greater responsiveness to stress may lead to an increased need to rely on parents for emotional support. The increased irritability and impulsivity of children may lead to more conflictual parent–child communication. The larger physical size and emerging adult physique of children in early adolescence may prompt parents to begin granting more autonomy through allowing decision-making input from the child and reducing their monitoring of children's whereabouts and activities. Indeed, Bumpas, Crouter, and McHale (2001) found that parents engage in less monitoring of the activities and whereabouts of postmenarcheal daughters than premenarcheal daughters. Attachment is positively related to levels of parental monitoring in preadolescents (Kerns, Aspelmeier, Gentzler, & Grabill, 2001), so the aforementioned decrease in monitoring after puberty may signal a related decrease in attachment.

This latter attachment-related behavior in the parent–child relationship may be especially important for early-maturing girls. "Early maturing" refers to girls who complete the process of pubertal change, including full breast development and onset of menarche, before most of the other girls in her age cohort (generally, before the age of 12 or by the end of middle childhood). Research on timing of puberty has documented a number of negative effects of early maturation for girls. These include a greater risk of depressed mood, negative body image, eating disorders, substance use, delinquency, school problems, conflicts with parents, early sexual activity, and teenage pregnancy (Steinberg, 2002). One reason for these problems is that early physical development draws the attention of older boys, who then introduce these girls to an older group of friends and to some of the problem behaviors more typical of older adolescents (Petersen, 1993). Parental monitoring can play an important role in the prevention of some of these problem behaviors (Jacobson & Crockett, 2000). Parental monitoring in later middle childhood is more likely to occur when there is a secure attachment, partially because securely attached children are more cooperative with parents' monitoring attempts (Kerns et al., 2001). That is, when children have experienced their parents as a secure base and a safe haven, they may be less likely to resist parents' attempts to supervise their activities and whereabouts (Waters, Kondo-Ikemura, Posada & Richters, 1991, cited in Kerns et al., 2001).

Although, as summarized, some preliminary evidence shows that physical changes of early adolescence result in changes in the parent–child relationship, a developmental contextual perspective suggests that individual and contextual change are reciprocal. That is, attachment-related behaviors in the parent–child relationships may influence pubertal change. For example, Ellis and colleagues found that an absence of positive, harmonious parent–child relationships, and particularly low father investment in the family, was associated with earlier onset of puberty in girls (Ellis, McFadyen-Ketchum, Dodge, Pettit, & Bates, 1999). Similarly, more conflictual family interactions and greater relationship discord in the family have been found to forecast earlier menarcheal age in girls (Ellis & Garber, 2000; Graber, Brooks-Gunn, & Warren, 1995; Moffit, Caspi, Belsky & Silva, 1992). Although the underlying process is not clear, it has been suggested that distance in the family may produce a small amount of stress, which in turn may affect hormone secretions (Graber et al., 1995). Research has not assessed parent–child attachment in relation to pubertal timing, nor has onset of puberty in boys been considered, but these may be important directions for future research.

PARENTAL EXPECTATIONS AND BELIEFS ABOUT ADOLESCENCE

Certainly, not all parents have the same response to their child's entry into early adolescence, suggesting that individual characteristics of parents may play a role in influencing their behavioral responses. Variables such as parent gender, attachment style, and expectations or beliefs about adolescence are important.

Research on parents' beliefs about adolescence has distinguished between category-based beliefs (concerning adolescents as a group) and target-based beliefs (concerning individual adolescents; Buchanan et al., 1990). In terms of the former, parents of sixth graders typically believe that adolescence is a difficult time of life due largely to hormones (Bu-

Parental Beliefs

chanan et al., 1990). But they also believe there are things they can do to make their relationships with young adolescents good. In thinking about their own particular children, parents generally endorse positive expectations, such as that they will take on more responsibilities and be more serious about schoolwork (Buchanan et al., 1990). However, they also expect to have more difficulty getting along with their children and expect their children to be more concerned with what friends think than what parents think.

Parent expectations about adolescence may differ somewhat by gender. For instance, mothers have been found to be more concerned than fathers with potential difficulty, anticipating more conflict for their adolescents between what friends think and what adults think, and fearing that their adolescent would be more difficult to get along with. Fathers expected their children, sons in particular, to become closer to them and seek their advice more often. Mothers expected to become closer to daughters than to sons (Buchanan et al., 1990).

Amount of prior experience with adolescents affects parental beliefs. For example, inexperienced parents have higher expectations that their child will get closer to them in adolescence than experienced parents, but they also are more likely to expect that things will get more difficult (Buchanan et al., 1990). Additionally among mothers, recollections of one's own experiences during adolescence are related to beliefs about adolescence. Specifically, recalling one's own adolescence as difficult relates to holding more stereotypic notions of adolescents as risk taking and rebellious (Buchanan & Holmbeck, 1998).

Although parental beliefs about adolescence have not been examined in relation to attachment and attachment-related behaviors in later middle childhood, the preceding findings suggest directions for future research into this issue and two alternative sets of hypotheses. On the one hand, parental beliefs may be associated with positive changes. For example, it is possible that expectations of increased closeness to one's child in early adolescence might lead parents to be more intentional about spending time together or expressing acceptance of the child. Similarly, believing that adolescence is a difficult time of life may be associated with a greater willingness to provide emotional support or serve as a secure base for the child as he or she enters early adolescence. On the other hand, one can hypothesize about potential negative effects of parental expectations on attachment-related behaviors. For instance, expecting greater closeness to one's child as he or she moves into early adolescence may lead parents to be more disappointed by the feelings of distance and increased conflict typical of parent–child relationships at this time. Negative beliefs and expectations about adolescence may lead parents to become less accepting of their child and more inclined toward hostile, conflictual communication. As a result, parents' ability or willingness to serve as a safe haven may be negatively affected. And parental beliefs that adolescence is a difficult time of life may prompt parental anxiety about letting the child grow up.

In fact, by the time their children are in sixth grade, some parents exhibit separation anxiety in reaction to their child's entry into adolescence. Two dimensions of parental separation anxiety have been identified by Hock and colleagues (2001). Anxiety about Adolescent Distancing (AAD) refers to feelings of discomfort or loss associated with the adolescent's increasing affiliation with others and decreasing involvement and time spent with parents. Comfort with Secure-Base Role (CSBR) refers to parents' contentment with being accessible and serving as a source of security to their adolescents, who are expanding their social and physical worlds (Hock et al., 2001). Parents of sixth graders exhibit anxiety about adolescent distancing similar to that of parents of eighth, tenth, and twelfth graders, but they are more involved in providing a secure base. Although such findings suggest that parental attachment is at least partially related to a child's transition into adolescence, the extent to which parents' beliefs and expectations influence attachment remains a question for further inquiry.

Research does offer some clues as to what influences parental separation anxiety. Specifically, levels of AAD and CSBR are related to parents' mental representations of attachment. Parents who express healthy feelings about attachment relationships (i.e., have positive mental representations) report less anxiety about adolescent distancing and are more comfortable serving in the secure-base role. This contributes to higher adolescent attachment to parents and lower levels of conflict and negative communication in the parent–child relationship (Hock et al., 2001). There may be longer term implications, as well, in that mothers' comfort with providing a secure base and fathers' anxiety about distancing both have an impact on identity development in later adolescence (Bartle-Haring et al., 2002). Although there are more questions than answers at this time, it is clear that consideration of parent expectations and beliefs about adolescence is important when examining attachment in later middle childhood.

FAMILY CONTEXT

In describing the family microsystem of early adolescence, parental marital status and sibling configuration are important dimensions. With regard to the former, current statistics indicate that approximately 50% of U.S. children under the age of 18 live in intact two-parent families, whereas 28% live in households headed by a single parent and 14% live in remarried parent households (U.S. Bureau of the Census, 1998). Although children from divorced and remarried families, in contrast to those from never-divorced families, exhibit more problem behaviors and lower psychological well-being, there is little agreement about the extent, severity, and duration of these problems (Hetherington, Bridges, & Insabella, 1998). There is great diversity in children's responses to parental marital transitions, and research generally indicates that family process is more important than father absence, parental distress, economic deprivation, and stressful life experiences in predicting children's adjustment (Demo & Acock, 1996; Hetherington et al., 1998).

Levels of parent–child disagreement or conflict, parental supervision or monitoring of children, parental support such as expressions of affection, and spending time together in shared activities are components of family process important for children's adjustment (Demo & Acock, 1996; Hetherington et al., 1998). These relate to attachment functions of providing a safe haven (e.g., lack of conflict, expressions of affect) and secure base (supervision and monitoring). Furthermore, parental divorce and remarriage increase the probability that children will not obtain these from their families. For example, up to one third of young adolescents in divorced families become disengaged from their families, avoiding interactions, activities, and communication (Hetherington, 1993). And children in single-parent families may receive less monitoring and supervision of their activities and whereabouts (Kerns et al., 2001). Woodward and colleagues (2000) found that the younger the age of the child at the time of the parental separation, the greater the negative impact on child's attachment to parents by the time they reached age 15. Children who were less than 5 years old or between 5 and 10 years old scored lower on measures of parental attachment and bonding at age 15 than did children who were 10–15 years old at the time of the separation. It appears that parental separation in early adolescence has less impact on attachment than it does if the separation occurs at a younger age.

A portrait of impaired family process does not apply in every case of parental divorce or remarriage. Girls in particular often have close, companionate, confiding relationships with their divorced mothers, and early assignment of responsibilities may be associated with resilience and unusual social competence (Hetherington et al., 1998). Research on one sample of 10- to 14-year-olds found that compared with those in married-parent families, those in single-parent families spent less time with parents simultaneously but spent similar amounts of time with family overall when time with mothers and extended kin was included (Asmussen & Larson, 1991). Time spent with mothers was more likely to revolve around maintenance activities (e.g., chores, grocery shopping, meal preparation) in single-parent families but did not differ in emotional quality. In fact, youths in single-parent families experienced both parents as relatively more friendly than did youths in married-parent families (Asmussen & Larsen, 1991). Thus, although in some respects single-parent family status may be associated with less secure-base and safe-haven behavior (e.g., lower levels of parental monitoring, less parent–child communication), in other respects, particularly for children in later middle childhood, the outcome may be an increase in some attachment-related behaviors (e.g., affective bonds).

A second important dimension of family context for children is sibling configuration. This encompasses such features as the size of the sibling group (i.e., number of children in the family), ordinal position (i.e., the child's position in the age hierarchy of siblings in the family), sibling density (i.e., age spacing between siblings), and sex composition (i.e., relative number of boys and girls in the sibling group; Steelman, Powell, Werum, & Carter, 2002). Sibling configuration has been examined primarily with regard to status outcomes such as educational attainment, standardized test scores, and academic performance. There is a strong and virtually unequivocal negative relationship between family size and academic success. Close age spacing also is inversely linked to children's academic performance, whereas ordinal position has not been found to be universally related to status outcomes. Findings regarding the relative advantage of having brothers versus sisters have been mixed (Steelman et al., 2002).

In attempting to explain these sibling configuration influences, researchers have documented differences in family resource allocation. For example, as the number of children in a family increases, there is a dilution of resources, including not just economic resources but also interpersonal resources such as parental time and attention (Steelman et al., 2002). Firstborn children have an advantage over later-born siblings in access to parental time, energy, and engagement in children's lives (Powell & Steelman, 1990, 1993, as cited in Steelman et al., 2002). Wider spacing between children has been associated with greater parental reasonableness and supportiveness (Kidwell, 1981), and this benefit appears to be particularly evident in the father–child relationship (Richardson, Abramowitz, Asp, & Petersen, 1986). Sibling configuration has received very little attention in research on attachment in middle childhood. Ammaniti, Speranza, and Fedele (Chapter 6, this volume) have reported data showing that the number of younger siblings is a significant predictor of longitudinal change in children's attachment classification from ages 1 to 5. Specifically, they have found that the introduction of additional children into the family is associated with a shift from insecure to secure attachment. But family size effects on attachment in middle childhood have not been investigated.

With regard to ordinal position, Bumpas and colleagues (2001) examined adolescents' decision-making input and parental knowledge of adolescents' daily experiences in relation to birth order and found that firstborns were granted more autonomy than second-borns. It should be noted, however, that birth order and age were confounded in this sample, in that the mean age for the firstborn participants was 15 and that the majority of the second-born participants were younger, with a mean age of 12.5. Thus it is not clear whether the finding reflects an effect of birth order or an effect of child age. More recent research disentangling effects of birth order and age indicates that within the same family second-born children reported more conflict with their parents at age 11 than did their firstborn siblings when they were the same age (Whiteman, McHale, & Crouter, 2003). In these same families, parents were more knowledgeable about their second-born children's activities at age 11 than about their firstborn children's activities at the same age (Whiteman et al., 2003). Such effects of birth order on attachment-related behaviors may be at least partially due to the fact that experiences with firstborn children shape the responses of parents to their subsequent children. Some evidence in support of this comes from Whiteman and Buchanan (2002), who looked at mothers' expectations for their children's adolescence and found that experienced mothers who had a positive experience with earlier-born adolescents had higher expectations for prosocial and positive behavior in their second-born children. As discussed earlier in this chapter, it is possible that these parental expectations influence attachment-related behaviors.

Sex composition of sibling pairs also is important to consider when examining attachment-related behaviors in the parent–child relationship. For instance, Bumpas and colleagues (2001) found that the differences in decision-making input and parent knowledge of adolescents' daily experiences were most evident in sibling dyads with firstborn girls and second-born boys, such that parents were more knowledgeable about the activities of second-born boys. In contrast, however, Whiteman and colleagues (2003) reported that parents differed more in their treatment of second-born versus firstborn children when the siblings were of the same biological sex.

Obviously, much remains to be learned about the significance of various aspects of sibling configuration for parent–child attachment in middle childhood. Attachment researchers may want to include measures of family size, birth order, spacing, and sex composition when considering family context variables in relation to measures of attachment and parental caregiving behaviors.

TRANSITION TO MIDDLE SCHOOL

During the later middle childhood years, the school context changes significantly. Children move from an elementary school to a middle school, and there are a number of differences in the social and academic environments of these two. Middle schools are larger, both in terms of physical structure and number of students. In addition, students typically change classrooms and classmates for each course. As a result, students encounter much larger peer groups in middle school than in elementary school. This can contribute to disruptions in previous friendships, as there are fewer opportunities for interaction with the same peers (Hardy, Bukowski, & Sippola, 2002). Lack of recess time and multiple lunch periods can further contribute to estrangement from former elementary school friends. Additionally, the social environment is characterized by more impersonal student–teacher relationships and teachers who are less friendly, supportive, and caring toward their students (Eccles et al., 1993). The academic environment of middle school includes greater emphasis on teacher control and fewer opportunities for student decision making, more whole-class task organization, more between-classroom ability grouping, and more public evaluation of work (Eccles et al., 1993). In addition, higher standards for evaluation and grading student academic performance contribute to a decline in grades (Eccles et al., 1993).

Collectively these differences between elementary and middle school make the transition to middle school stressful for many youngsters. Numerous investigations have looked at changes in self-esteem, academic performance, and motivation as a function of the transition to middle school (e.g., Wigfield, Eccles, MacIver, Reuman, & Midgley, 1991). Declines in self-esteem have been found fairly consistently among students from urban, large suburban, and small community socioeconomically heterogeneous settings (Seidman, Lambert, Allen, & Aber, 2003). Similarly, research has consistently documented declines in academic performance (i.e., GPA or standardized achievement test scores), as well as motivation and attitudes toward school (Seidman et al., 2003). Most of these declines have been explained in terms of the previously noted characteristics of middle schools, which provide a poor developmental fit for children in early adolescence (Eccles et al., 1993). For example, school strain, such as too much homework and lack of feedback from teachers, contributes to declines in self-worth (Fenzel, 2000).

Although the importance of attachment has not been directly assessed, there is evidence that family relationships can influence the transition to middle school. A study of 500 racially and ethnically diverse urban children attending public schools found that perceptions of daily hassles or conflicts with families before the transition to middle school were associated negatively with changes in self-esteem and preparation for class (doing homework and working hard in school; Seidman et al., 2003). The researchers suggest that under conflictual living arrangements parents may have difficulty noticing children's needs for support and assistance and thus may fail to respond with appropriate social support. This seems to describe a case in which parents are failing to serve as a secure base for their children during a difficult transitional time.

Fenzel (2000) examined the role of parental support in moderating the effects of school strain. Parental support was defined as perceiving that parents understand, like, care about, and are available to help and listen to the child. Fenzel's findings indicated that support from parents reduces school strain and thus diminishes declines in self-worth during the first year of middle school. Studies such as this provide preliminary evidence that parental attachment-related behaviors may be important for helping children respond to school context changes in the later middle childhood years. Children's attachment to parents may also be important, as it is generally understood that secure attachment is associated with a more comfortable approach to new situations.

CHANGES IN PEER GROUP

Concurrent with the transition to middle school, multiple changes in peer relations take place during later middle childhood. One of these changes is in the sheer amount of time children spend with friends. As children move into early adolescence at age 10, they begin to spend more time with friends and less time with family (Larson, Richards, Moneta, Holmbeck, & Duckett, 1996). To some degree, the amount of time spent with friends is a function of attachment, in that children with insecure attachments tend to become more peer-oriented by the time they are 17 years old (Freeman & Brown, 2001). Additionally, during later middle childhood, time spent with friends is less likely to be adult-supervised. For example, in the United States 10% of 9-year-old children, 14% of 10-year-olds, 24% of 11-year-olds, and 33% of 12-year-olds regularly spend time in self-supervision during the after-school hours (U.S. Bureau of the Census, 2000). Undoubtedly, some of this self-supervised time is spent in the company of friends. A recent study of students' use of time outside of school revealed that 60% of seventh graders in an urban sample spend at least one hour per day going out with friends (Shann, 2001). Implications of this change in the structure of peer relations for attachment-related behaviors in the parent–child relationship include the obvious fact that there is a reduction in time spent in shared activities, as well as a need for parents to become more intentional about monitoring their children's whereabouts. It also contributes to the decreases in feelings of closeness between parent and child that were discussed earlier.

The transition to middle school typically results in other changes in friendships, as well. The availability of previously unfamiliar peers in the new middle school setting results in changes in friendship choices. Both boys and girls have been found to lose old friendships and acquire new ones during the first year of middle school (Hardy et al., 2002). Whereas boys maintain the same number of friends, girls exhibit more instability in the number of reciprocated friendships. That is, girls with many friendships at the end of elementary school tend to have fewer friendships during the first year of middle school, and girls with fewer elementary school friendships tend to develop more when they get to middle school (Hardy et al., 2002). Several researchers have documented the connection between parent–child attachment and children's friendship competence (Kerns, Klepac, & Cole, 1996; Schneider, Atkinson, & Tardif, 2001). Lieberman and colleagues (1999) found that during early adolescence, children who view their parents as more available and who rely on them more in times of stress report higher positive qualities in their close same-sex friendships. Securely attached youths probably approach new social relationships with confidence and positive expectations, and these youths may therefore be better equipped to handle the friendship changes that accompany the transition to middle school. Interestingly, Verschueren and Marcoen (Chapter 10, this volume) and Steele and Steele (Chapter 7, this volume) all have found that it is early experiences with and attachments to fathers, but not mothers, that are correlated with peer relations and acceptance in middle childhood. Similarly, Lieberman and colleagues concluded that father availability was particularly important for predict ing lower conflict in friendships among 9- to 14-year-old children.

The link between attachment and peer relationships becomes important in another way during later middle childhood. Bullying and social aggression, although not limited to this age group, become more prevalent as children move through early adolescence (Haynie et al., 2001). In their sample of over 4,000 sixth-, seventh-, and eighth-grade students, Haynie and colleagues (2001) found that 47% reported bullying a peer at least once during the previous year and that 44% had been victimized at least once. Among boys, bullying predominantly takes the form of physical aggression, whereas girls tend to adopt methods of social manipulation or relational aggression such as gossiping, spreading rumors, and social ostracism (Crick, Bigbee, & Howes, 1996). Parenting characterized by lack of warmth and involvement, low levels of monitoring, and either overprotection or neglect may contribute to a tendency to bully peers (Haynie et al., 2001). These parenting behaviors are often indicative of insecure attachment. Indeed, recent research has linked quality of attachment and aggressive behavior among middle school students (Simons, Paternite, & Shore, 2001). This link is mediated by social cognition and self-esteem, such that those youngsters with more insecure attachments to their mothers exhibit lower self-esteem and greater hostile attributional bias. These more negative working models of self and social relationships are predictive of higher rates of aggressive responses to peers (Simons et al., 2001).

Finally, one other area of change in peer relations with potential links to parent–child attachment is increased contact with members of the opposite sex. In early adolescence, the sex segregation typical of childhood peer groups begins to diminish, and boys and girls become more interested in interacting with one another, although there are distinct gender boundaries prescribing when and in what manner contact may occur (Sroufe, Bennett, Englund, Urban, & Shulman, 1993). For most youngsters in the later years of middle childhood, cross-gender contact consists of casual interaction in a group setting, with no element of psychological intimacy or romantic interest (Sroufe et al., 1993). Although some middle school students do claim to be "going with" a member of the opposite sex, these relationships are typically very superficial connections of short duration (a week or two) with limited face-to-face contact (Merten, 1996). Some young adolescents do enter into early steady dating relationships, and research evidence suggests that this has a number of negative effects, such as early sexual activity, lower academic achievement and aspirations, involvement with deviant peers, and problem behaviors (Doyle, Brendgen, Markiewicz, & Kamkar, 2003).

Attachment history has been found to play a role in predicting the likelihood of violating gender boundaries in early adolescence. Sroufe and colleagues (1993) found that, for their sample of 10- and 11-year-old children, a history of secure attachment was associated with less gender boundary violation (i.e., physical contact, flirting, sexual gestures toward members of the opposite gender) and more gender boundary maintenance (e.g., limiting opposite-sex contact to brief, casual group interaction). Security of attachment also plays a role in moderating the negative outcomes of early romantic involvement. For example, those young adolescents who are well integrated into the same-sex peer group and have positive relationships with same-sex friends are less likely to be negatively influenced by steady dating relationships (Brendgen, Vitaro, Doyle, Markiewicz, & Bukowski, 2002). It is likely that these are youngsters who have positive working models of relationships stemming from secure attachment to parents. These positive working models may result in not only more positive relationships with same-sex peers but also more positive dating relationships. Recent research has directly examined the role of parental attachment in moderating effects of early romantic involvement. Doyle and colleagues (2003) studied a sample of seventh- and eighth-grade students and found that security of attachment to the mother serves a protective role against negative effects of steady dating on school grades. For other outcomes such as depression and externalizing behavior problems, however, attachment did not moderate the negative effects of early steady dating. Although this is another area in which much additional research is needed, it further illustrates the value of recognizing the microsystem contexts of early adolescence when investigating attachment.

CONCLUSION

The later years of middle childhood are a time of numerous developmental and contextual changes. Little research has directly examined implications of these changes for attachment in the parent–child relationship or the converse (i.e., implications of attachment for developmental and contextual changes). In describing the salient changes and contexts of early adolescence, this chapter has suggested a number of potentially important directions for future research. Physical and behavioral changes of early adolescence, parental expectations and beliefs about adolescence, parental marital status, sibling configuration, transition from elementary to middle school, and changes in relations with peers all may be connected to attachment-related behaviors in the parent–child relationship, and all are worthy of consideration by attachment researchers.

REFERENCES

Asmussen, L., & Larson, R. (1991). The quality of family time among young adolescents in single-parent and married-parent families. *Journal of Marriage and the Family, 53,* 1021–1030.

Bartle-Haring, S., Brucker, P., & Hock, E. (2002). The impact of parental separation anxiety on identity development in late adolescence and early adulthood. *Journal of Adolescent Research, 17,* 439–450.

Bowlby, J. (1982). *Attachment and loss: Vol 1. Attachment* (2nd ed.). New York: Basic Books.

Bradley, R. H., Whiteside-Mansell, L., Brisby, J. A., & Caldwell, B. M. (1997). Parents' socioemotional investment in children. *Journal of Marriage and the Family, 59,* 77–90.

Brendgen, M., Vitaro, F., Doyle, A. B., Markiewicz, D., & Bukowski, W. M. (2002). Same-gender peer relations and romantic relationships during early adolescence: Interactive links to emotional, behavioral, and academic adjustment. *Merrill-Palmer Quarterly, 48,* 77–103.

Bronfenbrenner, U. (1979). *The ecology of human development.* Cambridge, MA: Harvard University Press.

Brooks-Gunn, J., & Warren, M. (1989). Biological contributions to negative affect in young girls. *Child Development, 60,* 40–55.

Buchanan, C. M., Eccles, J. S., & Becker, J. B. (1992). Are adolescents the victims of raging hormones: Evidence for activational effects of hormones on moods and behavior at adolescence. *Psychological Bulletin, 111,* 62–107.

Buchanan, C. M., Eccles, J. S., Flanagan, C., Midgley, C., Feldlaufer, H., & Harold, R. D. (1990). Parents' and teachers' beliefs about adolescents: Effects of sex and experience. *Journal of Youth and Adolescence, 19,* 363–394.

Buchanan, C. M., & Holmbeck, G. N. (1998). Measuring beliefs about adolescent personality and behavior. *Journal of Youth and Adolescence, 27,* 607–627.

Bumpas, M. F., Crouter, A. C., & McHale, S. M. (2001). Parental autonomy granting during adolescence: Exploring gender differences in context. *Developmental Psychology, 37,* 163–173.

Crick, N. R., Bigbee, M. A., & Howes, C. (1996). Gender differences in children's normative beliefs about aggression: How do I hurt thee? Let me count the ways. *Child Development, 67,* 1003–1014.

Demo, D. H., & Acock, A. C. (1996). Family structure, family process, and adolescent well-being. *Journal of Research on Adolescence, 6,* 457–488.

DeWolff, M. S., & van IJzendoorn, M. H. (1997). Sensitivity and attachment: A meta-analysis on parental antecedents of infant attachment. *Child Development, 68,* 571–591.

Dorn, L. D., Susman, E. J., Nottelmann, E. D., Inoff-Germain, G., & Chrousos, G. P. (1990). Perceptions of puberty: Adolescent, parent and health-care personnel. *Developmental Psychology, 26,* 322–329.

Doyle, A. B., Brendgen, M., Markiewicz, D., & Kamkar, K. (2003). Family relationships as moderators of the association between romantic relationships and adjustment in early adolescence. *Journal of Early Adolescence, 23,* 316–340.

Eccles, J. S., Midgley, C., Wigfield, A., Buchanan, C. M., Reuman, D., Flanagan, C., & MacIver, D. (1993). Development during adolescence: The impact of stage-environment fit on young adolescents' experiences in schools and families. *American Psychologist, 48,* 90–101.

Ellis, B. J., & Garber, J. (2000). Psychosocial antecedents of variation in girls' pubertal timing: Maternal depression, stepfather presence, and marital and family stress. *Child Development, 71,* 485–501.

Ellis, B. J., McFadyen-Ketchum, S., Dodge, K. A., Pettit, G. S., & Bates, J. E. (1999). Quality of early family relationships and individual differences in the timing of pubertal maturation in girls: A longitudinal test of an evolutionary model. *Journal of Personality and Social Psychology, 77,* 387–401.

Fenzel, L. M. (2000). Prospective study of changes in global self-worth and strain during the transition to middle school. *Journal of Early Adolescence, 20,* 93–116.

Finnegan, R. A., Hodges, E. V. E., & Perry, D. G. (1996). Preoccupied and avoidant coping during middle childhood. *Child Development, 67,* 1318–1328.

Flannery, D., Torquati, J., & Lindemeier, L. (1994). The method and meaning of emotional expression and experience during adolescence. *Journal of Adolescent Research, 9,* 8–27.

Freeman, H., & Brown, B. B. (2001). Primary attachment to parents and peers during adolescence: Differences by attachment style. *Journal of Youth and Adolescence, 30,* 653–674.

Graber, J. A., Brooks-Gunn, J., & Warren, M. P. (1995). The antecedents of menarcheal age: Heredity, family environment, and stressful life events. *Child Development, 66,* 346–359.

Hardy, C. L., Bukowski, W. M., & Sippola, L. K. (2002). Stability and change in peer relationships during the transition to middle-level school. *Journal of Early Adolescence, 22,* 117–142.

Haynie, D. L., Nansel, T., Eitel, P., Crump, A. D., Saylor, K., Yu, K., & Simons-Morton, B. (2001). Bullies, victims, and bully-victims: Distinct groups of at-risk youth. *Journal of Early Adolescence, 21,* 29–49.

Herman-Giddens, M. E., Slora, E. J., Wasserman, R. C., Bourdony, C. J., Bhapkar, M. V., Koch, G. G., & Hasemeier, C. M. (1997). Secondary sexual characteristics and menses in young girls seen in office practice: A study from the Pediatric Research in Office Settings Network. *Pediatrics, 88,* 505–512.

Herman-Giddens, M. E., Wang, L., & Koch, G. (2001). Secondary sexual characteristics in boys. *Archives of Pediatrics and Adolescent Medicine, 155,* 1022–1028.

Hetherington, E. M. (1993). An overview of the Virginia Longitudinal Study of Divorce and Remarriage with a focus on early adolescence. *Journal of Family Psychology, 7,* 39–56.

Hetherington, E. M., Bridges, M., & Insabella, G. M. (1998). What matters? What does not? Five perspectives on the association between marital transitions and children's adjustment. *American Psychologist, 53,* 167–184.

Hill, J. (1983). Early adolescence: A framework. *Journal of Early Adolescence, 3,* 1–21.

Hock, E., Eberly, M., Bartle-Haring, S., Ellwanger, P., & Widaman, K. F. (2001). Separation anxiety in parents of adolescents: Theoretical significance and scale development. *Child Development, 72,* 284–298.

Holmbeck, G. N., & Hill, J. P. (1991). Conflictive engagement, positive affect, and menarche in families with seventh-grade girls. *Child Development, 62,* 1030–1048.

Jacobson, K. C., & Crockett, L. J. (2000). Parental monitoring and adolescent adjustment: An ecological perspective. *Journal of Research on Adolescence, 10,* 65–98.

Kerns, K. A., Aspelmeier, J. E., Gentzler, A. L., & Grabill, C. M. (2001). Parent–child attachment and monitoring in middle childhood. *Journal of Family Psychology, 15,* 69–81.

Kerns, K. A., Klepac, L., & Cole, A. K. (1996). Peer relationships and preadolescents' perceptions of security in the mother–child relationship. *Developmental Psychology, 32,* 457–466.

Kerns, K. A., Tomich, P. L., Aspelmeier, J. E., & Contreras, J. M. (2000). Attachment-based assessments of parent–child relationships in middle childhood. *Developmental Psychology, 36,* 614–626.

Kidwell, J. S. (1981). Number of siblings, sibling spacing, sex, and birth order: Their effects on perceived parent–adolescent relationships. *Journal of Marriage and the Family, 53,* 325–332.

Larson, R. W., Richards, M. H., Moneta, G., Holmbeck, G., & Duckett, E. (1996).

Changes in adolescents' daily interactions with their families from ages 10 to 18: Disengagement and transformation. *Developmental Psychology, 32,* 744–754.

Laursen, B., Coy, K. C., & Collins, W. A. (1998). Reconsidering changes in parent–child conflict across adolescence: A meta-analysis. *Child Development, 69,* 817–832.

Lerner, R. M. (1995). *America's youth in crisis.* Thousand Oaks, CA: Sage.

Lieberman, M., Doyle, A. B., & Markiewicz, D. (1999). Developmental patterns in security of attachment to mother and father in late childhood and early adolescence: Associations with peer relations. *Child Development, 70,* 202–213.

Merten, D. (1996). Going-with: The role of a social form in early romance. *Journal of Contemporary Ethnography, 24,* 462–282.

Moffit, T. E., Caspi, A., Belsky, J., & Silva, P. A. (1992). Childhood experience and onset of menarche: A test of a sociobiological model. *Child Development, 63,* 47–58.

Molina, B., & Chassin, L. (1996). The parent-adolescent relationship at puberty: Hispanic ethnicity and parent alcoholism as moderators. *Developmental Psychology, 32,* 675–686.

Ogletree, M. D., Jones, R. M., & Coyl, D. D. (2002). Fathers and their adolescent sons: Pubertal development and paternal involvement. *Journal of Adolescent Research, 17,* 418–424.

Petersen, A. C. (1993). Creating adolescents: The role of context and process in developmental trajectories. *Journal of Research on Adolescence, 3,* 1–18.

Petersen, A. C., Crockett, L., Richards, M., & Boxer, A. (1988). A self-report measure of pubertal status: Reliability, validity, and initial norms. *Journal of Youth and Adolescence, 17,* 117–133.

Resnick, G. (1993). *Measuring attachment in early adolescence: A manual for the administration, coding, and interpretation of the Separation Anxiety Test for 11- to 14-year-olds.* Unpublished manuscript.

Richardson, R. A., Abramowitz, R. H., Asp, C. E., & Petersen, A. C. (1986). Parent–child relationships in early adolescence: Effects of family structure. *Journal of Marriage and the Family, 48,* 805–811.

Sagrestano, L., McCormick, S., Paikoff, R., & Holmbeck, G. (1999). Pubertal development and parent–child conflict in low-income, urban, African American adolescents. *Journal of Research on Adolescence, 9,* 85–107.

Salt, R. E. (1991). Affectionate touch between fathers and preadolescent sons. *Journal of Marriage and the Family, 53,* 545–554.

Schneider, B. H., Atkinson, L., & Tardif, C. (2001). Parent–child attachment and children's peer relations: A quantitative review. *Developmental Psychology, 37,* 86–100.

Seidman, E., Lambert, L. E., Allen, L., & Aber, J. L. (2003). Urban adolescents' transition to junior high school and protective family transactions. *Journal of Early Adolescence, 23,* 166–193.

Shann, M. H. (2001). Students' use of time outside of school: A case for after school programs for urban middle school youth. *Urban Review, 33,* 339–356.

Simons, K. J., Paternite, C. E., & Shore, C. (2001). Quality of parent–adolescent attachment and aggression in young adolescents. *Journal of Early Adolescence, 21,* 182–203.

Spear, P. (2000). The adolescent brain and age-related behavioral manifestations. *Neuroscience and Biobehavioral Reviews, 24,* 417–463.

Sroufe, L. A., Bennett, C., Englund, M., Urban, J., & Shulman, S. (1993). The significance of gender boundaries in preadolescence: Contemporary correlates and antecedents of boundary violation and maintenance. *Child Development, 64,* 455–466.

Steelman, L. C., Powell, B., Werum, R., & Carter, S. (2002). Reconsidering the effects of sibling configuration: Recent advances and challenges. *Annual Review of Sociology, 28,* 243–269.

Steinberg, L. (2002). *Adolescence.* New York: McGraw-Hill.

Tanner, J. M., & Davies, P. S. W. (1985). Clinical longitudinal standards for height and height velocity for North American children. *Journal of Pediatrics, 107,* 317–329.

U.S. Bureau of the Census. (1998). Marital status and living arrangements. *Current Population Reports* (Series P20–514). Washington, DC: U.S. Government Printing Office.

U.S. Bureau of the Census. (2000). *Grade school children in self-care: Fall 1995.* Retrieved July 18, 2003, from http://www.census.gov/Press-Release/www/2000/childcare.pdf

Wigfield, A., Eccles, J. S., MacIver, D., Reuman, D. A., & Midgley, C. (1991). Transitions during early adolescence: Changes in children's domain-specific self-perceptions and general self-esteem across the transition to junior high school. *Developmental Psychology, 27,* 552–565.

Whiteman, S. D., & Buchanan, C. M. (2002). Mothers' and children's expectations for adolescence: The impact of perceptions of an older sibling's experience. *Journal of Family Psychology, 16,* 157–171.

Whiteman, S. D., McHale, S. M., & Crouter, A. C. (2003). What parents learn from experience: The first child as a first draft? *Journal of Marriage and Family, 65,* 608–621.

Woodward, L., Fergusson, D. M., & Belsky, J. (2000). Timing of parental separation and attachment to parents in adolescence: Results of a prospective study from birth to age 16. *Journal of Marriage and the Family, 62,* 162–174.

CHAPTER 3

◆ ◆ ◆

Assessing Attachment in Middle Childhood

KATHRYN A. KERNS
ANDREW SCHLEGELMILCH
THERESA A. MORGAN
MICHELLE M. ABRAHAM

A tremendous amount of research over the past 30 years has focused on the definition, measurement, antecedents, and correlates of child–parent attachment. Most of this work has examined attachment in young children (5 years of age and under), with a more specific focus on children's attachments to their mothers. This work has confirmed several tenets of attachment theory. First, responsive and sensitive care has been identified, in both correlational and intervention designs, as a factor related to secure attachment (DeWolff & van IJzendoorn, 1997; van IJzendoorn, Juffer, & Duyvesteyn, 1995). Second, attachment has been linked to several indicators of social and emotional competence (Belsky & Cassidy, 1994; Contreras & Kerns, 2000; Thompson, 1999). Third, attachments to particular caregivers show some stability and specificity (i.e., attachments to different figures are consistent over time but not always the same across partners; Thompson, 1998).

An important achievement that allowed for tests of the theory was the development of research methods to index the quality of child–parent attachment. Substantial progress has been made for the infancy and early childhood years. The development of the Strange Situation (Ainsworth, Blehar, Waters, & Wall, 1978) was crucial in that it provided researchers the first highly reliable and well-validated measure of infant–parent attachment, and it has become a "gold standard" against which other infancy and early childhood measures could be compared. Other measures (e.g., Attachment Q-Sort; separation–reunion procedures for older children) were developed to assess attachment in infancy and early childhood, and consequently the study of attachment in young children is no longer simply the study of the Strange Situation (for reviews of infancy and early childhood measures, see Solomon & George, 1999; Thompson, 1998). The development of the Adult Attachment Interview (Main, Kaplan, & Cassidy, 1985) and other, similar interview measures for adults and adolescents (see Crowell, Fraley, & Shaver, 1999, for a review) has also led to new research on attachment in the teen and adult years.

By contrast, despite children's need for attachment figures in middle childhood, the latter has been a relatively neglected period for attachment research. This has been partly due to a lack of validated attachment measures for children 8–12 years of age, although recently a number of measures have been developed. The goal of this chapter is to evaluate progress that has been made toward developing tools for measuring attachment in middle childhood. The chapter begins with a discussion of the nature of attachment during the middle childhood years. Next, we discuss the common approaches to assessing attachment. Third, we describe available attachment measures that can be used with children 8–12 years of age. In the final section we evaluate progress and identify theoretical challenges that still need to be solved.

THE NATURE OF ATTACHMENT IN MIDDLE CHILDHOOD: IMPLICATIONS FOR MEASUREMENT

Measurement of constructs is, of course, dependent on having clear definitions of the constructs of interest. Attachment (in children) is typically referred to as an emotional and long-lasting bond that a child forms with (or to) an attachment figure and that provides the child with feelings of security and comfort (see Ainsworth, 1989; Cassidy, 1999). The child organizes his or her attachment behavior (e.g., crying, smiling) around the set goal of retaining proximity to the attachment figure (Ainsworth, 1990; Bowlby, 1982). Once mobile, the child uses the attachment figure as a haven of safety when distressed and as a secure base to support exploration when threats are absent (Ainsworth et al., 1978). Attachment is usually measured with reference to the organization of a child's affect, behavior, and cognitions in relation to the attachment figure.

Although this definition may seem clear, there are ambiguities. Sometimes attachment is described as a characteristic of a relationship dyad (Waters, 1981), whereas other times it is discussed as the internalization of the relationship within the child (Ainsworth, 1990). A second issue is whether attachment refers to relationship-specific or generalized behaviors and beliefs in reference to attachment figures. In early childhood, the term "attachment" is usually used to refer to the quality of a specific relationship, whereas many adult and adolescent measures of attachment assess a person's general state of mind regarding attachment rather than the quality of particular bonds. These issues of definition are discussed more in the last section, but for now one can see how different researchers might adopt different measurement approaches, depending on their conceptualization of attachment.

To construct middle-childhood attachment assessments, it is important to delineate more specifically how attachment might operate within middle childhood. One question concerning attachment in middle childhood is who children rely on as their primary attachment figures. In early childhood, children form attachments to caregivers (e.g., parents, day-care providers). By contrast, most authors suggest that attachments to peers do not emerge until adolescence (Allen & Land, 1999; Bowlby, 1982; Marvin & Britner, 1999), when they supplement attachments to parents. A different view is offered by Hazan and colleagues (Hazan & Shaver, 1994; Hazan & Zeifman, 1994, 1999), who have claimed that the emergence of attachments to peers is a gradual process that begins in middle childhood, when children begin to direct proximity maintenance behaviors toward peers. However, their research has not clearly delineated seeking out partners for companionship versus seeking out partners when the attachment system is activated (e.g., child is scared). When we asked third- and sixth-grade children whom they wanted to be with in different contexts, children clearly preferred peers for companionship but parents for fulfillment of attachment needs (Kerns, Tomich, & Kim, 2003). Thus, although peers might be used as safe havens in an emergency when parents are not readily available (Crowell & Waters, 1994) and may be ancillary attachment figures in middle childhood (see Mayseless, Chapter 1, this volume), children seem to rely primarily on parents to fulfill attachment needs. Thus, measures of *attachment* in middle childhood need to address parent–child rather than peer relationships, because it is unclear what a measure of "peer attachment" would be a measure of (e.g., perhaps it is better labeled as a measure of friendship quality). Of course, peers are important relationship partners in middle childhood, even if they do not clearly fulfill the role of attachment figure to one another. Once well-validated measures of parent–child attachment are available for middle childhood, it may be easier to develop tests of whether peer relationships at this age share any of the features of parent–child attachment (i.e., we first need a good idea of what secure-base utilization looks like in middle childhood, and for this initial step it is important to examine relationships that are unequivocally attachment relationships).

The definition of attachment offered earlier in this chapter is adevelopmental. Bowlby (1982) hypothesized that there are some changes in attachment from early to middle childhood. First, there may be a decline in the frequency and intensity of specific attachment behaviors directed toward the attachment figure. This decline might be due to changes in the attachment system whereby, as children get older, the system develops toward increased self-reliance on the part of the child (Marvin & Britner, 1999). As Marvin and Britner (1999) note, older children are better at coping with dangers and are less dependent on parents, and therefore they may need to utilize or rely on parents less often. A second hypothesized change is that, in many circumstances, attachment behavior may be terminated in older children by a wider range of conditions (Bowlby, 1982). For example, although physical proximity may be necessary to terminate attachment behaviors in younger children, an older child's attachment behavior might also be terminated by a phone call or by seeing a photograph of the attachment figure (Bowlby, 1982). Third, there may be a change in the set goal of the attachment system, with availability rather than proximity of the attachment figure becoming the set goal of the system (Bowlby, 1987, cited in Ainsworth, 1990). Availability of the figure is reflected by open communication between parent and child, parent responsiveness to child needs, and the parent's physical accessibility to the child. When availability becomes the set goal of the attachment system, children's expectations and beliefs regarding attachment figures become important markers of attachment (Kerns, Tomich, Aspelmeier, & Contreras, 2000).

Taken together, these ideas suggest that children will want parent attachment figures available but that they may exhibit attachment behavior less frequently and in fewer situations as they get older. These hypotheses have now been supported in studies of 8- to 14-year-old children's perceptions of attachment (Kerns et al., 2003; Lieberman, Doyle, & Markiewicz, 1999). Because of these changes, it is difficult after early childhood to infer attachment quality from secure-base behavior in everyday naturalistic settings or laboratory separation–reunion procedures (Main & Cassidy, 1988, noted that reunion behavior in 5- and 6-year-olds is difficult to observe and presumably would be even more subtle in an older child). It would probably be unethical to expose preadolescents to situations sufficiently stressful to elicit secure-base behavior, although behavioral measures may be useful in some naturalistic contexts (e.g., when a child and parent reunite after several days apart). As will be seen in the review of available measures for 8- to 12-year-olds, to date investigators have relied instead on self-report measures to index attachment in middle childhood.

REVIEW OF AVAILABLE MEASURES

Solomon and George (1999) have reviewed the attachment measures developed for 1- to 7-year-old children (see also Green, Stanley, Smith, & Goldwyn, 2000, for a newer measure not included in the Solomon & George review). To avoid duplication, this chapter focuses on measures available to assess attachment in 8- to 12-year-old children. Table 3.1 provides summary information about the measures included in this review. All of the available measures are based on children's self-reports and are categorized into three types: standardized questionnaires, narrative discourse techniques, or family drawings.

Questionnaires have been developed to assess who children identify as attachment figures and their perception of the quality of attachments to parents. The questionnaires to identify attachment figures (Kerns et al., 2003; Kobak, Esposito, & Serwik, 2003) ask whom children would seek out in attachment-relevant situations (e.g., when a child is feeling scared). The questionnaires that assess perceived quality of attachment (i.e., Security Scale and Avoidant and Preoccupied Coping Scales) ask children to rate statements that refer to the child's expectations, affect, and behavior in relation to a specific attachment figure (mother or father). As with all questionnaires, a concern is that children's responses might be influenced by demand characteristics or response biases. Because of these concerns, relating child reports of attachment to other questionnaire self-reports from the child does not provide strong evidence for the validity of attachment questionnaires (Kerns, Klepac, & Cole, 1996). Rather, it is important for questionnaire measures to be validated against information obtained from individuals other than the target child (e.g., teachers, trained observers, peers).

A second assessment approach is the use of narrative discourse techniques, involving storytelling or answering questions about one's relationships. The child participates in an open-ended interview that is recorded, and the child's discourse is later evaluated by trained raters. On questionnaires children are reporting beliefs and feelings in regard to the attachment figure that they are able to bring into conscious awareness. Discourse techniques are designed to tap conscious and unconscious at-

TABLE 3.1. Attachment Measures for 8- to 12-Year-Olds

Measure	Description
Identification of attachment figures	
Important People Interview (Kobak et al., 2003)	Interview to obtain attachment hierarchy and hierarchy violations
Attachment Figure Interview (Kerns et al., 2003)	Interview to identify primary and secondary attachment figures
Perceptions of attachment quality	
Security Scale (Kerns et al., 2001)	Questionnaire assessing dimension of security for mother–child and father–child relationships
Avoidant and Preoccupied Scales (Finnegan et al., 1996)	Questionnaire assessing Avoidant and Preoccupied attachment styles (as dimensions)
Narrative discourse measures	
Doll Story Completion Task (Granot & Mayseless, 2001)	Story-stem interview to assess four attachment patterns (ratings and classifications): Secure, Avoidant, Ambivalent, Disorganized
Separation Anxiety Test (Resnick, 1993)	Picture-based interview that classifies children into three groups: Secure (Autonomous), Dismissing (Avoidant), Enmeshed (Ambivalent)
Attachment Interview for Childhood and Adolescence (Ammaniti et al., 2000)	Interview regarding childhood relationships, with scoring that classifies children into four groups: Secure, Dismissing, Preoccupied, Unresolved
Friends and Family Interview (Steele & Steele, Chapter 7, this volume)	Interview regarding self and childhood close relationships with scoring for narrative coherence and secure-base availability of parents
Analysis of drawings	
Family Drawing (Fury et al., 1997)	Child's drawing of family that is scored for attachment category (Secure, Avoidant, Resistant) and for ratings that reflect the child's representation of self and attachment figure

tachment attitudes because they evaluate both what is said and how the information is communicated. This includes an analysis of narrative coherence. A coherent narrative is truthful, succinct but complete, relevant, and clear and orderly (Main, 1996; see also Steele & Steele, Chapter 7, this volume). For example, individuals who are secure may or may not report positively about their experiences with attachment figures, but in all cases they are expected to provide fluent and open yet reasonably concise descriptions of attachment phenomena (Main, 1996). A third assessment approach, analysis of family drawings, is also thought to tap unconscious attitudes and beliefs. Thus an important question is whether attachment questionnaires and projective techniques are assessing the same construct. Some studies have found the two measurement approaches to be related in middle childhood (e.g., Granot & Mayseless, 2001; Kerns et al., 2000), but their overlap needs further study.

As can be seen from Table 3.1, a number of different instruments have been developed. We have provided a short description of each measure (please contact scale authors for a fuller description of the instrument and scoring procedures). In addition, where available, we have included information about the measure's reliability, validity, associations with other attachment measures, and associations with theoretically related constructs.

IDENTIFICATION OF ATTACHMENT FIGURES

Important People Interview

The Important People Interview (IPI; Kobak et al., 2003; Kobak, Rosenthal, & Serwik, Chapter 4, this volume) assesses a child's attachment hierarchy. Children first identify the four most important people in their lives. Then they are asked whom (of the four) they would want to be with in different attachment-relevant situations (e.g., if the child was really upset and crying). The situations were picked to assess four components of attachment identified by Hazan and Zeifman (1999): proximity seeking, safe haven, secure base, and separation protest. For each situation, the child indicates whom he or she would go to first, second, and so forth.

The interview questions are scored so that the highest scores are assigned to individuals whom the child would seek out first in a situation. Scores are then summed to identify a child's primary and secondary attachment figures. Finally, violations in the attachment hierarchy are calculated. A violation is defined as a failure to nominate the primary or secondary attachment figure in the top two choices for a question. Such a violation reflects a lack of consistency as to whom a child would want to

be with in attachment-relevant situations. A total score for violations of
the hierarchy is calculated based on the number and severity of the violations. Test–retest data are not available, and the IPI has not yet been examined in relation to other attachment measures. In a study of fifth graders, Kobak and colleagues (2003) reported that most children showed a
stable attachment hierarchy (i.e., they did not show violations of the hierarchy), with parents nominated most often as primary attachment figures.
Further, they found that children who lacked a stable hierarchy were rated
by teachers as experiencing more adjustment problems.

Attachment Figure Interview

The Attachment Figure Interview (Kerns et al., 2003) asks children whom
they would want to be with in two types of situations: when attachment
needs are invoked (e.g., feeling scared) and when companionship is desired (e.g., wanting to play). Children are allowed to nominate up to two
people whom they would seek out in a given situation.

The measure is scored by coding whether children seek out an adult
or a peer for each situation. Third- and sixth-grade children most frequently nominated adults (usually parents) for attachment situations,
whereas peers were most frequently nominated for companionship situations (Kerns et al., 2003). Test–retest data have not been collected, and
scores have not yet been examined in relation to other attachment measures or indices of child adjustment.

PERCEPTIONS OF ATTACHMENT QUALITY

Security Scale

The 15-item Security Scale (Kerns, Aspelmeier, Gentzler, & Grabill, 2001)
measures the child's perception of his or her relationship with a parent.
Items tap the degree to which children perceive an attachment figure (i.e.,
parent) as responsive and available, tend to rely on an attachment figure
in times of stress, and report an ease and interest in communicating with
an attachment figure. Bowlby (1982) identified these as three key components of attachment in middle childhood (cited in Ainsworth, 1990).
Children complete the items separately for mother and father, and thus
the measure is relationship specific.

The items are presented in the Harter (1982) "Some kids . . . other
kids . . . " format, in which children are presented statements about two
types of children and asked to pick which type of kids they are more like.
The child then indicates strength of endorsement ("really like" or "sort of

like" one group of kids). This format is used, rather than a Likert scale, because Harter has argued that this approach decreases socially desirable responding by allowing a child to respond affirmatively that he or she is like a certain group of kids. For example, it may be easier for a child to say that he or she is like kids who don't like to share what they are thinking with their moms (vs. those who like to share), rather than having to rate him- or herself low on a single dimension of sharing thoughts and feelings with a parent. Items scores are summed so that a higher score indicates greater perceived security of attachment.

The questionnaire has been used in several studies of 8- to 12-year-old U.S. children. The Security Scale has been found to have adequate internal consistency (Cronbach's alphas around .80 or higher; Kerns, 1996; Kerns et al., 1996, 2000), except that alphas are sometimes lower for third graders (8- to 9-year-olds) than for older children (Kerns et al., 2000). Two-week test–retest reliability was also adequate ($r = .75$) in a sample of fourth and fifth graders (Kerns et al., 1996). The Security Scale has shown associations with other measures of attachment. It appears to measure a security–avoidance dimension in that security scores correlate positively with other measures of security (e.g., narrative coherence, Kerns et al., 2000; interviewer ratings of security, Granot & Mayseless, 2001), correlate negatively with questionnaire and interview measures of avoidance (Granot & Mayseless, 2001; Kerns et al., 2000), and do not correlate consistently with measures of ambivalence or preoccupation (Granot & Mayseless, 2001; Kerns et al., 2000). Child reports of security have also been associated with parent reports of willingness to serve as a secure base (Kerns et al., 1996, 2000) and, for sixth graders, with child and parent reports of monitoring (Kerns et al., 2001). Perceptions of security are also related, as expected, to children's reports of loneliness, self-esteem, social, and academic competence; to sociometric ratings obtained from peers; and to friendship quality as rated by observers (Kerns et al., 1996). There is some evidence of discriminant validity in that attachment is not related to grade point average or perceptions of athletic competence (Kerns et al., 1996) or to parent ratings of child temperament (Abraham, Kerns, Morgan, & Schlegelmilch, 2004).

Lieberman and colleagues (1999) have suggested that the items on the Security Scale tap two dimensions—perceived availability and perceived dependence on (i.e., utilization of) attachment figures. They reported adequate internal consistency for the two subscales and further found that perceptions of availability and dependency showed some associations with self-reports of friendship quality. However, Verschueren and Marceon (Chapter 10, this volume) explicitly tested this two-dimensional scoring of the Security Scale and did not find evidence for the two dimensions.

Avoidant and Preoccupied Coping Scales

The original 36-item Avoidant and Preoccupied Coping Scales (Finnegan, Hodges, & Perry, 1996) was designed to assess children's perceptions of preoccupied and avoidant coping in relation to a particular attachment figure. Children are presented with a situation and asked to choose how they would respond. Preoccupied coping items reflect the child's experience of high distress, difficulty in being calmed, and continued proximity to the attachment figure when coping with problems. Avoidant items indicate whether the child would or would not need or seek assistance or comforting from the attachment figure to cope with problems. Like the Security Scale, items are presented using Harter's "Some kids . . . Other kids . . . " format (see Finnegan et al., 1996, for information about scoring). Higher scores indicate higher avoidance or preoccupation. More recently, a 20-item version (10 items per scale) has been developed. The newer version has briefer items and is labeled a measure of preoccupied and avoidant attachment styles (see Chapter 5 by Yunger, Corby, and Perry, this volume).

The Preoccupied and Avoidant Scales have been evaluated in several studies of U.S. children 8–13 years of age (see also Yunger et al., Chapter 5, this volume). Both scales consistently show high internal consistency for children in grades 3 through 7 (typically Cronbach's alphas of .80 or higher; Finnegan et al., 1996; Hodges, Finnegan, & Perry, 1999; Kerns et al., 2000). Two-week test–retest correlations, based on data from third through seventh graders, were .83 for the Preoccupied scale and .76 for the Avoidant scale (Finnegan et al., 1996). One study evaluated how the coping scales are related to other measures of attachment. The Avoidant scale was consistently and negatively correlated with indicators of security and parental responsiveness, but the Preoccupied Scale did not show a consistent pattern of associations with the other attachment measures (Kerns et al., 2000). Both concurrent and longitudinal analyses have shown that the scales are related to peer evaluations of behavior. More specifically, avoidant coping is related to peer reports of externalizing behavior, whereas preoccupied coping is related to internalizing behavior (Finnegan et al., 1996; Hodges et al., 1999).

Comments on Questionnaire Measures of Attachment

Both the Security Scale and the Preoccupied and Avoidant Coping Scales have shown evidence of reliability and validity. Two issues remain. First, there is a need for additional evidence of both convergent and discriminant validity (especially for self-reports of other constructs to establish discriminant validity). Second, more studies are needed to examine whether the two questionnaires are related to narrative assessments of attachment and parental behavior.

NARRATIVE ASSESSMENT TECHNIQUES

As noted earlier, narrative assessment techniques are based on children's self-reports, but the tasks elicit from children their discussion of attachment events. The interview format allows for more detailed responses than can be obtained from questionnaires, and the open-ended questions allow for substantial variability in responding. Two types of narrative techniques have been employed in middle childhood. One approach, based on procedures initially developed for children in early childhood (see Page, 2001), involves having an interviewer begin a story and then having the child finish the story (either verbally or by enacting the story with dolls and props). In this case, children are not directly queried about their own experiences, but it is assumed that their stories will reflect their thoughts, feelings, and actions in relation to their own attachment figures. The other approach, based on the Adult Attachment Interview (which was developed for adults and has been used with older adolescents), involves asking the child a number of open-ended questions about his or her actual experiences in family relationships. With both techniques, trained coders later evaluate how relationships are portrayed (e.g., whether there is ready comforting by attachment figures and open expression of emotion) and whether the child can provide coherent answers (e.g., whether description of actions is logical and coherent and relevant to the topic). The latter is considered an important indicator of a person's "state of mind in regard to attachment" (Main, 1996) and thus an indicator of security (i.e., a secure child can provide a coherent discussion of attachment-related events). In the following sections, story methods are described first, followed by AAI-type interview techniques.

Doll Story Completion Task

The Doll Story Completion Task (Granot & Mayseless, 2001) is designed to assess a child's representations of attachment to a parent in terms of security, avoidance, ambivalence, and disorganization. The measure is an adaptation of Bretherton, Ridgeway, and Cassidy's (1990) story-stem technique in which an interviewer begins to tell a story and the child uses dolls and props to complete the story. The target child, one parent, and siblings are represented as characters in the story. Five stories that had been used with younger children (3- to 6-year-olds) were adapted to make the stories appropriate for children 9–12 years of age. The themes of the stories are: child spills juice at dinner, child gets hurt after falling off a rock, child sees something after going to bed, parent departs for 3 days, and reunion of parent and child after 3-day separation.

Coders first judge whether each story is secure or insecure, using four criteria: whether there is open expression of emotion, the nature of the child–parent relationship (e.g., is parent responsive and sensitive), whether events are resolved in a positive way, and the coherence of the narrative. Then, after considering the entire interview, raters rate each child on security, avoidance, ambivalence, and disorganization and choose a best fitting classification.

The Doll Story Completion Task was initially developed and validated with Israeli samples. Granot and Mayseless (2001) examined mother–child attachment in a sample of fourth and fifth graders (9- to 11-year-olds). They reported good observer agreement (80% category agreement, scale rs .78 to .85) and high test–retest reliability (94%) over a 3-month interval. In addition, scores from the interview were related to children's scores on the Security Scale, with children who were rated higher on security and lower on avoidance reporting greater security on the Security Scale. The Doll Story Completion Task was also significantly related to teacher ratings of school adjustment and to peer dislike nominations, with children classified as secure showing better adjustment than children classified as avoidant or disorganized. There was some evidence of discriminant validity in that attachment classifications were not related to logical reasoning and language test scores. Additional data with a U.S. sample are presented later in the chapter.

Separation Anxiety Test

The Separation Anxiety Test (SAT; Klagsbrun & Bowlby, 1976) is a semiprojective technique in which children are shown pictures depicting parent–child interaction and asked to talk about the pictures. The instrument was initially developed for adolescents (Hansburg, 1972), then later adapted for 6- to 7-year-olds (Main et al., 1985). Children are shown a series of six pictures that vary from mild to severe in intensity and are asked to talk about the feelings and actions of the targets. Additional details regarding the procedures and validity of the SAT for 6-year-olds is provided in Solomon and George (1999).

One version of the SAT has been developed for 10- to 14-year-old children (Resnick, 1993). This version combines elements from both the adolescent and age-6 versions. The situations depicted were taken from the adolescent version, and the administration and scoring procedures were based on versions developed for both age groups. For example, like the version for 6-year-olds, the coding focuses on the child's ability to express emotions openly and to propose constructive solutions for the situation; but, like the adolescent version, there are both open- and closed-ended questions regarding the pictures. The scoring system was also based on the scoring system developed for the Adult Attachment Interview (Resnick, 1993).

In the Resnick (1993) version, children are shown six separation pictures that vary in intensity (e.g., child is transferring to a new school; child's parent is being taken away to the hospital in an ambulance). The child is asked how the target child feels, using both open- and close-ended questions. Then the child is asked what the target child would do next. Coders rate the child's responses to each story on nine 9-point scales (e.g., emotional openness, devaluing of attachment, coherence). Then overall scale ratings are made, taking into account the child's responses across the stories. Finally, children are assigned to a single best fitting classification, using a three-category system: secure/valuing of attachment, dismissing/avoidant, or enmeshed/preoccupied/ambivalent. Later, an alternative scoring system was developed. With the Automated Separation Anxiety Test (ASAT), the interview is computer administered and then analyzed by a neural network that was developed based on 200 hand-scored interviews (Contreras, Kerns, Weimer, Gentzler, & Tomich, 2000).

Observer agreement was adequate in two studies (Kerns et al., 2000, U.S. sample; Resnick, 1997, Israeli sample). SAT classifications and some of the ratings scales were related to child reports of attachment in one study (Kerns et al., 2000) but not another (Resnick, 1997). In a longitudinal analysis, Strange Situation classifications were obtained at age 1, separately with mother, father, and metapelet (i.e., kibbutz caregiver). In addition, SAT classifications were collected at age 11. SAT classifications were not related to infancy assessments of attachment to mother or to metapelet but did show a marginally significant association ($p < .06$) with father–infant attachment (children secure with father in infancy tended to be secure on the later SAT). SAT scores were significantly related to child reports of friendship quality (Howes & Tonyan, 2000) but were not related to child reports of self-concept (Resnick, 1997) or to teacher ratings of children's school adjustment (Kerns et al., 2000).

Attachment Interview for Childhood and Adolescence

The Attachment Interview for Childhood and Adolescence (AICA; Ammaniti, van IJzendoorn, Speranza, & Tambelli, 2000; Ammaniti, Speranza, & Fedele, Chapter 6, this volume) is an adaptation of the Adult Attachment Interview (AAI; Main et al., 1985) for children in late childhood and early adolescence. Thus, like the AAI, the measure is designed to assess a person's state of mind in regard to attachment rather than the quality of a particular relationship. The interview structure and questions follow the AAI, but the language was simplified, and some questions were dropped to make the interview appropriate for younger children. As with the AAI, the target is asked to discuss autobiographical family memories and the effects of their experiences on their current views of relationships.

The coding of the interview is similar to the AAI. Coders rate each interview on twelve 9-point scales that capture the quality of earlier relationships (e.g., whether parents are loving or rejecting) and the nature of current representations (e.g., idealization, coherence of transcript). In addition, coders assign participants to one of four categories: Secure (valuing of attachment), Dismissing, Preoccupied, and Unresolved (with respect to past trauma). The coding of coherence was modified from the AAI because certain violations of coherence occur more often in preadolescents and early adolescents than in adults (Ammaniti et al., 2000).

The AICA has been administered to a sample of 31 Italian children residing in two-parent families (Ammaniti et al., 2000). The children were interviewed twice at ages 10 and 14 years. Observer agreement was adequate (82% agreement on classifications and correlations of .60 to 1.00 for the rating scales). Stability of the four category placements over 4 years was 71%, with stability highest for participants who were initially secure or dismissing. In a second longitudinal study (Ammaniti et al., Chapter 6, this volume), children completed the AICA at age 11. AICA classifications were not related to observational measures of attachment collected at ages 1 and 5, but they were related to a narrative attachment assessment from age 5 and to maternal AAIs collected when children were 5 years old. Although there is some evidence for the discriminant validity of the AAI (see Ammaniti et al., 2000), comparable data have not yet been collected for the AICA.

Friends and Family Interview

The Friends and Family Interview (FFI; Steele & Steele, Chapter 7, this volume) is an open-ended interview designed to tap children's feelings concerning self, parents, siblings, and friends. Children are asked, for each domain, to describe what they like best and least about themselves. Specific probes are used to clarify answers and to request supporting memories. Scoring for the interview is similar to the AAI in that trained raters score both narrative coherence and reported experience with parents (more specifically, secure base availability of each parent).

The FFI has been administered in a longitudinal study of families recruited prior to the birth of the target child (Steele &, Steele, Chapter 7, this volume). FFI scores were significantly related to parental AAIs collected prior to the birth of the child. When mothers were secure on the AAI, at age 11 both boys and girls scored higher on availability of mother and some measure of coherence of discourse. Fathers secure on the AAI subsequently had sons (but not daughters) who were more coherent and who perceived parents as more available. FFI coherence and perceptions of parental availability were related, for boys, to having formed a secure attachment to their fathers in infancy. There was some evidence of discriminant validity in that FFI coherence scores were not related to a measure of verbal IQ.

Comment on Narrative Assessment Techniques

The SAT has produced the weakest evidence of validity (see also Ammaniti et al., Chapter 6, this volume). The other measures seem more promising, having shown evidence of test–retest reliability, associations with measures of attachment from earlier age periods or concurrent measures of child functioning, and some evidence of discriminant validity. Note, however, that only some of this information is available for each of the measures. In addition, none of the measures has shown consistent associations with behavioral measures of attachment. Finally, additional discriminant validity data are needed to assess the degree to which the interviews are tapping related constructs such as self-concept or peer relationships (see especially the interview content of the FFI).

FAMILY DRAWING TECHNIQUES

Only one study of children 8–12 years of age has included an analysis of a family drawing as a measure of attachment representations (Fury, Carlson, & Sroufe, 1997). Using an approach initially developed for younger children, Fury and colleagues (1997) asked 8- to 9-year-old children to draw pictures of their families. Trained raters scored the drawings for: (1) attachment classification (secure, avoidant, resistant); (2) particular signs thought to reflect security (e.g., placement of arms); and (3) ratings reflecting the quality of the drawings (e.g., emotional distancing).

Coder agreement was adequate. The measure was administered in a longitudinal study in which children had been seen in the Strange Situation (SS) at 12 and at 18 months. SS classifications were related to attachment classifications and ratings of quality based on the drawings (fewer associations were found for specific signs). Some ratings scales were associated with particular forms of insecurity as reflected in the drawings (e.g., avoidance with emotional distancing, resistance with vulnerability).

There was some evidence of discriminant validity in that interviewer ratings were not related to child IQ.

Thus this study did provide some evidence for using an analysis of family drawings as a measure of attachment in middle childhood, although additional validity data are needed (including evidence of associations with measures of current relationships with parents and discriminant validity in relation to child adjustment).

QUESTIONS AND CHALLENGES CONCERNING THE ASSESSMENT OF ATTACHMENT IN MIDDLE CHILDHOOD

As can be seen from the previous section, investigators have recently developed a number of tools for assessing attachment during the later middle childhood years. Thus progress has begun toward the goal of developing an assessment battery for this age period. Nevertheless, a number of important challenges remain. One challenge is that the available validity data for the measures reviewed is rather limited. It would certainly be ideal to obtain all of the following for each measure: internal consistency or observer agreement, test–retest information, associations with other attachment measures, correlations with measures of parenting (especially sensitive/responsive care) and parent representations of attachment, and associations with theoretically important indices of child social and emotional adjustment. Also, longitudinal studies allow for examining associations with measures from other developmental periods and continuity of attachment into, across, and after middle childhood. At least some of the aforementioned data are available for each of the measures reviewed earlier. In our opinion, one of the most critical needs is for studies that include multiple, contemporaneous assessments of attachment to examine whether the different approaches are in fact iterating on a common construct. In addition, much more attention needs to be paid to questions of discriminant validity. As well as establishing the correlates of attachment measures, we also need to know what they do *not* measure to rule out other (perhaps even more parsimonious) explanations for the correlates of attachment. In addition, sampling issues need attention. Most of the measures have been used only in one culture and/or within samples with limited range on income and ethnicity, and thus their applicability in more diverse samples is not known. Administration and scoring procedures of the measures may need to be adapted to make them applicable to samples other than those on which they were developed.

A second challenge is to understand how normative changes in children's social, emotional, and cognitive development affect attachment (see Mayseless, Chapters 1, and Richardson, Chapter 2, this volume). The influence of normative social developmental processes on attachment has received limited discussion. Marvin and Britner (1999) speculate that normative changes in children's social capabilities and striving for independence may affect how children talk about and view the need for the attachment figure. As another example, even in adolescence children may lack the physical and psychological distance from parents that is needed to evaluate parent–child relationships fully, which would limit their ability to reflect on parent–child relationships (Black, Jaeger, McCartney, & Crittenden, 2000). Thus a consideration of normative changes can inform how we conceptualize and assess attachment in middle childhood.

An analysis of how cognitive development may affect attachment (including how children construct representations of attachment relationships) is also needed (see also Raikes & Thompson, Chapter 12, this volume; Steele & Steele, Chapter 7, this volume). For example, it is not clear when children begin to construct generalized representations of attachment, although they may emerge in middle childhood. One can ask, What kinds of cognitive abilities would be necessary for a child to construct a general model of attachment relationships? As another example, if children engage in more defensive processing in adolescence than in middle childhood, as suggested by Ammaniti and colleagues (2000), then how does this affect our understanding and measurement of avoidance in middle childhood? And if children are less defensive in middle childhood, then might questionnaire and interview measures of attachment be more highly related in middle childhood than in adolescence or adulthood? Another example pertains to the importance of narrative coherence in evaluating attachment. The AAI is predicated on the notion that how one talks about attachment relationships is as important as whether caregivers are portrayed in a positive or negative light (Main, 1996; Main et al., 1985; Steele & Steele, Chapter 7, this volume). Thus an adult who has had difficult relationships with parents but has been able to reflect on and integrate the experiences into an open and coherent understanding of attachment relationships can nevertheless be secure (termed "earned secure"; Main et al., 1985). Main and colleagues (1985) suggest that the capacity to reflect on and to change one's cognitive models of relationships emerges in adolescence, suggesting that the concept of "earned security" would not be relevant in middle childhood. Thus it may be that in middle childhood, as in early childhood (Bretherton, 2003), secure children's narratives are marked by both positive descriptions of family relationships and coherence. One can also ask whether coherence might be manifested differently in middle childhood than later (see Ammaniti et al., 2000). Collaboration between social and cognitive developmentalists would likely provide new approaches to addressing the meaning of attachment in middle childhood.

Perhaps the most important challenge for the field is to answer the question, What are middle childhood measures of attachment measures of? All of the attachment measures created for children in middle childhood rely on children's self-reports, and they are thought to reflect children's understanding of attachment. Not yet settled is the exact nature of children's attachment representations, or what are sometimes referred to as "working models" of attachment (Bowlby, 1973). Are they relational schemas, defined as "cognitive structures representing regularities in patterns of interpersonal relatedness" (Baldwin, 1992), which then guide how children process and organize relationship information (Baldwin, 1992; Bowlby, 1973)? Or could they be conceptualized as scripts, that is, knowledge of the sequence of elements that typically occur in a situation, with attachment scripts organized around how the child uses the attachment figure as a secure base and safe haven (Waters, Rodrigues, & Ridgeway, 1998)? Alternatively, to what degree do responses during attachment interviews reflect children's ability to construct and relate to others emotionally laden narratives (Oppenheim & Waters, 1995)?

Another aspect of defining the meaning of attachment assessments is to consider whether the various measures are tapping a child's general orientation to attachment relationships or are relationship-specific assessments. Early childhood assessments are typically described as relationship-specific assessments (e.g., the Strange Situation is treated a measure of a child's attachment to a particular caregiver). By contrast, measures for older adolescents and adults (e.g., the AAI) are often designed to assess a person's "state of mind" toward attachment and are thus measures of an individual's general style across relationships rather than indicators of the quality of a specific relationship. Both of these conceptualizations have been used to guide the development of middle childhood measures. It is critical for investigators to be clear about the conceptualization that guides their measurement approach (i.e., whether it is a measure of a specific relationship or of general style). In addition, if a measure is conceptualized as relationship specific, then it is important to specifically test this claim by examining the concordance of a child's attachments to different attachment figures.

Of course, it is possible for attachment to be an aspect of personality and to retain a relationship component, as well. That is, children may eventually develop a general style of relating within attachment relationships, but because relationships are dyadic, they may nevertheless have somewhat qualitatively different relationships with different attachment figures. This perspective is consistent with Cook's (2000) examination of attachments in families with adolescent children. Every family member (mother, father, two adolescent children) completed questionnaires asking about their relationship with every other family member. Then, using a social relations analysis, Cook estimated actor, partner, and relationship contributions to family members' perceptions of their relationships with each other. Actor and partner effects represent consistency in behavior across relationships, whereas relationship contributions identify unique components of particular relationships. Cook found that all three were significant, and thus: (1) people tended to form somewhat similar attachments to different family members (actor effect); (2) individuals tended to elicit/create similar relationships with different partners (partner effect); and (3) there was a unique component to attachment relationships that could not be explained by individual characteristics (relationship effect). Across measures and type of relationship, actor and relationship effects were larger than partner effects.

In a recent study we examined the stability and specificity of attachment in 9- to 11-year-old children using the Doll Story Completion Task (Granot & Mayseless, 2001). Three published studies have examined the stability of attachment within middle childhood. Using a separation–reunion procedure with a U.S. sample of fifty 6-year-old children, Main and Cassidy (1988) reported a 62% stability rate over a 1-month interval. Using the Doll Story Completion Task in an Israeli sample of 27 fourth and fifth graders, Granot and Mayseless (2001) reported 94% stability over a 3-month interval. A third study used the child version of the AAI to assess attachment. In a sample of 31 Italian children (Ammaniti et al., 2000), interviewed at 10 and 14 years of age, there was a 71% stability rate. Given these findings and our 3-month test–retest interval, we expected to find evidence for stability of attachment.

Second, we examined the concordance of children's attachments to mother and to father. In the interview stories, only one parent is included in the story. The child's interview responses are thought to reflect the quality of a child's attachment to that particular parent (Granot & Mayseless, 2001). We were able to find only one published study of children in middle childhood in which mother–father concordance was assessed. Verschueren & Marcoen (1999) used a story-stem interview to assess, separately, mother–child and father–child attachment in a sample of seventy-six 6-year-olds. They found significant mother–father concordance, with 47% of the children receiving the same attachment classification to mother and to father. We therefore expected to find moderate concordance for mother–child and father–child attachment in our study.

We examined these questions in a sample of 49 fourth- and fifth-grade children (24 girls and 25 boys). The sample was 84% white, with the remaining a mix of ethnicities. Thirty-six children resided in two-parent households, with the other 13 children in single-mother families. Children made two visits, scheduled 3 months apart, to a university lab to be interviewed. In 25 of the two-parent families, both mothers and fathers agreed to participate. Thus there was an n of 25 for the concordance analyses. In the other 11 two-parent families, only the mother participated. These children, and children in single-mother households, were assigned to the test–retest condition, for an n of 24.

A trained interviewer administered the Doll Story Completion Task (Granot & Mayseless, 2001; see description earlier in chapter). The interviews were scored in two different ways. One set of coders rated the entire interview on four 5-point scales, measuring security, avoidance, ambivalence, and disorganization, and made a best fitting classification, based on the Granot and Mayseless (2001) coding manual. Coders were trained by David Granot and Ofra Mayseless. A second set of coders followed procedures outlined by Waters and colleagues (1998) for a script analysis of attachment narratives. They developed the expected secure script for each story and then ranked each set of stories on scriptedness. Thus children received one score per story, reflecting the degree to which the child's story was similar to the script expected for a securely attached child. Agreement for both sets of coders was adequate.

In the stability and concordance analyses, correlation coefficients were calculated for the pattern ratings, and chi-square and kappa were calculated for classifications. Beginning with the traditional scoring of the interviews, there was significant stability of attachment, although the level of stability was low. Specifically, for classifications, the chi-square test was significant (13.46, $p < .05$), with 50% stability, and rs for pattern ratings ranged from .25 to .54. In the 12 cases without stability, there were two common mismatches: disorganized versus other categories (5) and secure versus avoidant (7). Modest stability was also found when test–retest correlations for secure scriptedness scores were calculated. Scriptedness scores for all but one of the stories were significantly correlated, with significant rs ranging from .34 to .54.

We also found significant levels of mother–father concordance. Using traditional scoring methods, mother–father concordance for classifications was 72% (chi-square test = 24.32, $p < .01$), and rs for pattern ratings were .51 to .78. When mother and father scriptedness scores were correlated for each of the five stories, correlations ranged between .50 and .66. Thus, mother–father concordance was high and exceeded test–retest reliability estimates.

Given the evidence of high mother–father concordance, we suspect that the interview is tapping a generalized script or a child's state of mind in regard to attachment, rather than providing information about a specific attachment relationship. Then why was stability so low for the test–retest group? One possibility is that preadolescence may be the period during which more generalized models of attachment emerge. The process of constructing a generalized script or state of mind in regard to attachment may occur more easily for children who experience stable and consistent family relationships. On the other hand, this process may take more time for children who have a more diverse set of attachment experiences. The stability sample included children in two-parent homes in which only the mother participated ($n = 11$), but it also included all of the children in single-parent families ($n = 13$), and thus it includes some children who have experienced important changes in the reorganization of their families. What we are measuring as lack of consistency in interview responses may occur with some children because they have not yet been able to integrate a diverse set of attachment-related experiences into a coherent and consistent view of attachment relationships. The question would then become, Under what conditions might a preadolescent be able to form a consistent and coherent view of attachment relationships?

CONCLUSIONS

Substantial progress has been made in developing new approaches to assessing attachment during the later middle childhood years. The new methods have adopted different measurement techniques and different definitions of attachment, and a key task for future research is to determine the conceptual overlap of the measures. The construct of attachment also needs to be embedded within a broader developmental context to provide a more developmental approach to the assessment of attachment in middle childhood.

ACKNOWLEDGMENTS

This research was supported by a grant from the Kent State University Research Council. We thank the families who participated in this study. In addition, we thank Josefina Contreras and Rhonda Richardson for their comments on an earlier version of this chapter.

REFERENCES

Abraham, M. A., Kerns, K. A., Morgan, T. A., & Schlegelmilch, A. (2004, April). *Associations between attachment and emotion regulation in preadolescence.* Paper presented at the Conference on Human Development, Washington, DC.

Ainsworth, M. D. S. (1989). Attachments beyond infancy. *American Psychologist, 44,* 709–716.

Ainsworth, M. D. S. (1990). Epilogue: Some considerations regarding theory and assessment relevant to attachments beyond infancy. In M. T. Greenberg, D.

Cicchetti, & E. M. Cummings (Eds.), *Attachment in the preschool years* (pp. 463–488). Chicago: University of Chicago Press.

Ainsworth, M. D., Blehar, M. C., Waters, E., & Wall, S. (1978). *Patterns of attachment: A psychological study of the Strange Situation.* Hillsdale, NJ: Erlbaum.

Allen, J. P., & Land, D. (1999). Attachment in adolescence. In J. Cassidy & P. R. Shaver (Eds.), *Handbook of attachment: Theory, research, and clinical applications* (pp. 319–335). New York: Guilford Press.

Ammaniti, M., van IJzendoorn, M. H., Speranza, A. M., & Tambelli, R. (2000). Internal working models of attachment during late childhood and early adolescence: An exploration of stability and change. *Attachment and Human Development, 2,* 328–346.

Baldwin, M. W. (1992). Relational schemas and the processing of social information. *Psychological Bulletin, 112,* 461–484.

Belsky, J., & Cassidy, J. (1994). Attachment: Theory and evidence. In M. L. Rutter, D. F. Hay, & S. Baron-Cohen (Eds.), *Development through life: A handbook for clinicians* (pp. 373–402). Oxford, UK: Blackwell.

Black, K. A., Jaeger, E., McCartney, K., & Crittenden, P. M. (2000). Attachment models, peer interaction behavior, and feelings about the self. In P. M. Criteenden & A. H. Claussen (Eds.), *The organization of attachment relationships: Maturation, culture, and context* (pp. 300–324). New York: Cambridge University Press.

Bowlby, J. (1973). *Attachment and loss: Vol. 2. Separation, anxiety, and anger.* New York: Basic Books.

Bowlby, J. (1982). *Attachment and loss: Vol. 1. Attachment* (2nd ed.). New York: Basic Books.

Bretherton, I. (2003, April). *Discussant comments.* Paper presented at the biennial meeting of the Society for Research in Child Development, Tampa, FL.

Bretherton, I., Ridgeway, D., & Cassidy, J. (1990). Assessing internal working models of the attachment relationship: An attachment story completion task for 3-year olds. In M. T. Greenberg, D. Cicchetti, & E. M. Cummings (Eds.), *Attachment in the preschool years* (pp. 273–308). Chicago: University of Chicago Press.

Cassidy, J. (1999). The nature of the child's ties. In J. Cassidy & P. R. Shaver (Eds.), *Handbook of attachment: Theory, research, and clinical applications* (pp. 3–20). New York: Guilford Press.

Contreras, J. M., & Kerns, K. A. (2000). Emotion regulation processes: Explaining links between parent–child attachment and peer relationships. In K. A. Kerns, J. M. Contreras, & A. M. Neal-Barnett (Eds.), *Family and peers: Linking two social worlds* (pp. 1–25). Westport, CT: Praeger.

Contreras, J. M., Kerns, K. A., Weimer, B. L., Gentzler, A. L., & Tomich, P. L. (2000). Emotion regulation as a mediator of associations between mother-child attachment and peer relationships in middle childhood. *Journal of Family Psychology, 14,* 111–124.

Cook, W. L. (2000). Understanding attachment security in family context. *Journal of Personality and Social Psychology, 78,* 285–294.

Crowell, J. A., Fraley, R. C., & Shaver, P. R. (1999). Measurement of individual differences in adolescent and adult attachment. In J. Cassidy & P. R.

Shaver (Eds.), *Handbook of attachment: Theory, research, and clinical applications* (pp. 434–465). New York: Guilford Press.

Crowell, J. A., & Waters, E. (1994). Bowlby's theory grown up: The role of attachment in adult love relationships. *Psychological Inquiry, 5,* 31–34.

DeWolff, M. S., & van IJzendoorn, M. H. (1997). Sensitivity and attachment: A meta-analysis of parental antecedents of infant attachment. *Child Development, 68,* 571–591.

Finnegan, R. A., Hodges, E. V. E., & Perry, D. G. (1996). Preoccupied and avoidant coping during middle childhood. *Child Development, 67,* 1318–1328.

Fury, G., Carlson, E. A., & Sroufe, L. A. (1997). Children's representations of attachment relationships in family drawings. *Child Development, 68,* 1154–1164.

Granot, D., & Mayseless, O. (2001). Attachment security and adjustment to school in middle childhood. *International Journal of Behavioral Development, 25,* 530–541.

Green, J., Stanley, C., Smith, V., & Goldwyn, R. (2000). A new method of evaluating attachment representations in young school-age children: The Manchester Child Attachment Story Task. *Attachment and Human Development, 2,* 48–70.

Hansburg, H. G. (1972). *Adolescent separation anxiety: A method for the study of adolescent separation problems.* Springfield, IL: Thomas.

Harter, S. (1982). The perceived competence scale for children. *Child Development, 53,* 87–97.

Hazan, C., & Shaver, P. (1994). Attachment as an organizational framework for research on close relationships. *Psychological Inquiry, 5,* 1–22.

Hazan, C., & Zeifman, D. (1994). Sex and the psychological tether. In K. Bartholomew & D. Perlman (Eds.), *Attachment processes in adulthood* (pp. 151–178). Bristol, PA: Kingsley.

Hazan, C., & Zeifman, D. (1999). Pair bonds as attachments: Evaluating the evidence. In J. Cassidy & P. R. Shaver (Eds.), *Handbook of attachment: Theory, research, and clinical applications* (pp. 336–354). New York: Guilford Press.

Hodges, E. V. E., Finnegan, R. A., & Perry, D. G. (1999). Skewed autonomy-relatedness in preadolescents' conceptions of their relationships with mother, father, and best friend. *Developmental Psychology, 35*(3), 737–748.

Howes, C., & Tonyan, H. (2000). Links between adult and peer relations across four developmental periods. In K. A. Kerns, J. M. Contreras, & A. M. Neal-Barnett (Eds.), *Family and peers: Linking two social worlds* (pp. 85–113). Westport, CT: Praeger.

Kerns, K. A. (1996). Individual differences in friendship quality: Links to child–mother attachment. In W. M. Bukowski, A. F. Newcomb, & W. W. Hartup (Eds.), *The company they keep: Friendship in childhood and adolescence* (pp. 137–157). New York: Cambridge University Press.

Kerns, K. A., Aspelmeier, J. E., Gentzler, A. L., & Grabill, C. (2001). Parent–child attachment and monitoring in middle childhood. *Journal of Family Psychology, 15,* 69–81.

Kerns, K. A., Klepac, L., & Cole, A. (1996). Peer relationships and preadolescents' perceptions of security in the child–mother relationship. *Developmental Psychology, 32,* 457–466.

Kerns, K. A., Tomich, P. L., Aspelmeier, J. E., & Contreras, J. M. (2000). Attachment based assessments of parent–child relationships in middle childhood. *Developmental Psychology, 36,* 614–626.

Kerns, K. A., Tomich, P. L., & Kim, P. (2003). *Normative trends in perceptions of availability and utilization of attachment figures in middle childhood.* Unpublished manuscript.

Klagsbrun, M., & Bowlby, J. (1976). Responses to separation from parents: A clinical test for young children. *Projective Psychology, 21,* 7–28.

Kobak, R., Esposito, A. J., & Serwik, A. (2003, April). *Measuring the attachment hierarchy: Implications for child psychopathology and stress reactivity.* Paper presented at the biennial meeting of the Society for Research in Child Development, Tampa, FL.

Lieberman, M., Doyle, A., & Markiewicz, D. (1999). Developmental patterns in security of attachment to mother and father in late childhood and early adolescence: Associations with peer relations. *Child Development, 70,* 202–213.

Main, M. (1996). Introduction to the special section on attachment and psychopathology: 2. Overview of the field of attachment. *Journal of Consulting and Clinical Psychology, 64,* 237–243.

Main, M., & Cassidy, J. (1988). Categories of response to reunion with the parent at age 6: Predictable from infant attachment classification and stable over a 1–month period. *Developmental Psychology, 24,* 415–426.

Main, M., Kaplan, N., & Cassidy, J. (1985). Security of infancy, childhood, and adulthood: A move to the level of representation. In I. Bretherton & E. Waters (Eds.), Growing points of attachment theory and research. *Monographs of the Society for Research in Child Development, 50*(Serial No. 209).

Marvin, R. S., & Britner, P. A. (1999). Normative development: The ontogeny of attachment. In J. Cassidy & P. R. Shaver (Eds.), *Handbook of attachment: Theory, research, and clinical applications* (pp. 44–67). New York: Guilford Press.

Oppenheim, D., & Waters, H. S. (1995). Narrative processes and attachment representations: Issues of development and assessment. In E. Waters, B. E. Vaughn, G. Posada, & K. Kondo-Ikemura (Eds.), *Monographs of the Society for Research in Child Development, 60*(Serial No. 244).

Page, T. F. (2001). The social meaning of children's narratives: A review of the attachment-based narrative story stem technique. *Child and Adolescent Social Work Journal, 18,* 171–187.

Resnick, G. (1993). *Measuring attachment in early adolescence: A manual for the administration, coding, and interpretation of the Separation Anxiety Test for 11- to 14-year-olds.* Unpublished manuscript.

Resnick, G. (1997, April). *The correspondence between the Strange Situation at 12 months and the Separation Anxiety test at 11 years in an Israeli kibbutz sample.* Paper presented at the biennial meeting of the Society for Research in Child Development, Washington, DC.

Solomon, J., & George, C. (1999). The measurement of attachment security in infancy and childhood. In J. Cassidy & P. R. Shaver (Eds.), *Handbook of attachment: Theory, research, and clinical applications* (pp. 287–316). New York: Guilford Press.

Thompson, R. A. (1998). Early sociopersonality development. In W. Damon (Ed.), *Handbook of child psychology* (pp. 25–104). New York: Wiley.

Thompson, R. A. (1999). Early attachment and later development. In J. Cassidy & P. R. Shaver (Eds.), *Handbook of attachment: Theory, research, and clinical applications* (pp. 265–286). New York: Guilford Press.

van IJzendoorn, M. H., Juffer, F., & Duyvesteyn, M. G. C. (1995). Breaking the intergenerational cycle of insecure attachment: A review of the effects of attachment-based interventions on maternal sensitivity and infant security. *Journal of Child Psychology and Psychiatry, 36*, 225–248.

Verschueren, K., & Marcoen, A. (1999). Representation of self and socioemotional competence in kindergartners: Differential and combined effects of attachment to mother and to father. *Child Development, 70*, 183–201.

Waters, E. (1981). Traits, behavioral systems, and relationships: Three models of infant–adult attachment. In K. Immelman, G. Barlow, L. Petrinovitch, & M. Main (Eds.), *Behavioral development* (pp. 621–650). Cambridge, UK: Cambridge University Press.

Waters, H. S., Rodrigues, L. M., & Ridgeway, D. (1998). Cognitive underpinnings of narrative attachment assessment. *Journal of Experimental Child Psychology, 71*, 211–234.

CHAPTER 4

◆ ◆ ◆

The Attachment Hierarchy in Middle Childhood
Conceptual and Methodological Issues

ROGER KOBAK
NATALIE ROSENTHAL
ASIA SERWIK

The social world of middle childhood is extensive and complex. In addition to maintaining relationships with parents, elementary-age children are actively engaged in friendships, peer groups, and relationships with other adults, including relatives, teachers, and neighbors. Although peers often occupy much of the child's energies and attention, adults continue to provide an important source of guidance and security. Further, children's attachment relationships become more complex with their ability to use secondary or subsidiary attachment figures. The growing complexity of the child's social relationships raises a number of questions for attachment researchers. First, how do we define and identify attachment relationships in middle childhood? If attachment relationships in middle childhood can be clearly defined, a second question emerges. How does the child organize or prioritize multiple attachment relationships? Bowlby suggested that in fact the child would organize his or her attachment relationships by showing a clear preference for a primary attachment figure over subsidiary attachment figures. This organization has been termed an "attachment hierarchy" (Cassidy, 1999; Colin, 1996). Finally, how do children's attachment hierarchies develop and change during middle childhood?

In this chapter, we address three interrelated issues about attachment relationships in middle childhood. First, we consider criteria for identifying attachment relationships in middle childhood. We believe that this issue is best addressed by assessing the child's behavior in contexts that are likely to activate the child's attachment system. Threats to the self (accidents, illness, danger), threats to the availability of the attachment figure (separations, rejection, conflict), and exploratory challenges may all activate the attachment system and provide the opportunity to observe the child's preferences for attachment figures. Second, we explore the notion that school-age children have more than one attachment relationship and that these relationships are hierarchically organized. This hierarchy of attachment figures serves to guide the child's behavior when his or her attachment system is activated. Finally, we discuss a methodology for measuring the hierarchy of attachment relationships in middle childhood. After considering preliminary findings with this new measure, we conclude with directions for future research.

DEVELOPING A DESCRIPTIVE STRATEGY TO IDENTIFY ATTACHMENT RELATIONSHIPS

The growing diversity and complexity of the child's social relationships in middle childhood raises a number of questions about the child's attachment relationships. Although children can readily distinguish relationships with adults from relationships with peers, children clearly develop significant relationships with a variety of adults, including older siblings, teachers, stepparents, and relatives. However, at what point do these relationships qualify as attachments? Similarly, as development progresses, peer relationships occupy an increasingly important part of children's social networks. Can these peer relationships serve as "ad hoc" attachment functions (Waters & Cummings, 2000)? And when would a relationship with a peer qualify as an attachment relationship?

The study of attachment relationships has most often relied on a strategy that defines attachment relationships by categories of caregivers. Although mothers have been presumed to be the attachment figures in the vast majority of studies, other caregiver categories, such as fathers, grandmothers, day-care providers, and teachers (Berlin & Cassidy, 1999; Howes, 1999), should be considered as well. Cultural variations in childcare arrangements have also been investigated, with substantial attention given to the kibbutz arrangement, as well as to the role of grandparents in contexts involving poverty and teenage parents. Research in middle childhood has followed a similar strategy. To the extent that attachment relationships are considered, the presumption has been that children have attachment relationships with their mothers and fathers and perhaps to a lesser extent with stepparents, relatives, and possibly teachers.

Although the assumption that the child has an attachment to the mother is often correct and serves as a useful heuristic, there are exceptions to this rule that are likely to increase with the age of the child. Not only may the child experience disruptions in his or her relationship with a biological mother or father (Kobak, Little, Race, & Acosta, 2001), but he or she may also form significant new relationships with adults during the course of childhood. Development and experience create new possibilities for discontinuities in attachment relationships. By middle childhood most children have formed relationships with several adult caregivers, and many children have experienced divorce, remarriage, and other significant disruptions of their attachment relationships. By adolescence and early adulthood, children begin to transfer attachment functions from parents to close friends and romantic partners (Hazan & Zeifman, 1994).

The problem of defining attachment relationships is further complicated by other components of parent–child relationships. Attachment represents only one component of children's relationships with caregivers. Parents interact with their children in a variety of ways that can be distinguished from attachment, including serving as playmates and teachers (Colin 1996). As children mature, attachment becomes less pervasive in their relationships with parents (Ainsworth, 1991). Much of the child's attachment security derives from "cognitive–affective internalizations," or confident expectations that a parent would be accessible and responsive if needed. The child's internal expectations for attachment figures' availability are often supported by distal communication and are less dependent on immediate physical proximity. Together, these developmental changes reduce the frequency and intensity of attachment behavior and allow the child to attend to more salient developmental tasks (Mayseless, Chapter 1, this volume). As a result, it becomes more difficult to restrict attachment relationships to mothers and fathers. Not only may current parent–child attachments change, but new attachments may also begin to emerge, and attachment functions may be tested in relationships well beyond the biological family (Waters & Cummings, 2000). Furthermore, many aspects of parent–child relationships may be relatively independent of attachment functions. These developmental changes challenge researchers to develop both clearer conceptual definitions of attachment and more explicit contexts in which attachment behavior can be observed in middle childhood.

We propose an alternative to the categorical strategy for defining attachment relationships in middle childhood. Our strategy is guided by attachment theory and leaves questions about the organization of the child's attachment relationships open to descriptive information based on the child's attachment behavior and preferences (Colin, 1996). However, to observe the child's preferences for attachment figures, it is first necessary to identify contexts that activate and terminate the attachment behavioral system. The critical conditions for activating the attachment system involve the child's appraisals of threat and challenge (Kobak, 1999). These appraisals should activate the attachment system and provide an opportunity for researchers to describe attachment behavior and the child's preference for attachment figures.

APPRAISALS THAT ACTIVATE THE ATTACHMENT SYSTEM: DANGER, THREATS TO AVAILABILITY, AND CHALLENGE

Researchers who study attachment in older children and adults face a central problem. Whereas infant researchers can readily observe or create situations in which the attachment system is activated, researchers who study attachment at later periods of development have more difficulty observing attachment behavior (Kerns, Schlegelmilch, Morgan, & Abraham, Chapter 3, this volume; Mayseless, Chapter 1, this volume). Description and assessment of attachment behavior in childhood, adolescence, and adulthood requires a careful consideration of the conditions that activate and deactivate the attachment system and related attachment behavior. Bowlby's (1969/1982) control-systems model of attachment provides researchers with some valuable guidance. In Bowlby's view, the attachment system is regulated by ongoing appraisals of the environment and of the attachment figure (Bretherton 1980). These appraisals modulate the activation of the attachment system by combining perception of environmental cues with feeling evaluations of fear and safety.

Ainsworth (1991) and Bowlby (1969/1982) conceived of the attachment system as working in concert with other behavioral systems that include fear and exploration. Whereas the function of the attachment system is protection, the fear system alerts the individual to *clues of danger* in the environment. As a result, the fear system works in a synchronous relation with attachment. Thus, when the individual appraises cues in the environment as potentially threatening or dangerous, the fear system becomes active. This results in increased vigilance and possible responses that include freezing behavior, or fight-or-flight responses. Bowlby emphasized that appraisals of danger also activate the attachment system and attachment behavior. More subtle appraisals of danger, such as illnesses and periods of fatigue, could also activate the attachment system. Thus threat appraisals activate the attachment system and efforts by the individual to use the attachment figure as a safe haven.

In addition to perceived threats to personal well-being, Bowlby (1973) called attention to another class of appraisals that activate both the fear and the attachment systems. Perceived threats to the availability of the attachment figure could elicit intense anxiety and attachment behavior. In infancy, these threats to caregiver availability are often created by physical separations. At later periods of development, threats to availability can come from witnessing conflict (Davies & Cummings, 1994), threats of abandonment (Bowlby, 1973), and attachment disruptions (Kobak et al., 2001). This type of appraisal results in intense activation of the attachment system and a sequence of responses that Bowlby (1973) termed protest, despair, and detachment.

In addition to the emergency situations in which both fear and attachment systems are intensely activated, the attachment system may also be activated by less extreme situations involving the exploratory behavioral system (Waters & Cummings, 2000). Whereas the fear and attachment systems work in synchrony, exploration has an antithetical relation to the attachment system. For exploration to occur, the attachment system needs to operate at relatively low levels so as not to take precedence over the exploratory system. Yet appraisals of challenge and risk involved in exploration can be supported by the child's awareness that an attachment figure is available if needed. For Ainsworth (1991), a child's appraisals of challenge or uncertainty would also activate the attachment system. The child would not necessarily seek physical contact with the attachment figure in this situation but rather would use the attachment figure as a secure base for exploring the environment and gaining confidence in the face of challenge or uncertainty.

The child's growing cognitive abilities and coping capacities fundamentally alter appraisals of danger and threats to the availability of attachment figures (Mayseless, Chapter 1, this volume; Waters & Cummings, 2000). In infancy, an unfamiliar environment, presence of a stranger, and 2-minute separations from the caregiver can activate both the fear and attachment systems. By middle childhood, none of these conditions would necessarily activate the attachment systems. Several factors account for this profound change in how the child appraises danger. These factors include increased self-reliance and cognitive abilities and the capacity for joint planning with the attachment figure. These changes are illustrated by how the children appraise physical separations from attachment figures. During infancy, separations provide the most standard means of creating a threat to the availability of the caregiver that activates the attachment system. Yet the child's representations of the attachment figure and the linguistic ability to form joint plans reduce the likelihood that he or she will perceive separations as a threat to the caregiver's availability. As a result, physical absence of the attachment figure no longer elicits intense distress, and separation paradigms become less effective in activating the attachment system and eliciting attachment behavior.

The child's appraisal of challenge and uncertainty also changes dramatically with development. The child's growing competency and self-reliance produce many forms of exploration and learning independent of the attachment relationship. As a result, the parent's role increasingly shifts to monitoring the child's own ability to manage his or her stresses and intervening only when the child cannot manage a situation by him- or herself. The challenge for attachment researchers is to identify developmentally appropriate situations involving danger, a threat to the attachment figures' availability, or a challenge in which the child would likely use the attachment figure as a safe haven or secure base.

If attachment behavior is activated by appraisals of danger, threats to availability, and challenge, it becomes increasingly likely that peers and nonparental adults may serve attachment functions in contexts in which parents are not physically present. This creates a new set of questions. Does the child's use of an adult or peer as a safe haven or secure base mean that the child has an attachment relationship with that particular individual? For instance, many children use close friends to support their entry into challenging contexts at school. As the child develops a more differentiated understanding of social relationships, he or she may seek support or encouragement from individuals based on particular types of expertise. Peers' availability and expertise about peer-related threats or challenges might lead a child to prefer them as a safe haven or secure base over adult attachment figures. Would the use of the friend as a secure base or safe haven constitute an attachment relationship?

A definition of attachment relationships requires moving beyond a focus on attachment functions to identifying the special features of an attachment bond. In addition to serving attachment functions, an attachment relationship provides the individual with confidence that the attachment figure will be available in an enduring way despite changes that occur over time and place (Cassidy 1999). The enduring quality of an attachment bond provides the individual with the confident knowledge that an attachment figure can be counted on in a noncontingent or unconditional manner. In adult attachments, this knowledge has been measured as commitment, and it provides individuals with the confidence that their relationship will endure despite daily fluctuations (Duemmler & Kobak, 2001). In adult–child attachments, the child usually learns that the relationship will be maintained despite changes in residence and changes brought about by time. In this sense, an attachment bond can serve as a secure base and safe haven, which provides the individual with confidence in the unconditional nature of the bond.

In sum, theory suggests that the child's relationships with adults and peers must meet several criteria to be considered attachment relationships. First, the attachment figure needs to serve attachment functions, such as providing a safe haven when the individual appraises danger and a secure base when the individual appraises challenge. Second, the child's sense of safety and well-being must be linked to his or her appraisal of the availability of the attachment figure. The emotional significance of an attachment figure is tested when he or she perceives a threat to the attachment figure's availability (Kobak, 1999). Third, the child must view the attachment figure as having an enduring commitment to being available if needed regardless of changes in time or context. These criteria can guide researchers in identifying attachment relationships in middle childhood. However, if multiple attachment relationships are identified, another problem arises. Are the child's attachment figures equally significant, or does the child organize attachment relationships in a specific order of importance? A brief review of the theoretical and empirical literature on the attachment hierarchy in infancy and early childhood can help to guide considerations of how to approach this issue in middle childhood.

MULTIPLE ATTACHMENT RELATIONSHIPS AND THE ATTACHMENT HIERARCHY

If a child has multiple attachment relationships, a new issue arises. Are attachment figures interchangeable, or do children show clear preferences for one person over another? In the initial volume of his attachment trilogy (1969/1982), Bowlby proposed that children organize their relationships with caregivers into a hierarchy of attachment figures. The notion of a hierarchy was proposed to address several issues. First, it was meant to counter the notion that the child forms an attachment only with the maternal figure, thereby acknowledging the importance of multiple caregivers and cultural variations in caregiving arrangements. Second, the hierarchy concept suggested that not all caregivers play an equally significant role in meeting the child's attachment needs but rather that the child develops well-defined preferences for one caregiver over another at times when his or her attachment system is activated. Bowlby described the most preferred caregiver in the attachment hierarchy as a "principal" or primary attachment figure, and other caregivers were referred to as "subsidiary" (secondary, tertiary, etc.) attachment figures (Cassidy, 1999;

Colin, 1996). In spite of growing interest in the role of multiple caregivers (Colin, 1996; Howes, 1999) and cross-cultural variations in caregiving arrangements (Sagi et al., 1985; van IJzendoorn, Sagi, & Lambermon, 1992) the hierarchy construct has generated relatively little systematic research.

A child's attachment hierarchy consists of an organized set of preferences for whom the child would seek out at times when the attachment system is activated (Colin, 1996). This definition provides two major criteria for assessing a child's attachment hierarchy. First, the child's preferences for particular caregivers must be assessed. This suggests that children must be observed or interviewed in contexts in which they can choose between attachment figures. Second, the contexts in which the child's preferences are observed must be ones in which the attachment system is activated. As we have noted, the attachment system becomes most intensely activated in situations of danger or distress, challenge, or when the child perceives a threat to the caregiver's availability (Ainsworth, 1991). By assessing the child's preference for caregivers in each of these attachment-related situations, it becomes possible to assess the attachment hierarchy.

Several studies of infants and young children assessed young children's preferences in situations in which their attachment systems were activated. In her classic study of infants in Uganda, Ainsworth (1967), through extensive observation, could identify the caregivers around whom the child organized his or her attachment behavior. These observations led her to distinguish between primary and secondary attachment figures. Thus she could observe the child's preferences for caregivers in a range of naturally occurring situations in which the attachment system was activated. Similarly, observation of young children in a Scottish village allowed Schaffer and Emerson (1964) to identify children's attachment figures and assign them to primary or secondary status. However, not all studies suggest that children clearly prefer one parent over the other. Studies in the United States suggest that in families in which caregiving is shared between mothers and fathers, clear preference between the mother and father could not be readily observed (Lamb, 1978). Colin (1996) used a laboratory procedure similar to the Strange Situation with both the mother and father present. She observed that 70% of her sample showed clear preferences for the mother. However, 24% of her infants showed a preference for the father, and these infants had fathers who had been able to spend more time with them and had taken on more caregiving responsibilities.

Most studies of infant and toddler's caregivers have relied on Strange Situation assessment with different caregivers. For instance, van IJzendoorn and his colleagues (1992) focus on issues related to the validity of the Strange Situation categories. In order to decide whether a particular category of caregiver such as a day-care provider or metapelet was an attachment figure, they developed a set of validity criteria that can be applied to the Strange Situation paradigm. If a child's classifications with alternative caregivers (day-care providers, kibbutz metapelet) in the Strange Situation met similar validity criteria to those established with mothers, then it is assumed that the child had formed an attachment with the alternative caregiver. Howes (1999) proposed an alternative set of criteria for identifying attachment figures based on network analysis and assessment of the caregiver's provision of care, consistency, and emotional investment in the child. Although both approaches to identifying attachment figures can provide important data, neither approach provides an opportunity to observe the child's preferences for attachment figures or to determine the caregiver's place in the child's attachment hierarchy.

We believe that the lack of research on the attachment hierarchy stems from the difficulties in observing young children's preferences for caregivers in attachment-related contexts. However, as children become old enough to participate in interviews, investigators can adopt more approaches that allow children to identify or nominate the caregivers who constitute their attachment hierarchies. A number of investigators have employed such an approach with late adolescents and young adults (Fraley & Davis, 1997; Hazan & Zeifman 1994). These investigators developed a number of attachment-related contexts that included separation distress, proximity seeking, safe haven, and secure base and asked participants to name whom they would go to in each situation. Primary and secondary attachment figures were distinguished based on the number of situations in which they were nominated. The methodology used in these studies met two criteria for assessing the attachment hierarchy: They used a nomination procedure that was open ended as opposed to being based on researcher-defined categories, and the questions in the procedure were designed to elicit the participant's nominations in attachment-related contexts. However, the researchers did not use a ranking procedure, which can determine both the child's use of secondary or tertiary attachment figures and the consistency of the child's preferences across attachment situations.

The notion of having individuals order their preferences for caregivers in particular situations was a central feature of the Family and Friends measure developed by Reid, Landesman, Treder, and Jaccard (1989) to measure children's social support (Booth-LaForce, Rubin, Rose-Krasnor, & Burgess, Chapter 8, this volume; Booth, Rubin, & Rose-Krasnor, 1998). In this procedure, the interviewer asked the child to name, by category, potential sources of social support, including mother, father, siblings, a best friend, a relative, a teacher, and others. The child was then asked to rank who they would go to in five social-support situations that involved (1) talking about feelings, (2) telling something good that happened, (3) telling something bad that he or she did, (4) making the child feel good about him- or herself, and (5) knowing or understanding him or her. Children ranked their support figures based on the frequency with which they would go to each person. A support figure's ranking was determined by averaging his or her placement across the five support episodes. The Family and Friends offers a ranking procedure that allows researchers to consider the consistency of preference across situations requiring social support. Although social support may overlap with secure-base and safe-haven attachment functions, the situations were not specifically designed to assess attachment. In addition, nominations were structured by category in a way that may include individuals who are not likely to be attachment figures.

Developing situations that children will appraise as dangerous, as a threat to an attachment figure's availability, or as a challenge is a critical first step toward developing an attachment assessment. However, if these situations are to be useful in defining attachment relationships and assessing their hierarchical organization, several additional concerns need to be addressed. First, identifying the child's preference for particular attachment figures requires that the assessment context gives the child equal access to all possible caregivers. Various individuals need to be available in order to observe the child's preferences. Thus assessment contexts should not bias the child toward one figure or another. Finally, to consider secondary or subsidiary attachment figures, the context must be one in which the child's preference for a secondary attachment figure can be observed when access to a primary figure is blocked. This requirement may be met by asking children to rank their preferences for caregivers in an attachment-related context. In the next section, we describe the Important People Interview (IPI), a measure specifically designed to assess children's preferences for caregivers in attachment situations. This measure assesses children's preferences for attachment figures by using a ranking procedure similar to the Family and Friends measure. Preferences are assessed in response to questions designed to help the child identify attachment figures and his or her preferences in situations that are likely to activate his or her attachment system.

THE IMPORTANT PEOPLE INTERVIEW: ASSESSING CHILDREN'S PREFERENCES FOR CAREGIVERS IN ATTACHMENT SITUATIONS

We developed the IPI to assess a child's hierarchy of attachment figures (Kobak & Rosenthal, 2003). It is based on the three types of threat appraisals that may activate the attachment system: danger, threat to the attachment figure's availability, and challenge, as well as our fourth criteria, the idea that attachment bonds are enduring relationships that provide the individual with confidence in the availability of the attachment figure across time and place. The brief interview begins by asking the child to name the four most important people in his or her life and then to describe his or her relationship with each person. The child was asked to name four persons in order to allow us to test for the consistency of preferences across caregivers and to distinguish between the primary and secondary attachment figures. Each of the four people's names is written on an index card. The cards are then placed in front of the child for the next four questions. The experimenter then asks the child, "Of these people, who do you feel closest to?" After recording the child's response, the interviewer removes the card and then asks the child, "Of those people left, who do you feel closest to?" The procedure is repeated until all four people are ranked.

The interviewer repeats the same procedure for the three remaining questions: "Imagine something has really upset you and made you cry. Who would you go to for help?" "If you went on a trip across the country for several weeks, whom would you miss the most?"; and "Imagine you won a prize. Which of these people would feel the most proud of you?" Finally, children are asked several follow-up questions: "Who lives in your house?", "Which people do you see every day?", and, for any person the child does not list as seeing every day, "How often do you see (person)?"

The IPI is scored by assigning points for an individual's ranking on each of the five questions, beginning with the order in which the child names the important people in his or her life. Individuals listed first are given 4 points, those listed second receive 3 points, those listed third receive 2 points, and those listed fourth receive 1 point. If the child did not rank an individual on a particular question, that individual was given zero points for that question. Twelve children did not rank one or more individuals at some point during the task. The rankings of each of the four most important individuals were summed across the five questions in the IPI.

ASSESSING THE ATTACHMENT HIERARCHY:
THE CONSISTENCY OF PREFERENCES FOR ATTACHMENT FIGURES
ACROSS SITUATIONS

In our initial study, we administered the IPI to a total of 74 children who were included in the final data collection, ranging in age from 9 to 13, with a mean age of 11.34 years. The sample was 62% male and 51% white, with nonwhites being largely African American (88%). Fifty-one percent of the sample resided with both a biological mother and father, whereas 24% lived with a single parent, 16% lived in a household with a single parent and another adult, and 9% lived in a household with neither a biological mother nor a biological father. The rankings data from the IPI was used to address two descriptive questions. Our first question was whether children in late middle childhood organize their relationships into an attachment hierarchy. If children have a hierarchy, they would show consistency in their preference for a particular person across the five different attachment situations in the IPI. On the other hand, children with less hierarchical organization of their attachment relationships would change preferences for particular attachment figures with different situations. For example, they may miss a sibling more than a parent and yet report that they would go to the parent first when upset. We examined the consistency of the child's preferences for attachment figures by creating matrices for each child organized by person (the four most important people) and situation (the five attachment situations). If the child showed a consistent preference for a person (rows) across the five attachment situations (columns), a larger portion of the variance in rankings would be accounted for by person. Overall, children demonstrated a strong tendency to show consistent preferences for particular adults, with a mean of variance accounted for by attachment figure of 62% (range = 4–97%, SD = 23%), though we found considerable variability between children in the extent to which they showed hierarchical organization of the important people in their lives.

Categories of Primary and Secondary Attachment Figures

By adding the rankings of each person across the five situations, we could use the children's preferences for attachment figures to identify who they viewed as primary and secondary figures. Despite the common assumption that the mother is the primary attachment figure, only 73% of the children in our sample identified their biological mothers as their primary attachment figures; 14% identified their fathers as primary; and 13% identified someone other than a biological parent, usually a relative, as their primary figure. Persons occupying the position of secondary attachment figures proved to be more variable, with 48% of the sample identifying their biological fathers as their secondary attachment figure; 16% named their mothers; and 36% indicated some other individual in that role. Sixty-three percent of children with mothers as their primary figures had biological fathers as their secondary figures, whereas 82% of children with biological fathers as their primary figures had biological mothers as their secondary figures. These results suggest that even when a mother is not the primary figure, she is rarely out of the picture completely, whereas fathers tend to be somewhat more absent if they are not the primary figures. Our methodology for assessing children's attachment hierarchies opens the door to a wide variety of new questions about the role these hierarchies play in children's adaptation during middle child-hood. These questions fall into two broad categories. The first issue concerns normative development, and the second set of issues center on the influence that hierarchies have on an individual's adaptation.

NORMATIVE DEVELOPMENT AND THE ATTACHMENT HIERARCHY

By assessing the attachment hierarchy, researchers can further specify a number of issues related to normative development and the ontogeny of attachment relationships. First, the notion of an attachment hierarchy provides a way of differentiating between the many significant relationships that constitute the child's expanding social network. Peer and close-friend relationships clearly become a salient aspect of social relationships during middle childhood (Booth-LaForce et al., Chapter 8; Mayseless, Chapter 1, this volume). Do close friendships count as attachment relationships? Assessment of children's preferences in situations in which their attachment systems are activated provides a way of answering this question. Although none of the children in our sample identified a peer or sibling as a primary or secondary attachment figure, we suspect in specific contexts peers may serve attachment functions in middle childhood. There are many instances in which a child appraises a situation as moderately dangerous or challenging and in which peers would be more available than adults. These contexts provide the child with an opportunity to test peers as ad hoc attachment figures (Waters & Cummings, 2000). Furthermore, children are likely to have clear preferences in these situations that allow them to discriminate between friends and close friends. However, if situations involve more intense activation of the attachment system and if assessment contexts are constructed that hypothetically give the child equal access to significant peers and adults, we suspect that adult attachment figures are likely to be preferred over peers in middle childhood. This is even more likely when the enduring nature of the bond is considered and when participants are asked to identify their preferences for individuals who are "most important" or whom they can "always count on." By assessing the child's preferences for adults and peers in a variety of attachment and non-attachment-related situations, these types of predictions can be empirically tested.

Attachment researchers generally agree that by adulthood most individuals have replaced parents with an adult partner as the primary attachment figure (Weiss, 1982). This process of transferring attachment functions from parents to peers is likely to be a gradual process that begins in middle childhood with peers serving as ad hoc attachment figures. By adolescence, peers may begin to move toward the primary position in a child's attachment hierarchy. Hazan and Zeifman (1994), using a cross-sectional design, provided a general overview of changes in the attachment hierarchy across the lifespan. By adolescence, they report that children begin to transfer attachment from parents to peers, but these peers are nearly always romantic partners. By early adulthood, romantic relationships and parental ones continue to make up the majority of true attachment relationships (i.e., ones that meet their four criteria for an attachment bond). Assessing adolescents' preferences for adults, close friends, and romantic partners in attachment-related situations would provide valuable data for more clearly identifying these important developmental changes.

THE ATTACHMENT HIERARCHY AND ADAPTATION

The notion of monotropy has been one of the most controversial in the attachment literature and raises an important question about the hierarchy construct. Monotropy predicts that when a child's attachment system is activated, having a consistent set of preferences for a primary figure will lead to better adaptation. To answer this question, researchers need to be able to distinguish primary from secondary figures and to assess the security of attachment with each figure. Some studies lend support to the monotropy construct. For example, Howes and her colleagues found that children who were securely attached to their primary figures but insecurely attached to their secondary figures were more socially competent than children who were securely attached to their secondary but insecurely attached to their primary figures (Howes, Rodning, Galluzzo, & Myers, 1988).

Alternatives to the monotropy hypothesis have been proposed. Howes (1999) suggests three ways in which children could be influenced by multiple attachment relationships: hierarchical, independent, and integrative organization. The *hierarchical organization* model posits that a child's representation of one (the primary) attachment figure is the most influential in the child's developing models of self and others (Bretherton, 1985). Within this model, secondary attachment figures may serve as a secure base only when the primary attachment figure is unavailable. The theory of *independent organization* of multiple attachment figures suggests that each attachment figure may influence a different area of the child's development and that different attachment relationships influence different domains of functioning (Bretherton, 1985). Research on infants' security with mothers and fathers provides some support for this model (see Steele & Steele, Chapter 7, this volume). Finally, the theory of *integrative organization* proposes that a child integrates knowledge from multiple attachment relationships into a single model from which he or she attempts to understand him- or herself and others (van IJzendoorn et al., 1992). In this model, if one relationship is insecure, it may be compensated for by other, secure relationships; thus the overall quality of the child's entire attachment network should be predictive of the child's functioning.

Assessment of the attachment hierarchy is a critical step for testing these different models of how the organization of attachment relationships influences adaptation. Each of the models requires identifying multiple attachment figures, and the hierarchical model requires distinguishing a primary from a secondary attachment figure. Once attachment relationships are identified, each of the models requires an assessment of the quality or security of each relationship. In middle childhood, several measures of security in the context of a relationship are available (see Kerns et al., Chapter 3, this volume; Yunger, Corby, & Perry, Chapter 5, this volume). By combining measures of the attachment hierarchy with measures of attachment security, new types of analyses become possible. For instance, does a mother's status as a primary or secondary figure moderate the effect the child's security with that parent has on his or her adaptation? Are there families in which the distinction between primary and secondary is less hierarchically organized than in other families, and is this influenced by the quality of the marital relationship?

Finally, in addition to moderating the effects of attachment security on adaptation, the attachment hierarchy may have a direct effect on adjustment. Our hypothesis would be that children who show more consistent preferences for a primary attachment figure would have better adaptation. This suggests that children who demonstrate hierarchical organization of preferences would have more confidence about how to manage situations in which their attachment systems are activated. A longitudinal study of children age 4 to age 8 by Booth and her colleagues (1998) lends some support to our hypothesis. These investigators found that the child's security with mother at age 4, assessed with a reunion procedure, predicted the consistency with which the child ranked the mother across five social support situations at age 8. This suggested that children who had a more clearly defined set of preferences for their mothers at age 8 had been more secure with mothers at age 4.

SUMMARY AND FUTURE DIRECTIONS

We believe that the construct of an attachment hierarchy can contribute to more precise hypotheses about attachment in middle childhood and to methods that make these hypotheses subject to empirical test. First, it provides a way of accommodating the considerable diversity in caregiving practices in different cultural contexts. Although it is true that, in many cases in Western cultures, a child's primary attachment figure is his or her mother and the child's secondary attachment figure is his or her father (Ainsworth, 1967; Bowlby, 1969/1982; Howes, 1999; van IJzendoorn, et al., 1992), this is certainly not always the case. By assessing the attachment hierarchy, researchers can produce descriptive information about the diversity of adults who serve as attachment figures for children, adolescents, and adults. The hierarchy construct can also play an important role in testing hypotheses about normative development and the ontogeny of attachment relationships. By differentiating between attachment figures, it becomes possible to clearly specify when peers supplant adults in the attachment hierarchy. It may also be possible to identify occasions on which peers serve attachment functions but do not yet actually serve as attachment figures. Further refinement of our assessment of the attachment hierarchy may lead to new ways of testing hypotheses about the sequence through which attachment functions are transferred from parents to peers (Hazan & Zeifman, 1994). Finally, assessment of the attachment hierarchy makes it possible to specify and test hypotheses about how multiple attachment relationships contribute to children, adolescent, and adult adaptation. Not only can traditional questions of how security with mothers, fathers, and peers influence adaptation be refined, but also new questions about the importance of hierarchical organization to adaptation can be addressed.

ACKNOWLEDGMENTS

Preparation of this chapter was supported by Grant No. RO1-MH59670 from the National Institute of Mental Health to Roger Kobak.

REFERENCES

Ainsworth, M. D. S. (1967). *Infancy in Uganda*. Baltimore: Johns Hopkins Press.
Ainsworth, M. D. S. (1991). Attachments and other affectional bonds across the life cycle. In C. M. Parkes, J. Stevenson-Hinde, & P. Marris (Eds.), *Attachment across the life cycle* (pp. 33–51). London: Routledge.
Berlin, L. J., & Cassidy, J. (1999). Relations among relationships: Contributions from attachment theory and research. In J. Cassidy & P. R. Shaver (Eds.), *Attachment handbook: Theory, research, and clinical implications* (pp. 688–712). New York: Guilford Press.
Booth, C., Rubin, K. H., & Rose-Krasnor, L. (1998). Perceptions of emotional support from mother and friend in middle childhood: Links with social-emotional adaptation and preschool attachment security. *Child Development, 69*, 427–442.

Bowlby, J. (1973). *Attachment and loss. Vol. 2: Separation, anxiety and anger.* New York: Basic Books.

Bowlby, J. (1982). *Attachment and loss. Vol. 1: Attachment.* New York: Basic Books. (Original work published 1969)

Bretherton, I. (1980). Young children in stressful situations: The supporting role of attachment figures and unfamiliar caregivers. In G. V. Coelho & P. I. Ahmed (Eds.), *Uprooting and development* (pp. 179–210). New York: Plenum Press.

Bretherton, I. (1985). Attachment theory: Retrospect and prospect. *Monographs of the Society for Research in Child Development, 50*(1–2), 3–35.

Cassidy, J. (1999). The nature of the child's ties. In J. Cassidy & P. Shaver (Eds.), *Handbook of attachment, theory, research and clinical implications* (pp. 3–20). New York: Guilford Press.

Colin, V. (1996). *Human attachment.* New York: McGraw-Hill.

Davies, P., & Cummings, E. M. (1994). Marital conflict and child adjustment: An emotional security hypothesis. *Psychological Bulletin, 116,* 387–411.

Duemmler, S., & Kobak, R. (2001). The development of attachment and commitment in dating relationships: Attachment security as a relationship construct. *Journal of Adolescence, 24,* 401–415.

Fraley, C., & Davis, K. E. (1997). Attachment formation and transfer in young adults' close friendships and romantic relationships. *Personal Relationships, 4,* 131–144.

Hazan, C., & Zeifman, D. (1994). Sex and the psychological tether. In K. Bartholomew & D. Perlman (Eds.), *Attachment processes in personal relationships* (Vol. 5, pp. 151–177). London: Kingsley.

Howes, C. (1999). Attachment relationships in the context of multiple caregivers. In J. Cassidy & P. R. Shaver (Eds.), *Handbook of attachment: Theory, research, and clinical applications* (pp. 671–687). New York: Guilford Press.

Howes, C., Rodning, C., Galluzzo, D. C., & Myers, L. (1988). Attachment and child care: Relationships with mother and caregiver. *Early Childhood Research Quarterly, 3,* 705–715.

Kobak, R. (1999). The emotional dynamics of disruptions in attachment relationships: Implications for theory, research, and clinical intervention. In J. Cassidy & P. R. Shaver (Eds.), *Handbook of attachment: Theory, research, and clinical applications* (pp. 21–43). New York: Guilford Press.

Kobak, R., Little, M., Race E., & Acosta, M. (2001). Attachment disruptions in seriously emotionally disturbed children: Implications for treatment. *Attachment and Human Development, 3,* 243–258.

Kobak, R., & Rosenthal, N. (2003). *The important people interview.* Unpublished manuscript, Department of Psychology, University of Delaware.

Lamb, M. (1978). Qualitative aspects of mother– and father–infant attachments. *Infant Behavior and Development, 1,* 265–275.

Reid, M., Landesman, S., Treder, R., & Jaccard, J. (1989). "My family and friends": Six- to twelve-year-old children's perceptions of social support. *Child Development, 60,* 896–910.

Sagi, A., Lamb, M., Lewkowicz, K. S., Shoham, R., Dvir, R., & Estes, D. (1985). Security of infant-mother, –father and –metapelet attachments among kibbutz-reared Israeli children. In I. Bretherton & E. Waters (Eds.), Growing points in attachment theory and research. *Monographs of the Society for Research in Child Development, 50*(1–2, Serial No. 209), 257–275.

Schaffer, H. R., & Emerson, P. E. (1964). The development of social attachments in infancy. *Monographs of the Society for Research in Child Development, 29*(3), 1–77.

van IJzendoorn, M. H., Sagi, A., & Lambermon, M. W. (1992). The multiple caretaker paradox: Data from Holland and Israel. In R. C. Pianta (Ed.), *New directions for child development: Beyond the parent: The role of other adults in children's lives* (Vol. 57, pp. 5–24). San Francisco: Jossey-Bass.

Waters, E., & Cummings, E. M. (2000). A secure base from which to explore close relationships. *Child Development, 71*(1), 164–172.

Weiss, R. S. (1982). Attachment in adult life. In C. M. Parkes & J. Stevenson-Hinde (Eds.), *The place of attachment in human behavior* (pp. 171–184). New York: Basic Books.

CHAPTER 5

◆ ◆ ◆

Dimensions of Attachment
in Middle Childhood

JENNIFER L. YUNGER
BROOKE C. CORBY
DAVID G. PERRY

Although attachment theory is a theory of social development "from the cradle to the grave" (Bowlby, 1979, p. 129), research assessments of attachment are almost always limited to either quite young children (infants, toddlers, and preschoolers) or much older persons (adolescents and adults). Strategies for assessing attachment during the in-between period of middle childhood have been slow to develop, but they are necessary if we are to understand the full range of phenomena suggested by attachment theory. In this chapter, we argue that self-report questionnaires are useful for assessing attachment in middle childhood. We begin the chapter with a synopsis of prior research on attachment that highlights lacunae in our knowledge owing to the paucity of work in which attachment is assessed during middle childhood. We go on to describe the development of two self-report scales for assessing attachment, and we summarize preliminary evidence for the validity of the scales. We then present a new study offering more compelling support for the validity of the scales. Finally, we offer conclusions and suggestions for future research.

ATTACHMENT THEORY, RESEARCH, AND LACUNAE

Attachment theory distinguishes between secure and insecure attachments (Ainsworth, 1979; Bowlby, 1973). In infancy, a *secure* attachment is presumably promoted by a caregiver who is reliably available and effectively provides care and comfort. Secure infants are believed to form a cognitive representation of the relationship (an "internal working model") in which the caregiver is viewed as available if needed and the self is viewed as lovable and worthy of care. Infants are judged to be secure if they seek the caregiver at times of stress, effectively use the caregiver to allay distress, and use the caregiver as a secure base for exploration (by venturing out from the parent to explore novelty but returning for soothing when difficulties are encountered).

Other infants, however, are less fortunate. Perhaps their chosen caregivers are not consistently responsive, are insensitively responsive, or are even rebuffing. If so, these infants may develop insecure attachments by forming working models in which the caregiver is viewed as unavailable, unhelpful, or hurtful and the self is viewed as unloved. Insecure attachments can assume either an organized or a disorganized form. Two distinct, well-organized styles of coping with insecurity are the *preoccupied* and *avoidant* styles. The hallmark of preoccupied attachment (also called resistant or ambivalent) is excessive clinginess; preoccupied babies have a strong need for the caregiver in even mildly stressful and novel situations (which impedes exploration), have difficulty separating from the caregiver, and have difficulty deriving comfort from the caregiver when distressed, especially after a separation. Avoidant attachment (also called dismissing) is marked by limited affective engagement with the caregiver. Avoidant babies explore but avoid the caregiver while doing so; they do not seek the caregiver when distressed; and they ignore the caregiver after a separation. Thus both preoccupied and avoidant babies fail to use the caregiver as a secure base, but in opposite ways. An insecure infant is said to have a *disorganized* attachment when the infant fails to use the caregiver as a secure base but does not exhibit a consistent style of relating to the caregiver (e.g., the baby mixes preoccupied with avoidant behavior or simply freezes during crucial attachment contexts, such as stress). In this chapter, we focus on the two organized styles of insecure attachment, but the importance of disorganized attachment is also discussed.

The different internal working models and behavioral styles of secure, preoccupied, and avoidant infants presumably influence how the children adapt in later social contexts. Secure children are believed to carry positive social expectations (e.g., a belief that others are helpful) and competencies (e.g., the ability to calm oneself when distressed) into new relationships, thereby encouraging benign behavior from others and leading to positive social interactions and relationships. In contrast, inse-curely attached children are thought to possess less favorable expectations and competencies that undermine prospects for later social success.

Much of the evidence bearing on these hypotheses comes from stud-ies in which young children have been assessed for attachment using the Strange Situation procedure (Ainsworth & Wittig, 1969), or a variation thereof, and then assessed for adjustment a few years later. As expected, children with secure histories have more harmonious interactions with teachers and peers, are better liked, have more friends and higher quality friendships, and have fewer behavior problems (Berlin & Cassidy, 1999; Thompson, 1998).

An attachment style developed in infancy is believed to have a good chance of persisting for many years, for several reasons (Sroufe & Fleeson, 1986; Thompson, 1998). First, there may be continuity in the caregiving environment. Second, children's internal working models may promote expectancy-confirmation processes that reinforce the attachment style (e.g., an insecure child's expectation that others will be rejecting may cause the child to be accusatory toward a friend, leading to a new instance of rejection). Third, social skills (or deficits) may elicit behaviors from interaction partners that help maintain the attachment style. Fourth, at-tachment security may influence how well the child masters later develop-mental tasks (e.g., identity formation) that have the power to challenge earlier working models. Despite these bases for continuity, many children are likely to experience changes over time in the contextual conditions that support attachment styles (e.g., parental divorce may render a parent less supportive), and thus strong continuity in attachment style from in-fancy to middle childhood should not be expected (Fox, 1997; Lewis, Feiring, & Rosenthal, 2000).

To complete our synopsis of attachment theory and research, it is necessary to jump to adulthood. The literature on attachment in adult-hood is bifurcated into two traditions. The first focuses on adults' repre-sentations of their attachments to their parents. Even adults possess work-ing models of their relationships with their parents that can be classified (on the basis of the Adult Attachment Interview) as secure, preoccupied, or avoidant (Main, Kaplan, & Cassidy, 1985). Adults classified as preoccu-pied or avoidant exhibit problematic adjustment, as well as inept parent-ing of their own offspring (Crowell, Fraley, & Shaver, 1999). Several longi-tudinal studies show some (slight) continuity in attachment style from infancy to early adulthood (Carlson, 1997; van IJzendoorn, 1997; Waters, Merrick, Albersheim, & Treboux, 1995).

The other research tradition on adult attachment focuses on adults' styles of relating to romantic partners. Using self-report questionnaires, researchers have been able to identify secure, preoccupied, and avoidant romantic styles (Brennan, Clark, & Shaver, 1998; Hazan & Shaver, 1987). Secures are comfortable with intimacy and do not have undue fears of rejection; preoccupieds report intense needs for closeness but fear there is something wrong with them that will ultimately drive their partner away; avoidants report difficulty being close to and trusting others. Compared with adults with secure romantic styles, those with preoccupied and avoidant styles report more distressed relationships and are less able to use their partners to cope effectively with stressors (Feeney, 1999). Match-ups of romantic styles also matter. For example, preoccupied women tend to experience avoidant male partners as problematic (e.g., Kirkpatrick & Davis, 1994).

This synopsis highlights gaps in our knowledge owing to the lack of procedures for assessing attachment during middle childhood. First, it is impossible to identify determinants of change in attachment style between early and middle childhood, or between middle childhood and adulthood, without assessing attachment in middle childhood. In addition, attachment during middle childhood may have crucial consequences for children's later social adaptation. For example, Furman and Wehner (1994) have suggested that preadolescents tend to transfer their styles of attachment from family members to peers (e.g., a child who is preoccupied with the mother tends to be clingy with close same-sex friends) and, moreover, tend to carry their styles of relating to same-sex friends into later romantic relationships. Evaluating such a model requires assessing attachment during middle childhood.

DEVELOPMENT OF THE CHILDREN'S COPING STRATEGIES QUESTIONNAIRE

In recent years, there have been several attempts to measure attachment in preadolescence, but in our view the approach has been too limited. In most of these studies, assessment of attachment is restricted to children's perceptions of the global warmth, responsiveness, and supportiveness of the caregiver. Typical items on such scales assess children's perceptions of the caregiver's availability, affection, trustworthiness, helpfulness, openness to communication, and the like—qualities that should promote a basic sense of security. These studies show that such measures indeed predict several aspects of adjustment, including self-esteem, antisocial behavior, peer rejection, friendship formation and functioning, association with deviant peers, and academic performance (e.g., Armsden & Greenberg, 1987; Kerns, Klepac, & Cole, 1996). However, none of these studies assessed preoccupied and avoidant coping styles. This is unfortunate because conceptual definitions of attachment security refer not only to children's confidence in the caregiver's availability and responsiveness but also to children's skillful use of the caregiver as a secure base for exploration (Thompson, 1999; Waters & Cummings, 2000). Preoccupied and avoidant coping styles represent two well-organized and well-documented styles of failure to use the caregiver as a secure base and may have different implications for subsequent adjustment.

With these considerations in mind, Finnegan, Hodges, and Perry (1996) set out to develop measures of preoccupied and avoidant attachment in middle childhood. They opted to develop self-report scales to assess these two coping styles because they saw potential problems with narrative (interview) and behavioral observation approaches at these ages. Narratives are valuable because they can be scored on dimensions that allow inferences about unconscious processes (e.g., cohesiveness, defensiveness), but they are difficult to score reliably, they may be influenced by language competence, and (at least for some scoring schemes) they presuppose formal operational capabilities (Crowell et al., 1999). Behavioral observations are probably not suitable for children much older than 5 or 6 years of age, because it is difficult to implement age-appropriate stressors, and children begin to balk at the procedures (Lewis et al., 2000; Stevenson-Hinde & Shouldice, 1995).

In developing their items, Finnegan and colleagues (1996) looked carefully at the ways attachment researchers had described the fundamental difficulties of preoccupied and avoidant infants, and they wrote items that they thought represented conceptually similar modes of failure to use the caregiver as a secure base in middle childhood. Items require children to imagine that they are experiencing a relevant attachment event (e.g., stress, separation, reunion, challenge) and to indicate how likely they would be to make a specified response.

Each item on the scale that measures preoccupied coping describes two possible reactions to the hypothetical situation depicted in the item—a preoccupied response and a nonpreoccupied (i.e., more secure) response. Children must choose which response they would be more likely to make and then indicate how confident they are of that choice. Items that measure avoidant coping are structured in an analogous way. For items on the Preoccupied scale, the preoccupied response options describe children who are experiencing a strong need for the mother in stressful and novel situations, trouble separating from the mother, excessive concern for the mother's whereabouts, prolonged upset following reunion, and trouble exploring or meeting challenges owing to excessive need for the mother. On the Avoidant scale, the avoidant response options depict children who deny affection toward the mother (e.g., deny that they would miss her during a long separation), fail to seek the mother when upset, avoid the mother during exploration and reunion, and refuse to use the mother as a task-relevant resource. The scales have been used with third through eighth graders and show high internal and temporal reliability (Finnegan et al., 1996; Hodges, Finnegan, & Perry, 1999; Kerns, Tomich, Aspelmeier, & Contreras, 2000). The scales are negatively correlated, around −.40.

One benefit of using the two scales to assess attachment in middle childhood is that doing so represents a point of contact with other recent developments in the assessment of attachment in both adulthood and infancy. Researchers of adult romantic attachments are increasingly turning away from a categorical approach toward a dimensional approach, arguing that an individual's attachment style is best captured by the person's location in a two-dimensional space created by the variables of preoccupied (often relabeled "anxious") behavior and avoidant behavior (e.g., Brennan et al., 1998). Similarly, factor analyses of infants' attachment behaviors yield two factors akin to preoccupied and avoidant dimensions (Fraley & Spieker, 2003). Applying a common two-dimensional scheme to assess attachment across ages and relationship types carries many obvious advantages.

We believe that the two coping styles captured by the Preoccupied and Avoidant scales reflect distinctive sets of insecurity-motivated strategies (some unconscious) for processing information and regulating affect when the attachment system is activated. We also believe that these strategies sometimes carry over into children's new relationships (e.g., with friends at school). We summarize findings from our prior research using these scales. We then present the results of a new study that addresses some unresolved issues about the scales.

PRELIMINARY STUDIES USING THE CHILDREN'S COPING STRATEGIES QUESTIONNAIRE

Finnegan and colleagues (1996) furnished preliminary evidence for the scales' validity by showing that the scales relate to adjustment in theoretically predictable ways. Children who scored high on preoccupied coping were perceived by peers to have internalizing problems, whereas children high in avoidant coping were seen as having externalizing problems. To help sort out the direction of influence between coping style and adjustment, Hodges and colleagues (1999) readministered the coping and adjustment measures to Finnegan and colleagues' participants a year later. Analyses indicated support for the hypothesized coping-influences-adjustment model but not for an alternative adjustment-influences-coping hypothesis.

Hodges and colleagues (1999) also addressed several questions concerning continuity in children's coping style across different relationships.

First, children were assessed for preoccupied and avoidant coping with their fathers as well as their mothers. Considerable consistency across the mother and father relationships was found for both coping styles (r for preoccupied = .82, r for avoidant = .65).

Hodges and colleagues (1999) also developed new scales to assess preoccupied and avoidant coping in the child's relationship with his or her best same-sex friend at school. Items measuring preoccupied coping tapped excessive distress over separation from the friend, prolonged upset over minor threats to the relationship, strong need for the friend in novel and challenging situations, and hypervigilance to the possibility of rejection by the friend. Items measuring avoidant coping tapped denial of the emotional importance of the friendship, lack of feeling during separation and reunion, and avoidance of the friend when distressed or challenged.

Children's coping styles with their best friends were moderately predictable from their coping styles with their parents. Preoccupied coping with mothers (fathers) correlated .49 (.47) with preoccupied coping with friends; avoidant coping with mothers (fathers) correlated .48 (.37) with avoidant coping with friends. These data suggest that children with insecure attachments to their parents are also not coping optimally with everyday stressors in the best-friend relationship. To see if coping style with best friends mediates continuity between style of attachment to parents and style of attachment to romantic partners, as suggested by Furman and Wehner (1994), it would be useful to examine adolescents' attachments to their parents, same-sex best friends, and romantic partners all within a single study, preferably using a longitudinal design.

A final issue examined by Hodges and colleagues (1999) was whether children become friends with peers whose coping styles resemble their own. By selecting relationship partners who behave like oneself, people can create environments that allow them to act freely in accord with their existing dispositions. Furthermore, the behavioral compatibilities afforded by such choices serve to reinforce each partner's adaptation pattern, thereby helping to maintain stability in personality (Caspi, 1998). Indeed, the data of Hodges and colleagues revealed marked "homophily of coping style," or similarity between members of friendship pairs in both preoccupied and avoidant coping.

A NEW STUDY: ADDITIONAL EVIDENCE FOR THE VALIDITY OF THE CHILDREN'S COPING STRATEGIES QUESTIONNAIRE

We noted that attachment security is conceptualized not only in terms of felt security but also in terms of skillful secure-base behavior. The Preoccupied and Avoidant coping scales clearly capture alternative modes of failing to use the caregiver as a secure base, but do they reflect underlying insecurity? Answering this question was the first purpose of this study. Our approach was to see whether the coping scales relate to children's perceptions of their mothers in ways that suggest underlying insecurity.

Research with infants has suggested that preoccupied attachment derives from inconsistently responsive parenting by a caregiver who can sometimes be quite sensitive but who responds unpredictably on the basis of her own needs, whereas avoidant attachment stems from aversive and overstimulating treatment by an angry or rejecting caregiver (Belsky, 1999a; Isabella, 1993). There may exist some continuity over ages in the parenting qualities that promote preoccupied and avoidant coping, but it may be unwise to assume strong continuity in the determinants of coping style from infancy to middle childhood, given that much transpires during this period. As Thompson (1999, p. 61) notes, "Parent–child interaction changes over time as the child's emergent capabilities broaden the parent's role to include not only attachment figure but also mentor, teacher, mediator, and disciplinarian." As children age, effective parenting expands to include serving as a sensitive listener, granting autonomy for exploration while at the same time monitoring the child's activities and companions, participating in joint recreational activities, and maintaining respect for the child during conflicts and disciplinary encounters. Collectively, these elements constitute a pattern of "authoritative parenting" that is associated with positive developmental outcomes across childhood and adolescence (Baumrind, 1991; Maccoby & Martin, 1983). The diversification of the parenting role as children age makes it possible that the parenting correlates of preoccupied and avoidant coping, as well as the sources of insecurity underlying these two coping styles, change between infancy and middle childhood. We believe that there is some continuity in the parenting correlates of the two coping styles over this period but that the continuity is greater for avoidant than for preoccupied coping.

Avoidant attachment may originate in infancy as a consequence of rejecting parenting, but ensuing child–parent transactions are likely to ensure that parental rejection and child avoidant attachment continue to go hand in hand, in the manner of a vicious cycle. The child's avoidant behavior probably elicits further rejection, disinterest, and lax discipline from the parent, and these parental reactions are likely to strengthen the child's avoidant style (Rubin, Bukowski, & Parker, 1998). Thus, across a broad age span, avoidantly attached children should perceive their caregivers as inaccessible, uncaring, unhelpful, and even hurtful; these perceptions of the parent as unhelpful if needed are the source of the avoidant child's insecurity. Indeed, even adults who are emotionally avoidant of their parents construe their parents as unavailable and rejecting; they also tend to dismiss their own children's attachment needs, and their children are also likely to be avoidantly attached (George & Solomon, 1999; Hesse, 1999).

We believe, however, that quite different child–parent transactional processes occur in the case of the preoccupied child. In infancy, preoccupied attachment may result from inconsistent parental responsiveness, but over time parental oversolicitousness and curtailment of exploration may take center stage as prime motivators of preoccupied coping. We believe that for some mothers the toddler's increasing need for autonomy triggers a strong separation anxiety that leads the mother to attempt to keep the child close—to engulf the child with affection but also with expectations for reciprocated proximity seeking. The system eventually becomes fear-based for both partners. The mother's fear is that the child will leave her by growing up; the child's fear is, initially, that he or she will be punished by the mother for separation and exploration, and, later, that he or she will not be able to leave the mother or cope without her (because excessive proximity seeking has prevented the acquisition of autonomous competencies). In this scenario, the insecurity of the preoccupied child derives not from anticipated caregiver punishment of proximity seeking, which is the source of insecurity for the avoidant child, but rather from anticipated caregiver punishment of autonomy.

The literature on attachment is replete with observations consistent with this picture. Rubin and colleagues (1998) point out how preoccupied infants can encourage maternal infantilization and overprotection; Radke-Yarrow and colleagues (1995) and Thompson (1999) describe how even secure infants can become preoccupied if their autonomy seeking frightens their caregiver. Cassidy (1994) reports that parents of preoccupied children tend to overmonitor their children and suggests that the preoccupied child's excessive clinginess and fearfulness serve to reassure the mother that she will continue to be needed and that the child will stay close and remain a child. Similar observations about how the caregivers of preoccupied children act to delay the child's maturity have been offered by Belsky (1999b) and by George and Solomon (1999). Separation anxiety exists even among the parents of older children and appears sometimes to be transferred to children in the form of school phobia (Eisenberg, 1958; Hock, Eberly, Bartle-Haring, Ellwanger, & Widaman, 2001; Hock & Lutz, 1998; Waldfogel, 1957). Adolescents with preoccupied attachments also tend to represent their parents as loving but role reversing, suggesting that the parents rely on them for caregiving and thereby keep them close at hand (Kobak & Sceery, 1988). Even adults with preoccupied attachments exhibit enmeshed attachment representations; they also display the greatest anxiety when separated from their toddlers, and their own babies tend to be preoccupied, too (George & Solomon, 1999; Hesse, 1999). These observations suggest that by middle childhood preoccupied children are likely to perceive their caregivers as inhibiting their autonomy (e.g., through overprotectiveness). However, they may not view their caregivers as inaccessible or unloving.

Our suggestion that two different types of anxiety underlie insecure attachment (fear of autonomy in the case of preoccupied children, fear of proximity seeking in the case of avoidant children) is consistent with other recent theorizing. Other researchers have stressed that a secure working model of the self as valued and competent derives as much from sensitive support of exploration as from sensitive care during distress (Bretherton & Munholland, 1999; Grossmann, Grossmann, & Zimmermann, 1999; Thompson, 1999).

In this study, we examined associations between preoccupied and avoidant coping and children's perceptions of five aspects of maternal behavior. The first dimension of maternal behavior was the mother's provision of *reliable support* for proximity seeking. The measure we used to tap this variable was a shortened version of Kerns and colleagues' (1996) Security Scale, which assesses the degree to which the caregiver is perceived as loving, accessible, and sensitive when needed for help or communication. It must be kept in mind that the kind of support tapped by this measure is mainly support for proximity seeking and open communication, not support for exploration and autonomy. The second dimension of perceived parenting we assessed was *harassment* by the mother. This measure assesses children's perceptions of angry, rejecting, and humiliating behavior by the mother (e.g., yelling at the child, coming into the child's room without asking). The third dimension was the child's perception of the mother's *enjoyment of the child*. This variable taps children's perception that they and their mothers share positive affect and engage in joint recreational activities. A fourth dimension was perceived maternal *monitoring* of the child's activities, whereabouts, and companions. The final measure was perceived maternal *overprotectiveness*, which captures children's perception that the mother discourages separation and exploration and is afraid that the child will get sick or injured.

We hypothesized that avoidant children would perceive their mothers as low in reliable support, high in harassment, and low in enjoyment of the child. We expected that preoccupied children would perceive their mothers as high in overprotectiveness and monitoring.

The second purpose of this study was to determine whether preoccupied and avoidant coping contribute beyond perceived-parenting variables to the prediction of important child outcomes. According to attachment theory, children's attachment styles are organized patterns of social cognition, affect regulation, and behavioral tendencies that are influenced by parental behavior but that gradually assume a force of their own, coming to serve as independent influences on children's development and adaptation. Evaluating such a position requires seeing whether attachment styles account for variance in child outcomes when parenting influences are statistically controlled.

In this study, we included five adjustment indexes. For comparison with our previous results (Finnegan et al., 1996; Hodges et al., 1999), we included peer reports of *internalizing problems* (e.g., sadness, fearfulness, social withdrawal) and *externalizing problems* (e.g., aggression, dishonesty, disruptiveness). However, we also included peer reports of two kinds of positive conduct—*communal behavior* and *agentic behavior.* Communal behaviors, which are especially important for sustaining close relationships (e.g., Clark & Ladd, 2000), included helpfulness, friendliness, and empathy; agentic behaviors included assertiveness, leadership, and interest in sports. We expected both preoccupied coping and avoidant coping to undermine communal behavior. Preoccupied children are likely to be too worried about their own welfare to attend sensitively to the needs of others, whereas avoidant children may simply not notice, or may fail to be aroused, when another is in need. We expected agentic competencies to be more clearly undermined by preoccupied attachment than by avoidant attachment. Agency rests strongly on exploration, something clearly missing from the preoccupied child's repertoire, but not from the avoidant child's. Finally, we included a self-report measure of *global self-worth.* We expected both preoccupied and avoidant children to be at risk for low self-esteem. Self-esteem is largely a function of two kinds of perceptions—perceptions of acceptance by significant others, especially one's parents, and perceptions of one's competencies (Harter, 1998). If, as expected, avoidant children perceive their parents to be rejecting, and preoccupied children are lacking in agentic competencies, both should be at risk for low self-esteem.

Method

The participants were 502 fourth and fifth graders in Florida. About 50% of the children were white, 30% black, and 20% Hispanic. Most children came from middle- or working-class families. All of the correlations reported below are partial correlations (*pr*s) that control for participant age, sex, and ethnic group.

Three sets of measures were administered: coping measures, perceived-parenting measures, and adjustment measures. The coping measures were shortened versions of the Preoccupied and Avoidant coping scales. The perceived-parenting measures, described earlier, included children's perceptions of reliable support, harassment, enjoyment of the child, monitoring, and overprotectiveness. The final set of measures were five indexes of adjustment. The first four of these were based on a peer nomination inventory and assessed internalizing problems, externalizing problems, communal behavior, and agentic behavior. The fifth adjustment measure was Harter's (1985) measure of global self-worth. All measures were reliable.

Children were queried about their coping styles and about parental behavior with respect only to their mothers. The reason is that children tend to report a similar style of coping across their two parents (Hodges et al., 1999) and tend to perceive their parents as treating them similarly (e.g., Steinberg, Lamborn, Dornbusch, & Darling, 1992). Each of the two main questions of the study is considered in turn.

Do Preoccupied and Avoidant Coping Reflect Insecurity?

We believe the answer is yes. The top part of Table 5.1 gives the correlations between the coping measures and the perceived-parenting measures. Because of the moderate negative partial correlation between the two coping scales, $pr = -.48$, associations between a given coping dimen-

TABLE 5.1. Relations of Child Coping Measures with Perceived-Parenting Measures and with Adjustment Measures

Measure	Preoccupied Coping	Avoidant Coping
Perceived-parenting measure		
Reliable support	−.19***	−.46***
Harassment	.15***	.43***
Enjoyment of child	−.14**	−.53***
Monitoring	−.02	−.35***
Overprotectiveness	.42***	.05
Adjustment measure		
Before controlling for perceived parenting		
Internalizing problems	.17***	.12**
Externalizing problems	.06	.11**
Communal behavior	−.05	−.16***
Agentic behavior	−.14**	−.12**
Global self-worth	−.20***	−.20***
After controlling for perceived parenting		
Internalizing problems	.10*	.05
Externalizing problems	.07	.06
Communal behavior	−.07	−.15***
Agentic behavior	−.12**	−.13**
Global self-worth	−.13**	.00

Note. Entries are partial correlations that control for age, sex, ethnic group, and the other coping measure. Entries in the last five rows also control for all five perceived-parenting measures.
*p < .05; **p < .01; ***p < .001.

sion and other variables were always examined with the other coping variable controlled. As hypothesized, each coping measure is associated with a distinct set of perceived-parenting variables, and the pattern for each coping style may be interpreted as reflecting a form of underlying insecurity.

Avoidant Coping

Thompson (1999, p. 282) has suggested that when children are formulating their internal working models, they rely strongly on their answers to two key questions: "What do others do when I am upset?" and "What happens when I venture to explore?" The data in Table 5.1 suggest that avoidant children formulate an especially devastating answer to the first question. They clearly view their mothers as unloving, unavailable when needed, unhelpful, uninterested, and even aversive. The correlations suggest that the internal working model of the avoidant child takes the form of a clear "relational schema"—a perception of the other in relation to the self coupled with a perception of the self in relation to the other (Baldwin, 1992). Avoidant children view their mothers as repudiating them, and they view themselves as repudiating their mothers in return.

It is likely that a relational schema characterized by mutual avoidance is difficult to repair. Once established, the schema probably serves as an interpretive filter that causes the child to notice and remember parental behaviors that are consistent with it and to ignore or discount parental actions that are positive but schema inconsistent.

Preoccupied Coping

Although avoidant children may provide the most discouraging answer to Thompson's (1999) first question ("What do others do when I am upset?"), preoccupied children appear to generate the most debilitating answer to his second question, "What happens when I explore?" The data in Table 5.1 show clearly that preoccupied children perceive their mothers to be overprotective—to discourage exploration, risk taking, independence, and separation and to be worried about their children's welfare, safety, and health. Preoccupied children also tend to view their mothers as somewhat unloving, unavailable, and even harsh. They do not perceive their mothers as especially high in monitoring. Thus it is specifically by discouraging exploration and separation that the mothers are seen as overcontrolling.

The relational schema of the preoccupied child, then, is the one expected: The child perceives both mother and self as fearfully clinging to each other. It is likely that the preoccupied child comes to expect that the mother will react with dismay if the child tries to separate, explore, or act autonomously. Some overprotected children may sense a neediness and vulnerability on the mother's part, causing them to develop a sense of responsibility for the mother's welfare and to engage in compulsive caregiving and clingy behaviors to reassure the mother that she will not be deserted. If the mother is motivated to keep the child close for these purposes, she may subtly communicate crippling messages to the child, such as the notion that the mother–child relationship should be exclusive or that the child is too weak to cope without her. If the mother uses guilt-instilling psychological control, she may contribute to the child developing self-blaming tendencies.

Summary

Preoccupied and avoidant children have very different representations of their mother's caregiving, yet it is reasonable to think that both kinds of children are insecure. The avoidant child cannot count on the mother for affection and understanding; the preoccupied child cannot count on her for support of exploration and autonomy.

Do Preoccupied and Avoidant Coping Contribute Beyond Perceived Parenting to Children's Adjustment?

Given that preoccupied and avoidant coping styles are associated with unique patterns of perceived parenting, one might wonder whether there is anything to be gained by including the coping constructs in accounts of family influence on children's adjustment. Perhaps the perceived-parenting variables, capturing as they do components of a pattern of authoritative parenting that is well known to affect children's adjustment, are all that are needed to explain the impact of parent–child relationships on children's development.

To answer this question, it is first useful to consider the entries in the middle part of Table 5.1, which show the relations between the coping variables and the adjustment measures before controlling for perceived parenting. As in previous studies (Finnegan et al., 1996; Hodges et al., 1999), preoccupied coping is associated with internalizing problems, and avoidant coping with externalizing problems. However, in the present study, avoidant coping is also associated with internalizing problems. Several other studies have also found avoidant attachment to be linked to depression (e.g., Kobak, 1999; Weinfield, Sroufe, Egeland, & Carlson, 1999). The entries in the table also show that both coping styles are associated with reduced agentic behavior in the peer group, as well as with reduced self-esteem. Avoidant coping is also associated with reduced communal behavior.

Before examining the relations between coping and adjustment with perceived parenting controlled, we should note that there were a number of significant associations between the perceived-parenting measures and the adjustment measures. Thus it is possible that the significant associations between these adjustment variables and the coping variables might vanish if the perceived-parenting variables were to be controlled.

To determine whether any of the significant associations between the coping measures and adjustment reported in the middle part of Table 5.1 remain significant when perceived parenting is controlled, the coping adjustment correlations were recomputed with all five perceived-parenting variables included among the control variables. These associations are given in the bottom part of Table 5.1. As is apparent, many of the original coping-adjustment associations remained significant. Results for each coping style are summarized in turn.

Preoccupied Coping

Preoccupied children possess adjustment difficulties that cannot be accounted for by perceptions of parenting. These children were perceived by peers to have internalizing problems and to lack agentic competencies, and they admitted to low self-esteem. It seems likely that preoccupied attachment prevents children from developing the competencies that promote agentic behaviors (e.g., leadership, competitiveness). These deficits in agentic skills may—especially if the child has adopted a self-blaming attributional style—undermine self-esteem and promote internalizing behaviors (e.g., fearfulness, social withdrawal). That preoccupied coping did not predict externalizing problems is consistent with previous results. It is somewhat surprising, however, that preoccupied coping did not undermine communal behavior more strongly.

Avoidant Coping

The most striking unique contribution of avoidant coping to children's adjustment appears to take the form of deficits in social skills. Avoidant children were reported by peers to be deficient in both communal and agentic competencies. That avoidant coping undermines communal behavior is consistent with Eisenberg and Fabes's (1998) conclusion that children's prosocial tendencies (e.g., empathy, sharing, helping) are hampered when parents fail to interact with their child in ways that help the child learn to self-regulate distressed emotional states. Avoidant children are unlikely to participate in such interactions. It is interesting that avoidant children were also perceived by peers as lacking in agentic competencies. Apparently, the compulsive self-reliance that characterizes avoidant children does not guarantee the development of agentic behavior. Many agentic activities require social participation and cooperation, and these dispositions may be lacking in avoidant children's repertoires.

It is interesting that the links of avoidant coping to internalizing problems, externalizing problems, and global self-worth that were significant before the perceived-parenting measures were controlled (middle part of Table 5.1) became nonsignificant when perceived-parenting was controlled (bottom part of Table 5.1). This does not necessarily mean, however, that avoidant coping plays no role in the development of any of these outcomes. It may be that during preadolescence avoidant coping contributes to parenting behaviors (e.g., rejection) that then promote internalizing problems, externalizing problems, or low self-esteem (Rubin et al., 1998). In this case, avoidant coping would be an indirect influence on these outcomes. It is particularly interesting that avoidant coping is not a unique influence on self-esteem, given that avoidant coping is associated with deficits in communal and agentic competencies. Perhaps avoidant children have a defensive, externalizing attributional style that protects them from viewing their deficiencies as reflecting poorly on their self-worth.

Summary

Both preoccupied and avoidant coping accounted for variance in child adjustment that could not be explained by perceived parenting. The primary implications are that coping styles should be included in assessments of attachment in middle childhood and should be accorded an important place in theoretical accounts of the impact of parent–child relations on children's social development.

Conclusions

Preoccupied and Avoidant Coping Reflect Insecurity

Consistent with what has been hypothesized to cause avoidant attachment in infancy, avoidantly attached preadolescents reported their mothers to be relatively unloving, unhelpful, uninterested, and even aversive. It is reasonable to assume that these children are insecure, with their insecurity deriving from their sense that their mothers are unavailable or unhelpful when needed. In contrast, preoccupied children perceived their mothers to discourage exploration and other expressions of autonomy and agency.

These children may also be said to be insecure, but with their insecurity deriving from a sense that they are not allowed to grow up, develop competencies, become separate individuals, and function on their own. That the Preoccupied and Avoidant coping scales are correlated in meaningful ways with the two types of insecurity theorized to be central to attachment security is additional evidence for the scales' construct validity.

Assessments of Preoccupied and Avoidant Coping are Necessary for Understanding the Impact of Attachment on Adjustment

The fact that both preoccupied coping and avoidant coping predicted adjustment outcomes beyond the perceived-parenting variables (and, moreover, predicted different outcomes) is significant. First, it indicates that assessment of attachment in middle childhood needs to include measures of both preoccupied and avoidant coping. Among the perceived-parenting variables were two measures believed to capture two main sources of felt insecurity—failure of the caregiver to provide sensitive support for proximity seeking (reliable support) and failure of the caregiver to provide sensitive support for exploration (overprotectiveness). However, the measures of preoccupied and avoidant coping predicted adjustment outcomes when these security-related perceived-parenting measures were controlled. Thus it is clear that assessments of coping style are needed to achieve a full understanding of the relations of attachment to adjustment. Assessing only the feelings of insecurity is unlikely to be an adequate approach. Moreover, the fact that preoccupied and avoidant coping predicted different patterns of adjustment recommends against the practice of combining preoccupied and avoidant children into a single insecure group (for comparison with a secure group).

The fact that the two coping styles rest on different sources of insecurity, represent different relational schemas ("My mother and I can't stand to be around each other" in the case of the avoidant child; "My mother and I can't stand to be apart" in the case of the preoccupied child), and predict different adjustment difficulties suggests that each coping style is associated with a distinct set of cognitions, emotional reactions, and behavioral tendencies that influences the child's social adaptation outside of the mother–child relationship. A challenge for future research is to elucidate the nature of these presumed mediators and to describe how particular events occurring within new relationships elicit the mediators, causing shifts in ongoing relationship cognition, affect, and behavior that determine the course of the relationship for better or for worse. This will require supplementing the global, summary-type measures of adjustment that were employed in this study with measures that capture typical reactions to contextually embedded relationship events. How, for example, do preoccupied and avoidant children differ in their attributions for ambiguous relationship events (e.g., a friend is late for an appointment, expresses interest in playing with someone else, talks about plans for recess or the weekend without mentioning the child, or makes a critical comment that might be serious or might be a joke)? What are the children's perceptions of self-efficacy for crucial relationship skills and affect management competencies? How willing are the children to put up with negative partner behavior? How do the children cope with dissolution of a friendship (e.g., do the partners become enemies)? These are just some of the questions that need to be answered if we are to understand the legacy of preoccupied and avoidant attachments for adaptation within new relationships.

The fact that each coping style is associated with a clear relational schema may help us understand certain well-known but unexplained phenomena in the attachment literature. It is often said, for example, that preoccupied persons fear rejection by their relationship partners. But why should this be the case if they are used to being smothered by an overprotective parent? Perhaps preoccupied children's conception of relationships is one in which each partner closely monitors both self and other for cues portending separation and acts quickly to restore togetherness. The partner is expected to be as clingy as the self. Preoccupied persons may interpret potential new relationship partners' relatively casual attitude toward separations as disinterest or rejection. Unable to tolerate partner behavior that might mean loss of interest, they may annoyingly solicit reassurance. This may lead to rejection and sow concerns about rejection in the future. Furthermore, when committed to a relationship, preoccupied persons may work diligently and self-sacrificingly to sustain it, but their obsessive concern with the partner's welfare and needs may be experienced as irksome by the partner, precipitating dissolution (Bretherton & Munholland, 1999; Cicchetti & Toth, 1998). At this point in the relationship, the preoccupied partner may not be expecting breakup and may be surprised (Feeney & Noller, 1992), as well as resentful ("I have given you so much; how could you do this to me?"). In this and other ways, the relational schema of the preoccupied child may generate expectations and behavior patterns that cause them difficulty in later relationships with friends, lovers, and their own children.

Although preoccupied and avoidant coping styles are related to adjustment, the relations are not strong. However, the coping styles might represent vulnerabilities that interact with other factors, especially stressors (e.g., parental divorce, victimization by peers), to affect adjustment more strongly (Cicchetti & Toth, 1998; Finnegan et al., 1996; Kobak, 1999; Leadbeater, Kuperminc, Blatt, & Hertzog, 1999; Rudolph et al., 2000; Thompson, 1999).

Assessments of Preoccupied and Avoidant Coping Are Unlikely to Constitute a Complete Approach to the Assessment of Attachment in Middle Childhood

At the time we developed our measures of coping style (Finnegan et al., 1996), we thought these two scales were all that would be necessary to assess attachment style in middle childhood. We reasoned that children with high scores on just one of the scales were either insecure–preoccupied or insecure–avoidant and that children with low scores on both scales were secure. Similar reasoning is evidenced by researchers who use the two dimensions of anxious (preoccupied) style and avoidant style to assess romantic attachment style in adulthood. That is, it is assumed that individuals with low scores on both dimensions have a secure style (e.g., Rholes, Simpson, Campbell, & Grich, 2001).

Although it would certainly be convenient to limit the assessment of attachment in middle childhood to children's scores on the two dimensions of preoccupied and avoidant coping, certain additional findings of the present study suggest that this may be unwise. The central problem with limiting assessment to the two coping measures is that these two scales do not capture all the variance associated with felt insecurity. It is true that each coping measure is highly correlated with a perceived-parenting variable that, on conceptual grounds, implies insecurity (i.e., avoidant coping is associated with low perceived reliable support, and preoccupied coping is paired with high perceived overprotectiveness), and therefore the two coping scales collectively do capture much of the variance in children's felt security. However, as we elaborate subsequently, supplementary data analyses suggest that some children feel insecure yet do not manifest either a preoccupied or an avoidant coping style. Moreover, these feelings of insecurity that are not associated with either preoccupied or avoidant coping appear to have independent negative effects on children's adjustment. Consequently, assessing only the two coping styles is an insufficient approach to assessing attachment; measures that capture felt insecurity that is not associated with either coping style need to be included.

The foregoing conclusion follows from supplementary analyses of the present data that were conducted to determine whether the two coping variables entirely mediate the effects of the felt-security components of perceived parenting (i.e., perceived reliable support and perceived overprotectiveness) on adjustment. We had thought that they would. That is, we reasoned that the effects of underlying insecurity on adjustment are routed through coping style and therefore that no effects of felt security on adjustment would be found once the coping variables were controlled. However, we were wrong. It is useful first to appreciate that when we computed correlations between the perceived-parenting variables and the adjustment variables without controlling for preoccupied and avoidant coping, several associations between the felt-security dimensions and the adjustment measures were significant (perceived reliable support was negatively related to internalizing problems and to externalizing problems and positively related to global self-worth, and perceived overprotectiveness was positively related to internalizing problems and negatively related to global self-worth). The question we then asked was, Do any of these significant correlations between the felt-security measures and adjustment remain significant when the two coping measures are included among the control variables?

Of the several significant correlations between the felt-security measures (reliable support and overprotectiveness) and the adjustment measures, two were indeed still significant when both of the coping variables (as well as the other perceived-parenting variables) were controlled. Both of these relations involved the reliable-support measure. Perceived reliable support was negatively related to externalizing problems (pr = -.10, p < .03) and positively related to global self-worth (pr = .15, p < .001). These results indicate that the two coping styles do not completely mediate the impact of this type of felt security on these adjustment outcomes.

Clearly, perceived reliable support—a central source of felt security in attachment theory—bears relations to externalizing problems and to global self-worth that are over and above any contributions of preoccupied and avoidant coping to these outcomes. How might this occur? Perhaps some children feel that their caregivers are unavailable, unloving, and unhelpful (i.e., are insecure) yet are unable to develop a coherent, predictable pattern of coping. In fact, children with attachments characterized as disorganized or disoriented qualify for this description (Main & Hesse, 1990). Infants assigned to this relatively recently identified attachment category do not make good use of their caregivers as a secure base, but their behavior is neither consistently preoccupied nor consistently avoidant (e.g., during stress, they may exhibit helpless freezing). Such infants appear to be at risk for serious behavior problems, especially aggression, later on (e.g., Lyons-Ruth, Easterbrooks, & Cibelli, 1997). It is thought that the parents of these children exhibit abusive, frightening behavior and that the children cannot cope in an organized way.[1]

The fact that some children can be low on both preoccupied and avoidant coping and yet be insecure (and, quite possibly, disorganized)

---

[1]We suggested earlier that the attachments of preoccupied children are also fear based. However, the nature of the fear of preoccupied and disorganized children is likely to be quite different. Presumably, preoccupied children fear the caregiver's punishment for autonomy, whereas disorganized children fear abuse or neglect by the parent.

suggests that assessments of attachment in middle childhood should not be limited to measures of preoccupied and avoidant coping. Measures of underlying security should also be included. Researchers might, however, also try to develop self-report measures to capture disorganized attachment (items might assess self-perceived freezing or uncertainty over what to do in crucial attachment contexts). In addition, measures of perceived parenting might be expanded to include perceptions of frightening, unpredictable behavior by the caregiver. In such a way it would be possible to see whether the disorganized child possesses the hypothesized working model ("fear without solution"). It would also be possible to see whether disorganized behavior contributes beyond the preoccupied and avoidant coping measures to adjustment outcomes.

One question researchers who use self-report scales of attachment must face is whether, in data analyses, to retain the continuous nature of the variables and use multiple regression or, alternatively, to assign children to attachment categories based on cutoff scores on the various dimensions. Our preference is to retain the continuous nature of the measures and to use multiple regression when relating the variables to other factors, such as adjustment. One reason for this recommendation is that most attachment dimensions bear significant associations with one another. For example, the fact that preoccupied coping and avoidant coping are correlated (negatively) requires using regression to determine the impact of one coping variable uncontaminated by the influence of the other. We have found, in fact, that failure to control avoidant coping when examining the relations of preoccupied coping to other variables sometimes results in nonsignificant relations that then become significant once avoidant coping is controlled; thus, if left uncontrolled, avoidant scores can obscure or "suppress" relations of preoccupied coping to other variables.

TOWARD THE FUTURE

We close by summarizing the major directions for future research suggested by this chapter. First, additional work on the assessment of attachment in middle childhood is needed. Self-report questionnaires are one promising approach, but questions remain about the exact stock of scales that need to be included and about whether certain attachment phenomena (e.g., disorganized attachment) can be captured using this method. Other methods (e.g., narratives) may capture aspects of attachment (e.g., unconscious feelings) that self-report scales do not and should be explored as well.

Second, more work on the consequences of attachment in middle childhood is needed. Several of the other contributions to this volume are steps in this direction (e.g., Booth-LaForce, Rubin, Rose-Krasnor, & Burgess, Chapter 8; Verschueren & Marcoen, Chapter 10). Preoccupied and avoidant coping styles might interact with stressors to affect adjustment (e.g., depression, aggression), and they are likely to affect children's functioning in relationships beyond the family. The merits of more comprehensive developmental models—such as the idea that middle-childhood attachments to parents affect style of relating not only to close same-sex friends but also to romantic partners (and possibly to one's own children)—also need to be evaluated.

Finally, more research on the determinants of attachment during middle childhood is needed. Among the many potential influences on change in attachment style during childhood are real and perceived caregiving, interparental conflict, changes in family structure (e.g., divorce, remarriage), protracted separation, and parental psychopathology. It would also be interesting to see whether preadolescents' attachment styles are correlated with their parents' states of mind regarding attachment (as assessed with the Adult Attachment Interview) and, if so, to determine the patterns of parent–child interaction that mediate the link.

ACKNOWLEDGMENTS

Preparation of this chapter and the research described in it were supported by Grant Nos. R01HD38280 and F31MH067404 from the National Institutes of Health. We thank Ernest V. E. Hodges and Louise C. Perry for commenting on a previous version of this chapter.

REFERENCES

Ainsworth, M. D. S. (1979). Infant–mother attachment. *American Psychologist, 34,* 932–937.

Ainsworth, M. D. S., & Wittig, B. A. (1969). Attachment and exploratory behavior of one-year-olds in a Strange Situation. In B. M. Foss (Ed.), *Determinants of infant behavior* (Vol. 4, pp. 113–136). London: Methuen.

Armsden, G. C., & Greenberg, M. T. (1987). The Inventory of Parent and Peer Attachment: Individual differences and their relationship to psychological well-being in adolescence. *Journal of Youth and Adolescence, 16,* 427–454.

Baldwin, M. W. (1992). Relational schemas and the processing of social information. *Psychological Bulletin, 112,* 461–484.

Baumrind, D. (1991). Parenting styles and adolescent development. In J. Brooks-Gunn, R. Lerner, & A. Petersen (Eds.), *The encyclopedia of adolescence* (pp. 746–758). New York: Garland.

Belsky, J. (1999a). Interactional and contextual determinants of attachment security. In J. Cassidy & P. R. Shaver (Eds.), *Handbook of attachment: Theory, research, and clinical applications* (pp. 249–264). New York: Guilford Press.

Belsky, J. (1999b). Modern evolutionary theory and patterns of attachment. In J. Cassidy & P. R. Shaver (Eds.), *Handbook of attachment: Theory, research, and clinical applications* (pp. 141–161). New York: Guilford Press.

Berlin, L. J., & Cassidy, J. (1999). Relations among relationships: Contributions from attachment theory and research. In J. Cassidy & P. R. Shaver (Eds.), *Handbook of attachment: Theory, research, and clinical applications* (pp. 688–712). New York: Guilford Press.

Bowlby, J. (1973). *Attachment and loss: Vol. 2. Separation, anxiety, and anger.* New York: Basic Books.

Bowlby, J. (1979). *The making and breaking of affectional bonds.* New York: Methuen.

Brennan, K. A., Clark, C. L., & Shaver, P. R. (1998). Self-report measurement of adult attachment: An integrative overview. In J. A. Simpson & W. S. Rholes (Eds.), *Attachment theory and close relationships* (pp. 46–76). New York: Guilford Press.

Bretherton, I., & Munholland, K. A. (1999). Internal working models in attachment relationships: A construct revisited. In J. Cassidy & P. R. Shaver (Eds.), *Handbook of attachment: Theory, research, and clinical applications* (pp. 89–111). New York: Guilford Press.

Carlson, E. A. (1997, April). *A prospective longitudinal study of disorganized/disoriented attachment.* Paper presented at the annual meeting of the Society for Research in Child Development, Washington, DC.

Caspi, A. (1998). Personality development across the life span. In N. Eisenberg (Ed.), *Handbook of child psychology: Vol. 3. Social, emotional, and personality development* (pp. 311–388). New York: Wiley.

Cicchetti, D., & Toth, S. L. (1998). Perspectives on research and practice in developmental psychopathology. In I. E. Sigel & K. A. Renninger (Eds.), *Handbook of child psychology: Vol. 4. Child psychology in practice* (pp. 479–583). New York: Wiley.

Clark, K. E., & Ladd, G. W. (2000). Connectedness and autonomy support in parent–child relationships: Links to children's socioemotional orientation and peer relationships. *Developmental Psychology, 36,* 485–498.

Crowell, J. A., Fraley, R. C., & Shaver, P. R. (1999). Measurement of individual differences in adolescent and adult attachment. In J. Cassidy & P. R. Shaver (Eds.), *Handbook of attachment: Theory, research, and clinical applications* (pp. 434–465). New York: Guilford Press.

Eisenberg, L. (1958). School phobia: A study in the communication of anxiety. *American Journal of Psychiatry, 114,* 712–718.

Eisenberg, N., & Fabes, R. A. (1998). Prosocial development. In N. Eisenberg (Ed.), *Handbook of child psychology: Vol. 3. Social, emotional, and personality development* (pp. 701–778). New York: Wiley.

Feeney, J. A. (1999). Adult romantic attachment and couple relationships. In J. Cassidy & P. R. Shaver (Eds.), *Handbook of attachment: Theory, research, and clinical applications* (pp. 355–377). New York: Guilford Press.

Feeney, J. A., & Noller, P. (1992). Attachment style and romantic love: Relationship dissolution. *Australian Journal of Psychology, 44,* 69–74.

Finnegan, R. A., Hodges, E. V. E., & Perry, D. G. (1996). Preoccupied and avoidant coping in middle childhood. *Child Development, 67,* 1318–1328.

Fox, N. A. (1997, April). *Attachment in infants and adults: A link between the two?* Paper presented at the annual meeting of the Society for Research in Child Development, Washington, DC.

Fraley, R. C., & Spieker, S. J. (2003). Are infant attachment patterns continuously or categorically distributed? A taxonomic analysis of Strange Situation behavior. *Developmental Psychology, 39,* 387–404.

Furman, W., & Wehner, E. A. (1994). Romantic views: Toward a theory of adolescent romantic relationships. In R. Montemayor, G. R. Adams, & T. P. Gullotta (Eds.), *Personal relationships during adolescence* (pp. 168–195). Thousand Oaks, CA: Sage.

George, C., & Solomon, J. (1999). Attachment and caregiving: The caregiving behavioral system. In J. Cassidy & P. R. Shaver (Eds.), *Handbook of attachment: Theory, research, and clinical applications* (pp. 649–670). New York: Guilford Press.

Grossmann, K. E., Grossmann, K., & Zimmermann, P. (1999). A wider view of attachment and exploration: Stability and change during the years of immaturity. In J. Cassidy & P. R. Shaver (Eds.), *Handbook of attachment: Theory, research, and clinical applications* (pp. 760–786). New York: Guilford Press.

Harter, S. (1985). *The Self-Perception Profile for Children: Revision of the Perceived Competence Scale for Children (Manual).* Denver, CO: University of Denver.

Harter, S. (1998). The development of self-representations. In N. Eisenberg (Ed.), *Handbook of child psychology: Vol. 3. Social, emotional, and personality development* (pp. 553–617). New York: Wiley.

Hazan, C., & Shaver, P. (1987). Romantic love conceptualized as an attachment process. *Journal of Personality and Social Psychology, 52,* 511–524.

Hesse, E. (1999). The Adult Attachment Interview: Historical and current perspectives. In J. Cassidy & P. R. Shaver (Eds.), *Handbook of attachment: Theory, research, and clinical applications* (pp. 395–433). New York: Guilford Press.

Hock, E., Eberly, M., Bartle-Haring, S., Ellwanger, P., & Widaman, K. F. (2001). Separation anxiety in parents of adolescents: Theoretical significance and scale development. *Child Development, 72,* 284–298.

Hock, E., & Lutz, W. (1998). Psychological meaning of separation anxiety in mothers and fathers. *Journal of Family Psychology, 12,* 41–55.

Hodges, E. V. E., Finnegan, R. A., & Perry, D. G. (1999). Skewed autonomy-relatedness in preadolescents' conceptions of their relationships with mother, father, and best friend. *Developmental Psychology, 35,* 737–748.

Isabella, R. A. (1993). Origins of attachment: Maternal interactive behavior across the first year. *Child Development, 64,* 605–621.

Kerns, K. A., Klepac, L., & Cole, A. (1996). Peer relationships and preadolescents' perceptions of security in the child-mother relationship. *Developmental Psychology, 32,* 457–466.

Kerns, K. A., Tomich, P. L., Aspelmeier, J. E., & Contreras, J. M. (2000). Attachment-based assessments of parent–child relationships in middle childhood. *Developmental Psychology, 36,* 614–626.

Kirkpatrick, L. A., & Davis, K. E. (1994). Attachment style, gender, and relationship stability: A longitudinal analysis. *Journal of Personality and Social Psychology, 66,* 502–512.

Kobak, R. (1999). The emotional dynamics of disruptions in attachment relationships: Implications for theory, research, and clinical intervention. In J. Cassidy & P. R. Shaver (Eds.), *Handbook of attachment: Theory, research, and clinical applications* (pp. 21–43). New York: Guilford Press.

Kobak, R. R., & Sceery, A. (1988). Attachment in late adolescence: Working models, affect regulation, and presentation of self and other. *Child Development, 59,* 135–146.

Leadbeater, B. J., Kuperminc, G. P., Blatt, S. J., & Hertzog, C. (1999). A multivariate model of gender differences in adolescents' internalizing and externalizing problems. *Developmental Psychology, 35,* 1268–1282.

Lewis, M., Feiring, C., & Rosenthal, S. (2000). Attachment theory. *Child Development, 71,* 707–720.

Lyons-Ruth, K., Easterbrooks, M. A., & Cibelli, C. D. (1997). Infant attachment strategies, infant mental lag, and maternal depressive symptoms: Predictors of internalizing and externalizing problems at age 7. *Developmental Psychology, 33,* 681–692.

Maccoby, E. E., & Martin, J. (1983). Socialization in the context of the family: Parent–child interaction. In P. H. Mussen (Series Ed.) & E. M. Hetherington (Vol. Ed.), *Handbook of child psychology: Vol. 4. Socialization, personality, and social development* (4th ed., pp. 1–101). New York: Wiley.

Main, M., & Hesse, E. (1990). Parents' unresolved traumatic experiences are related to infant disorganized attachment status: Is frightened and/or frightening parental behavior the linking mechanism? In M. T. Greenberg, D. Cicchetti, & E. M. Cummings (Eds.), *Attachment in the preschool years* (pp. 161–183). Chicago: University of Chicago Press.

Main, M., Kaplan, N. E., & Cassidy, J. (1985). Security in infancy, childhood, and adulthood: A move to the level of representation. In I. Bretherton & E. Waters (Eds.), Growing points of attachment theory and research. *Monographs of the Society for Research in Child Development, 50*(1–2, Serial No. 209), 257–275.

Radke-Yarrow, M., McCann, K., DeMulder, E., Belmont, B., Martinez, P., & Richardson, D. T. (1995). Attachment in the context of high-risk conditions. *Development and Psychopathology, 7,* 247–265.

Rholes, W. S., Simpson, J. A., Campbell, L., & Grich, J. (2001). Adult attachment and the transition to parenthood. *Journal of Personality and Social Psychology, 81,* 421–435.

Rubin, K. H., Bukowski, W., & Parker, J. G. (1998). Peer interactions, relationships, and groups. In N. Eisenberg (Ed.), *Handbook of child psychology: Vol. 3. Social, emotional, and personality development* (pp. 619–700). New York: Wiley.

Rudolph, K. D., Hammen, C., Burge, D., Lindberg, N., Herzberg, D., & Daley, S. E. (2000). Toward an interpersonal life-stress model of depression: The developmental context of stress generation. *Development and Psychopathology, 12,* 215–234.

Sroufe, L. A., & Fleeson, J. (1986). Attachment and the construction of relationships. In W. W. Hartup & Z. Rubin (Eds.), *Relationships and development* (pp. 51–71). Hillsdale, NJ: Erlbaum.

Steinberg, L., Lamborn, S. D., Dornbusch, S. M., & Darling, N. (1992). Impact of parenting practices on adolescent achievement: Authoritative parenting, school involvement, and encouragement to succeed. *Child Development, 63,* 1266–1281.

Stevenson-Hinde, J., & Shouldice, A. (1995). Maternal interactions and self-reports related to attachment classifications at 4.5 years. *Child Development, 66,* 583–596.

Thompson, R. A. (1998). Early sociopersonality development. In N. Eisenberg (Ed.), *Handbook of child psychology: Vol. 3. Social, emotional, and personality development* (pp. 25–104). New York: Wiley.

Thompson, R. A. (1999). Early attachment and later development. In J. Cassidy & P. R. Shaver (Eds.), *Handbook of attachment: Theory, research, and clinical applications* (pp. 265–286). New York: Guilford Press.

Waldfogel, S. (1957). The development, meaning, and management of school phobia. *American Journal of Orthopsychiatry, 27,* 754–780.

Waters, E., & Cummings, E. M. (2000). A secure base from which to explore close relationships. *Child Development, 71,* 164–172.

Waters, E., Merrick, S. K., Albersheim, W., & Treboux, D. (1995, March). *Attachment security from infancy to early adulthood: A 20–year longitudinal study.* Poster presented at the annual meeting of the Society for Research in Child Development, Indianapolis, IN.

Weinfield, N. S., Sroufe, L. A., Egeland, B., & Carlson, E. A. (1999). The nature of individual differences in infant–caregiver attachment. In J. Cassidy & P. R. Shaver (Eds.), *Handbook of attachment: Theory, research, and clinical applications* (pp. 68–88). New York: Guilford Press.

van IJzendoorn, M. H. (1997, April). *Attachment in the balance: Progress and problems of attachment theory and research.* Paper presented at the annual meeting of the Society for Research in Child Development, Washington, DC.

CHAPTER 6

◆ ◆ ◆

Attachment in Infancy and in Early and Late Childhood

A Longitudinal Study

MASSIMO AMMANITI
ANNA MARIA SPERANZA
SILVIA FEDELE

CONTINUITY AND CHANGE OF ATTACHMENT

Why do some children maintain the same type of attachment during infancy and childhood, whereas in other children the type of attachment changes?

Whereas the evaluation of attachment in infancy is primarily based on behavioral observations, and in adolescence and adulthood on representational reports, which are the most relevant measures to evaluate attachment during childhood?

These are the central questions to be addressed in this chapter.

In the attachment framework a central question deals with the continuity and change of the attachment behavioral system from infancy through subsequent phases of development. Although substantial progress has been made toward understanding the developmental process of attachment in infancy, there are still open questions regarding transformation, development, function, expression, and outcomes of different attachment organizations during childhood and throughout the lifespan (Ainsworth, 1985, 1991; Cassidy & Shaver, 1999; Greenberg, Cicchetti, & Cummings, 1990; Greenberg, Siegel, & Leitch, 1983; Kobak & Sceery, 1988; Kotler & Omodei, 1988; Main, Kaplan, & Cassidy, 1985; Mayseless, Chapter 1, this volume).

The continuity of attachment could be justified primarily by the repeated interactions with significant caregivers, which later become incorporated into specific mental representations or "internal working models" (IWM) of these relationships. These mental representations, which contain both cognition and affect, would influence the appraisal of behavior in later different social situations involving intimacy with others and threats to self (van IJzendoorn, 1995).

A large body of evidence documents long-term stability of attachment from infancy through later phases of development. It has been shown that from infancy through middle childhood there is a substantial stability of attachment, as Main and Cassidy (1988) have shown in the Berkeley Study, demonstrating that the A, B, and D categories of attachment to mother in a sample of children at age 1 were highly predictive (84%) of 6th-year attachments. These data have been replicated in subsequent studies in Germany by Wartner, Grossmann, Fremmer-Bombik, and Suess (1994) with a stability of 82% for the four types of attachment status (A, B, C, D) and more recently by Gloger-Tippelt, Gomille, Koenig, and Vetter (2002) with a stability of 85% based on the distinction of secure (B) and insecure attachment (A, C, D). In Italy, Ammaniti and Speranza (2002) have demonstrated a significant correlation between attachment in infancy and in early childhood, with a stability of 71% considering the three categories (A, B, C) and 74% when using the secure–insecure distinction. As far as the disorganized category (D) is concerned, in the last sample no stability has been confirmed.

Considering a longer period, between infancy and adolescence, the continuity is still high, as it has been documented by Hamilton (2000) with a stability of 77% (secure–insecure) and Waters, Merrick, Treboux, Crowell, and Albersheim (2000) with a stability of 72% (secure–insecure).

These studies, of course, support the hypothesis that attachment across infancy, childhood, and adolescence is quite stable, although no studies have yet determined the relative contributions of different factors and their interactions that play a role in promoting stability, based either on mental representations of attachment or on the caregiving system.

Contextual factors, especially negative life events, play an important role in the discontinuity of attachment, as demonstrated in the study by

Waters and colleagues (2000). They found that the attachment category changed in 44% of children whose mothers reported negative life events, such as loss of a parent, parental divorce, parent's or child's life-threatening illness, parental psychiatric disorder, and physical or sexual abuse by a family member. However, among the contextual factors it would be important to also consider changes in family organization and circumstances that could influence and interfere with the relationship between parents and children, such as a change in maternal employment status, the arrival of a new sibling (Teti, Sakin, Kucera, Corns, & Das Eiden, 1996), maternal and family stress, financial difficulties, deeper maternal depression, and less social support (Belsky & Pasco Fearon, 2002).

This stability paradigm of attachment, however, has not been accepted by all scholars in the field, starting with the critique of Lamb, Thompson, Gardner, and Charnov (1985), who argued that the environment in which the child was raised has been neglected both theoretically and empirically in longitudinal studies of attachment. The predictive association between early attachment and later socioemotional functioning could be more a function of the child's environment at the time of the subsequent assessment than, as is frequently presumed, of early attachment security. Recently Lewis, Feiring, and Rosenthal (2000) have given further support to this critique with the empirical evidence that the stability of attachment from age 1 to age 11 in the insecure sample was only 38%, whereas 43% of secure children became insecure. Also longitudinal studies in north and south Germany (Becker-Stoll & Fremmer-Bombik, 1997; Zimmermann, Fremmer-Bombik, Spangler, & Grossmann, 1995) and a Minnesota longitudinal study (Weinfield, Sroufe, & Egeland, 2000) do not confirm the correspondence of attachment from 1 to 16–18 years of age.

More recently, Belsky and Pasco Fearon (2002, p. 364) have emphasized that, although a large body of evidence documents the connection between maternal sensitivity and a child's attachment security (De Wolff & van IJzendoorn, 1997), "the specific role of the IWM has been less subject to empirical scrutiny, often being used primarily as an interpretative heuristic in accounting for discerned relations between early attachment and later psychological functioning" (see also Belsky & Cassidy, 1994; Hinde & Stevenson-Hinde, 1991).

Research has sought to understand the complex and interactive role of security in subsequent caregiving. Erickson, Sroufe, and Egeland (1985) theorized that problematic behavior evidenced by preschoolers would be a function of both their early attachment history and their subsequent developmental experience with mothers. It was found that the predictive power of attachment security was contingent on the quality of maternal care that children received after the assessment of security. Children with secure attachment experience whose subsequent care was not sensitive and supportive did not develop as well as it might have been predicted on the basis of their secure attachment. Insecure children who received sensitive and supportive subsequent care did not develop as poorly as might have been expected on the basis of early insecurity. In conclusion, the developmental benefits of security and the disadvantages of insecurity were correlated with the maintenance of care that initially promoted secure and insecure attachments.

A recent investigation by Belsky and Pasco Fearon (2002), which sought to replicate these observations, confirmed that "early insecure attachment followed by later sensitivity was associated with more positive developmental outcomes at three years than early attachment security followed by later insensitive care" (p. 386). These observations tend to emphasize at the same time both the attachment theory and the current understanding of the determinants of parenting (Belsky, 1984). Those families in which the children were secure at 15 months but in which later assessment of parent–child interaction indicated maternal insensitivity showed a greater rate of family life stress, deeper maternal depression, and less social support than the families in which infants were secure at 15 months and later received highly sensitive care. Similarly, families of children classified as insecure at 15 months but whose later assessment of sensitivity indicated high-quality interactions showed lower scores on family distress.

These results are consistent with Lewis's (1997) view, which greatly emphasizes the influence of later experiences on development rather than earlier ones, thus opening the possibility of transformation during development when the contextual and caregiving circumstances change.

Indeed, the quality of care that mothers provide their infants, which is causally related to attachment security, seemed crucial, as it not only could explain the construction of the child's IWM but also could directly contribute to the child's later functioning. This perspective has recently been further developed (Lewis, 1997; Lewis et al., 2000), demonstrating that concurrent experiences, rather than developmentally antecedent ones, could shape psychological and behavioral development.

An interesting question raised by van IJzendoorn (1995) deals with the mechanisms through which the maternal representations of attachment would influence the development of infantile attachment, as the relation between the two is quite strong. It has been demonstrated that maternal attachment intervenes in mother's responsiveness to the child and, in so doing, helps the child to build a secure attachment. But this is not the only mechanism implied, and, as has been discussed by van

IJzendoorn (1995), there are other dynamics of transmission that could play a greater role than responsiveness.

An interesting perspective in broadening the conceptual framework of attachment is the organizational–relational perspective of attachment proposed by Sroufe (1979; Sroufe, Carlson, Levy, & Egeland, 1999). This perspective regards attachment as an organized behavior within a relationship, taking into account those developmental tasks that are salient and specific to each period, in order to evidence the continuity of personality functioning over time expressed in different patterns of behavior.

ATTACHMENT IN CHILDHOOD

Once the attachment bonds are stabilized during infancy and early childhood, they tend to persist in subsequent years, especially in stable child-rearing environments (Bowlby, 1988), although they may undergo transformations and reintegrations during later years.

On the basis of the primary attachment system, the child develops specific attachment relationships with the primary caregivers, expressed at the procedural level. Previous experiences with the caregivers inform the implicit knowledge, and the child knows but at the same time does not know what to do (Nelson, 1999) when distressed or threatened by internal or external stimuli. An important question relating to the implicit IWM (which are never consciously constructed) is: Are they subsequently brought into consciousness, reflected upon, and changed as language becomes available, or, alternatively or in addition, does implicit learning continue to take place, thus changing the original models?

Transformations probably include further elaborations at the same level of implicit knowledge, which informs the early processes of attachment, but also at a different level—that is, of explicit knowledge, which reorganizes the attachment experiences in terms of mentalization (Spangler & Zimmermann, 1999). At this level the knowledge becomes available to the cognitive system. In this perspective, shared stories between parents and children bring out previously hidden experiences, emotions, and knowledge states that were inaccessible to children prior to the acquisition of narrative capacity. It is possible to suggest that the child could achieve new insights into him- or herself and others and into relationships. The implicit experiential level is not split off from the explicit linguistic/narrative level, but it is brought into consciousness through the latter. However, this process can fail in some cases because of defensive processes activated by anxiety connected with attachment relationships, excluding information from consciousness and keeping IWM levels and memories split and segregated. In the case of very young children, the defensive processes are quite active because of the frequency and intensity with which attachment behavior is activated during early years (Bretherton & Munholland, 1999). Bowlby (1969/1982) has stressed that defensive exclusion, which sometimes has a self-protective function, could also interfere with adequate updating of IWM. When illustrating the defensive mechanisms, Bowlby underlined that they are not necessarily unconscious, as there could be a deliberate suppression or avoidance of perceptions, behaviors, and thoughts. The family context could as well explain the convergence between defensive processes in children and parents who could have facilitated a specific behavior and emotional regulation.

Of course, the acquisition of language, the development of cognition and theory of mind, and the integration into more complex motivational systems (Bowlby, 1969/1982) further contribute to complex transformations of the quality of significant relationships and of cognitive and emotional representations of caregiving and support.

In this context the increasing structuring of the child's self, strictly connected to caregiving relationships, promotes "the inner organization of attitudes, expectations and feelings" (Sroufe, 1989, p. 79) that develops throughout infancy and childhood and guarantees the maintenance of personal stability, continuity, and integration (Kohut, 1971; Stern, 1985). Recent literature has stressed the link between attachments and the self. Although in infancy and toddlerhood secure attachments promote self-recognition, in later school years there are evident connections between self and attachment. The self has a developmental consistency (Sroufe, 1989) due to such factors as the active role that individuals play in structuring of experience, the inaccessibility of early experience to conscious awareness, and the resistance of modification of early structures. The research with 5- and 6-year-old children has evidenced an association between secure attachment and a positive view of the self (Cassidy, 1988; Verschueren & Marcoen, 1999; Verschueren, Marcoen, & Schoefs, 1996), although the dimension and the importance of the self-system in childhood has been discussed mostly in theoretical terms.

At the same time, during childhood, the relationship with parents remains a close one, based on a mutual goal-corrected partnership. It is for this reason that children still need to know where their parents are and need to have a secure sense of their parents' availability. During the school years most children develop other close and mutual relationships with a range of other children and adults, including older relatives, teachers, and day-care workers.

In our research we explore the following hypotheses:

1. Considering that internal working models express themselves in terms of behavior strategy, as well as in representations of attachment conveyed by narratives, there is a convergence between measures of attachment behaviors and representations during early childhood.
2. Attachment shows significant stability from infancy to middle childhood, especially when we consider stability of maternal attachment as a concurrent factor.
3. Some changes in attachment may occur from infancy through middle and late childhood as a consequence of changes in maternal attachment and family context, such as the birth of one or two siblings.

Sample

Thirty-five children (16 girls, 19 boys) served as participants in the longitudinal study. Participants were recruited through pediatricians or schoolteachers. The children's mean age upon entry to the study was 12 months; the mean age of their mothers was 29 years. All children were in good health, and they lived with both parents. Families were middle-class, and 80% of the mothers were employed. Employment status remained the same in the follow-up periods. Twenty-one families were able to take part in the third assessment. The mean ages of the children at the second and third assessments were 5.3 and 11.5 years, respectively. For the first two assessments, children and their mothers were seen in a laboratory setting, whereas the third assessment was conducted at the participants' homes.

Procedure and Measures

First Assessment (12–15 Months)

Children. The Strange Situation procedure (Ainsworth, Blehar, Waters, & Wall, 1978) was used to assess the quality of the infant–mother attachment. The infants' patterns of attachment behavior were classified as secure (B), avoidant (A), resistant (C), or disorganized/disoriented (D).

Mothers. On the same occasion, all mothers were administered the Adult Attachment Interview (AAI; George, Kaplan, & Main, 1996). The interviews were audiotaped, and transcripts were rated according to the Main and Goldwyn (1998) coding system, which includes the following categories: secure–autonomous (F), dismissing (Ds), preoccupied (E), and unresolved with respect to trauma or loss (U). Three interviews were lost due to technical problems.

Second Assessment (5 Years)

Children. At the second assessment, children's attachment behaviors were assessed through the Main and Cassidy (1988) attachment classification system for kindergarten-age children. Classification is based on the child's behavior during the first 3 minutes of two reunions following separations of 15 minutes and 1 hour, respectively. Security and insecurity of attachment were rated on a 9-point observational security scale, whereas avoidance was rated on a 7-point avoidance scale. Reunion behavior was also classified according to the four patterns of parent–child attachment at age 5: secure (B), avoidant (A), ambivalent (C), and controlling (D).

During the second separation, 31 children completed the Attachment Story Completion Task (ASCT; Bretherton, Ridgeway, & Cassidy, 1990), a doll-play procedure for assessing attachment security. For each narrative assessment theme, the interviewer began a story using doll play, and the child was asked to complete it as in a game. The child's spontaneous verbal and behavioral responses were followed by nondirective prompts. We used seven story stems that probe for narrative themes in the area of family relationships and attachment themes. Each narrative was coded according to the thematic content it was designed to elicit, and the raters assigned a main category (secure, avoidant, hostile/negative). Afterward, the Separation Anxiety Test (SAT; Klagsbrun & Bowlby, 1976; Slough & Greenberg, 1990) was administered to 29 children. This procedure consists of a set of six photographs depicting attachment-related scenes ranging from mild (a parent says good night to a child in bed) to stressful (a child watches parents leave for 2 days). Each picture is introduced by the interviewer, and the child is asked to describe how the child in the picture feels and what that child will do. Responses were scored using the scoring indices for the Seattle version of the Separation Anxiety Test (Slough, Goyette, & Greenberg, 1988). Three summary scales (Attachment, Self-Reliance, and Avoidance) were computed by summing scores across the appropriate stories.

Mothers. During the same laboratory visit, mothers were administered the AAI once again. Three of 35 interviews were lost due to technical problems.

Third Assessment (11–12 Years)

Children. At the third assessment, the Attachment Interview for Childhood and Adolescence (AICA; Ammaniti et al., 1990) was administered individually to the children at home. The AICA is a revised version of the AAI for participants in late childhood and early adolescence

(Ammaniti, van IJzendoorn, Speranza, & Tambelli, 2000). The structure of the interview and the sequence of the questions were unchanged, but the language was simplified and adjusted to age. Explanations were added to clarify some questions. However, these changes did not modify the structure of the interview, which provided enough information to rate overall states of mind. A set of questions about current relationships with friends was added, but the answers were not taken into account during the coding.

The AICA was transcribed verbatim and coded by two independent raters following Main and Goldwyn's coding system (1998) for the AAI. In order to adjust the coding system to children's narratives, a group of experts trained in the AAI rating scales produced specific criteria for the Coherence scale and the other "state of mind" scales (Dazzi, De Coro, Ortu, & Speranza, 1999; Muscetta, Bovet, Candelori, Mancone, & Speranza, 1999). The coding system was used to classify children into one of four categories: secure, freely valuing of attachment (F), dismissing of attachment relationships (Ds), preoccupied with attachment relationships (E), and unresolved with respect to past loss or trauma (U).

Mothers. On the same occasion, the AAI was administered to mothers again. Sixteen mothers also completed the Child Behavior Checklist (CBCL; Achenbach, 1991), a standardized rating scale designed to assess a child's competencies and behavioral and emotional problems.

Follow-up at 11 years included 21 children and 15 mothers.

Results and Discussion

The results of this study are presented in three parts. As a first step, we discuss how the use of both observational and representational measures may improve the study of attachment in the preschool period. As a second step, we discuss stability and change of children's attachment as assessed in infancy and in early and late childhood. Finally, we explore factors that could be related to continuity and discontinuity, specifically, mothers' state of mind with respect to attachment as related to children's attachment across this 10-year period.

Assessment of Attachment in Early Childhood: Behavioral and Representational Measures

One of the aims of our study was to assess the quality of attachment relationships in childhood through both behavioral and representational measures, testing their efficacy and relatedness. Results showed a strong, significant concordance between the reunion pattern and the Story Completion classification, ranging from 74.2% in the four-way categories to 83.9% (kappa = .64, p < .001) in the secure-versus-insecure classification, as shown in Table 6.1. Moreover, we converted story classification scores into security scores, using a 4-point scale previously employed by Maslin, Bretherton, and Morgan (1986), on which B3 = 4; B1, B2, and B4 = 3; A2 and C1 = 2; and A1, C2, and D = 1. The story security scores were significantly related to the reunion Security scale ($r = .45$, $p < .01$) and to the reunion Avoidance scale ($r = -.50$, $p < .004$). Our data supported the use of narrative technique related to attachment issues as a possible assessment tool to explore IWMs of attachment at the age of 5. Secure children, who showed warm and intimate relationships with their mothers during the reunions, tended to describe doll-family interactions as positive, supportive, and warm and themselves as accepted and valued. Their narratives were coherent, and frequently the stories had good endings: The child was looked after, helped, and taken care of. It should be pointed out that in all the stories secure children were able to recognize the existence of a conflict by facing it; they never referred to themselves or to the family as perfect and problem free. On the contrary, avoidant children, who tended to be focused on play and to reduce physical and psychological intimacy on reunion with the mother, tended to show difficulties in getting involved or interested in the stories. The child described in the narratives was often depicted as isolated and unloved and frequently punished. At other times, conflicts in the stories were simply not accepted, and, as a consequence, no action was taken toward possible solutions. On the whole, in avoidant children the issues related to attachment seemed to raise emotional difficulties that, in turn, activated defensive mechanisms.

The features of secure and avoidant children's stories represented a significant marker of their own representational world. The IWMs ex-

TABLE 6.1. Concordance between Behavioral and Representational Measures in Childhood

Laboratory reunion (5 years)	Story Completion (5 years)			
	Avoidant (A)	Secure (B)	Hostile/ Bizarre (D)	Total
Avoidant (A)	**15**	2	1	18
Secure (B)	2	**8**		10
Ambivalent (C)	2	1		3
Total	19	11	1	31

Note. Stability is indicated by **bold** numbers.

pressed through the narratives seem to be at the forefront of attachment behaviors exhibited during the reunion. This relation is particularly important because it leads to regarding attachment as a complex motivational system. In this way, it becomes possible to understand its evolution over time, despite the substantial changes that occur during childhood, when language comes to play a preeminent role within the overall child's experience and behavior.

On the contrary, we didn't find any significant relations between SAT scales and both story and reunion classifications. Other studies (Kerns, Tomich, Aspelmeier, & Contreras, 2000; Resnick, 1997; Slough & Greenberg, 1990; Wright, Binney, & Smith, 1995) found inconsistent findings using SAT in the preschool or middle childhood periods. It could be argued that the way children describe emotions and solutions to feelings engendered by separation pictures might not be related to IWMs of attachment. As Solomon and George (1999) argued, we should "consider the degree to which representational procedures activate the attachment system" (p. 306) at different ages: For example, an overnight separation from the parents might not be a very disturbing stimulus for a 5- or 6-year-old. Moreover, as with adult self-report measures, we should carefully distinguish between attachment questionnaires such as the SAT and narrative technique such as the ASCT. Narrative assessment evaluates not only the content of the narrative but also the coherency and the structure of the discourse. It could be assumed that the organization of the discourse might reflect the implicit knowledge and its defense processes for regulating emotions (Jacobvitz, Curran, & Moller, 2002).

Continuities and Changes from Infancy to Late Childhood

The most important aim of our longitudinal study was to explore the stability and change of IWMs of attachment from infancy to late childhood.

In regard to the preschool period, we found that classifications of early attachment to the mother were significantly related to attachment classifications at 5 years. Table 6.2 contains the cross-tabulation of infant and child attachment classifications. Using three-way classifications at each age, 25 out of 35 children (71.4%, kappa = .48, $p < .001$) were assigned to corresponding classifications in infancy and childhood. Twenty-six out of 35 (74.2%, kappa = .46, $p < .01$) received the same classification using the secure–insecure dichotomy. On the contrary, we didn't find stability for the Disorganized/Controlling classification. At 5 years, none of the 7 children who were disorganized at 1 year received a primary Controlling (D) classification. Other studies (Lyons-Ruth, Repacholi, McLeod, & Silva, 1991; van IJzendoorn, Schuengel, & Bakermans-Kranenburg,

**TABLE 6.2. Stability of Children's Attachment Classifications
(12 Months–5 Years)**

Strange Situation (12 months)	Laboratory reunion (5 years)			
	Avoidant (A)	Secure (B)	Ambivalent (C)	Total
Avoidant (A)	**15**	3	1	19
Secure (B)	4	**9**	2	15
Ambivalent (C)			**1**	1
Total	19	12	4	35

Note. Stability is indicated by **bold** numbers.

1999) found that the stability of the Disorganized pattern may vary in relation to time of follow-up (12 to 48 months) and kind of sample (maltreated vs. normal).

Strange Situation classification also predicted avoidant and secure behaviors in childhood. Children classified as secure in infancy (both as primary classification and as secondary to disorganization) showed significantly higher mean scores on the Security scale at 5 years ($M = 4.8$, $SD = 0.8$) than insecure children ($M = 3.8$, $SD = 1.0$) ($t = 3.1$, $p < .01$). Secure infants showed positive and reciprocal interactions or conversations with the mother at age 5, and their proximity-seeking behaviors were relaxed and confident. Moreover, the most salient characteristic of secure children's behavior at 5 years seemed to be their ability to openly discuss feelings and emotions about recent separation. On the contrary, children classified as insecure in infancy showed significantly more avoidant behaviors ($M = 4.0$, $SD = 1.3$) than secure infants ($M = 3.1$, $SD = 1.0$) at 5 years ($t = 1.91$, $p < .05$). They tended to maintain affective neutrality, limiting opportunities for interaction or giving only impersonal responses to their mothers' discourse. The mother–child dialogue seemed to be so poor that these children frequently continued to do what they were doing without showing any apparent interest in their mothers' return.

Classifications of early attachment to mothers at 12 months were also significantly related to attachment representations at 5 years (Table 6.3). Using the secure–insecure classification, 23 out of 31 children (74.2%, kappa = .45, $p < .01$) retained the same category: Attachment behaviors during the Strange Situation significantly predicted the IWMs assessed through the ASCT.

At the 11-year follow-up, 21 of 35 families participated in the study. There was no significant difference in the 12-month or 5-year secure–insecure distribution between children who participated in the follow-up

TABLE 6.3. Stability of Attachment (12 Months–5 Years) (Behavioral-Representational Measures)

Strange Situation (12 months)	Story Completion (5 years)		
	Secure	Insecure	Total
Secure	**8**	5	13
Insecure	3	**15**	18
Total	11	17	31

Note. Stability is indicated by **bold** numbers.

and those who dropped out. The distribution of AICA classifications was 13 (61.9%) Secure, 6 (28.6%) Dismissing, and 2 (9.5%) Preoccupied.

In regard to stability of children's attachment classifications from infancy through late childhood, results showed that only 12 out of 21 children (57.1%, kappa = .26, n.s.) retained the same three-way attachment classification over time (Table 6.4). Thirteen out of 21 (61.9%, kappa = .26, n.s.) received the same secure–insecure classification. In the same way, we found only a moderate stability in attachment classification from 5 to 11 years (52.3%, kappa = .21, n.s., for the three-way distribution; 57.1%, kappa = .19, n.s., for secure vs. insecure) when we used patterns of reunion as an observational measure. Stability increased to 68.4% (kappa = .39, $p < .06$) when we considered representational rather than observational assessment at age 5. Six of 7 (85.7%) children classified as secure in

TABLE 6.4. Stability of Children's Attachment Classifications (12 Months; 5 Years; 11 Years)

	AICA (11 years)			
	Dismissing (Ds)	Secure (F)	Preoccupied (E)	Total
Strange Situation (12 months)				
Avoidant (A)	**5**	5	1	11
Secure (B)	1	**7**	1	9
Ambivalent (C)		1		1
Laboratory Reunion (5 years)				
Avoidant (A)	**5**	6		11
Secure (B)		**6**	2	8
Ambivalent (C)	1	1		2

Note. Stability is indicated by **bold** numbers.

the ASCT at 5 years remained secure at 11 years, and 7 of 12 (58.3%) inse-cure children were also classified as insecure across this period.

Data concerning competencies and behavioral problems, assessed with the Child Behavior Checklist (CBCL) at 11 years, didn't show signifi-cant differences related to attachment classification as assessed at age 11.

These results, as well as those of other studies (Lewis et al., 2000; Weinfield et al., 2000), suggested that other experiences beyond infancy could play a significant role on attachment stability. Change in attachment status could not be ascribed to the method, because AICA was found to be accurate in discriminating between different states of mind with re-spect to attachment (Ammaniti et al., 2000).

In order to clarify the moderate stability, we explored whether nega-tive life events, family changes, and mothers' attachment classification could account for it.

Factors That Affect Continuity and Discontinuity

In order to assess the influence of several variables on continuity–discontinuity of children's attachment, multiple regression analyses were used. Stressful life events (presence vs. absence), infant attachment classi-fication (secure vs. insecure), and concordance between mother and in-fant attachment, both at 1 year and at 5 (presence vs. absence), were not statistically significant predictors of whether infants' attachment classifi-cations changed or remained the same in the two follow-up assessments.

In regard to the infancy–early childhood period, we found that both stability of maternal attachment (R^2 = .23, $F(1,28)$ = 7.9, p < .01, beta = .47, p < .01) and the number of younger siblings (R^2 = .30, $F(1,28)$ = 11.4, p < .01, beta = –.54, p < .01) significantly predicted stability of children's attachment. Infants whose mothers showed stability in their IWMs of at-tachment were more likely to maintain the same attachment classification (95.5%, 21 of 22) than were infants whose mothers changed attachment classification over time (57.1%, 4 of 7). At the same time, children with no siblings were more likely to retain attachment classification (100%, 15 of 15) than children with one younger sibling (81.8%, 9 of 11) or with two (33.3%, 1 of 3). Finally, because these two variables were not correlated, the interaction between them was also significant to predict stability (R^2 = .47, $F(1,28)$ = 11,6, p < .001).

In regard to children's attachment classifications from 12 months through 11 years, the number of younger siblings was the only variable that significantly predicted continuity or discontinuity of attachment (R^2 = .29, $F(1,20)$ = 7.9, p < .01, beta = –.54, p < .01). Number of siblings was sig-nificantly related to the likelihood of changing attachment classification from infancy to age 11 (16.7%, 1 of 6, for only children; 36.4%, 4 of 11, for children with one younger sibling; 100%, 4 of 4, for children with two younger siblings). Interestingly, most children with siblings (6 of 8) changed from insecure to secure attachment classifications.

The stability of our sample in the infancy–early childhood period corresponds to other studies that have used the same observational measure (Main & Cassidy, 1988; Wartner et al., 1994). Based on predictions from attachment theory and previous studies on continuity, it could be hypothesized that stability of mother's mental representation of attachment promotes continuity in the quality of children's attachment relationships (van IJzendoorn, 1995). As the child grows up, maternal attachment representations and behaviors continuously influence the mother–child relationship and, in turn, the child's behaviors and IWMs of attachment enhance stability. This could be especially true in the preschool years, when the mother still represents the child's primary attachment figure. Afterward, in late childhood, other experiences and relationships could widen the child's social world and exert their influence. The birth of new siblings and the reorganization of family relationships may affect the mother–child relationship, as well as the child's IWM (Touris, Kromelow, & Harding, 1995). This could be the result of changes in maternal sensitivity in the direction of a decreasing responsiveness to the firstborn child if the mother is confronted with challenging and demanding younger children, as well as in the direction of an increasing ability to interpret and respond to the child's signals (Dunn, Plomin, & Daniels, 1986; Dunn, Plomin, & Nettles, 1985; van IJzendoorn et al., 2000). Moreover, it is possible to suggest that if a mother is able to give every child his or her own space by recognizing his or her individual mind, the child will feel more sure about his or her relationship with the mother.

As noted earlier, stability of maternal state of mind with respect to attachment significantly affected the likelihood of a child maintaining the same attachment classification in the preschool period. Twenty-two out of 29 (75.8%) mothers retained the same classification at 12-month and at 5-year follow-ups, both for the three-way classification (kappa = .53, p < .001) and for the secure–insecure classification (kappa = .47, p < .01; Table 6.5). Moreover, 9 out of 14 (64.3%) mothers were classified in the same three-way category across the 10-year period (kappa = .38, p < .05). Similarly, stability of maternal attachment was found between the two follow-ups (5 and 11 years): 73.3% of mothers (11 of 15) retained the same classification (kappa = .55, p < .003). The stability of this sample over the long-term period is about the same as found in some short-term test–retest studies (78%; Bakermans-Kranenburg & van IJzendoorn, 1993). About 25% of mothers changed their IWMs in the two follow-up periods. Some of them were working through their attachment experiences as a consequence of specific life events: the loss of a rejecting mother, a new approach and co-

TABLE 6.5. Stability of Maternal Attachment Classification

AAI (12 months)	AAI (5 years)				AAI (11 years)			
	Ds	F	E	Total	Ds	F	E	Total
Dismissing (Ds)	**5**	3		8	**2**	1	1	4
Secure (F)	1	**15**	2	18	1	**6**	1	8
Preoccupied (E)		1	**2**	3		1	**1**	2
Total	6	19	4	29	3	8	3	14

Note. Stability is indicated by **bold** numbers.

habitation with very involved parents, the solution of a very difficult relationship with the father. It is possible that such emotionally significant experiences could induce representational and behavioral changes that
affect, as a result, the mother–child relationship. In fact, we observed an
increased concordance between maternal IWM and child attachment as
the child grew up, especially in the case of mother's stability. Three-way
classification matches were found for 17 of the 32 dyads (53.1%, kappa =
.21, n.s.), whereas secure-versus-insecure concordance reached 62.5%
(kappa = .29, p < .06) when the infant was 12 months old. At the 5-year
follow-up, correspondence between mother and child attachment classification was 53.1% (kappa = .30, p < .01), and it increased to 65.6% for the
secure–insecure dichotomy (kappa = .38, p < .01). In the same way,
matches in the 15 dyads who were assessed at age 11 was 66.7% (kappa =
.44, p < .01) and 80% (kappa = .59, p < .02), respectively, for the three-way
and for the secure-versus-insecure attachment classification.

CONCLUSION

This study examined the stability of attachment between infancy and late
childhood.

In regard to the infancy–early childhood period, we found a substantial stability both for three-way and for secure–insecure categories. Data
indicated also that behavioral and representational assessments were
strongly related in early childhood, representing two faces of the same
IWM. Results suggested that maternal attachment plays a role in continuity or discontinuity of child attachment in early childhood. When mothers
showed stability in their IWMs, attachment stability in children increased
from 74 to 95% in the infancy–early childhood period, especially for secure children. Moreover, instability in mothers' IWMs was significantly re-

lated to the likelihood of a secure infant becoming insecure in childhood. Data supported the hypothesis that ongoing mother–child interactions continue to influence the nature of the child's attachment to mother beyond early infancy. At the same time, the birth of a sibling seemed to be an important factor of change, not necessarily for the worse. Other studies emphasized the transition to siblinghood as a significant factor of attachment instability (Teti et al., 1996; Touris et al., 1995). As in the study by Touris and colleagues (1995), our results showed that the birth of a second child led to instability in the mother–firstborn-infant attachment relationship but not to specific changes toward increased security or insecurity.

In regard to the infancy–late childhood period, we found a moderate stability in attachment classification. Examining possible factors associated with instability, we found that in the long-term period mothers' attachment classifications, as well as stressful events, were not important factors of change. The only significant factor was the birth of one or two siblings. Number of siblings was significantly related to the likelihood of an infant changing attachment classification (16.7% for only children; 36.4% for children with one sibling; 100% for children with two siblings). The change for most of the children was toward security. The impact of a sibling's birth on relational patterns in the family may be considerable, and it may constitute a life event that changes the mother's sensitivity and responsiveness to children.

We conclude with some open questions that have been raised concerning the results of the research.

1. The research in the area of attachment tends to focus on the mother as the central figure in the organization of attachment. In our research we have demonstrated a limited stability between infancy and late childhood, which probably occurs because other attachment figures intervene as well as the mother: fathers, grandparents, siblings, and teachers.

2. This study has highlighted the role of the birth of siblings in changing attachment status toward security. Nevertheless, our data should be replicated, because other studies emphasize that the birth of a sibling has a worsening role. Future studies should more deeply explore the psychological mechanisms that could intervene in changing the type of attachment.

3. During childhood there is an important process of integration and complex reorganization of the attachment representational models, which assume a hierarchical structure with a dominant categorical attachment and subordinate attachments. In this period it is important to address the process of integration and hierarchical organization between the behavioral and the representational domains.

REFERENCES

Achenbach, T. M. (1991). *Manual for the Child Behavior Checklist/4–18 and 1991 Profile.* Burlington: University of Vermont, Department of Psychiatry.

Ainsworth, M. D. S. (1985). Attachment across the life span. *Bulletin of the New York Academy of Medicine, 61,* 792–812.

Ainsworth, M. D. S. (1991). Attachment and other affectional bonds across the life cycle. In C. M. Parkes, J. Stevenson-Hinde, & P. Marris (Eds.), *Attachment across the life-cycle* (pp. 35–51). London: Routledge.

Ainsworth, M. D. S., Blehar, M. C., Waters, E., & Wall, S. (1978). *Patterns of attachment: A psychological study of the Strange Situation.* Hillsdale, NJ: Erlbaum.

Ammaniti, M., Candelori, C., Dazzi, N., De Coro, A., Muscetta, S., Ortu, F., et al. (1990). *A.I.C.A. Attachment Interview for Childhood and Adolescence.* Unpublished manuscript, University of Rome.

Ammaniti, M., & Speranza, A. M. (2002). I modelli di attaccamento dalla prima infanzia alla pre-adolescenza: Uno studio longitudinale [Patterns of attachment from infancy through late childhood: A longitudinal study]. *Psichiatria dell'Infanzia e dell'Adolescenza, 69*(1), 5–18.

Ammaniti, M., van IJzendoorn, M. H., Speranza, A. M., & Tambelli, R. (2000). Internal working models of attachment during late childhood and early adolescence: An exploration of stability and change. *Attachment and Human Development, 2,* 328–346.

Bakermans-Kranenburg, M. J., & van IJzendoorn, M. H. (1993). A psychometric study of the Adult Attachment Interview: Reliability and discriminant validity. *Developmental Psychology, 29,* 870–879.

Becker-Stoll, F., & Fremmer-Bombik, E. (1997, April). *Adolescent–mother interaction and attachment: A longitudinal study.* Poster presented at the biennal meeting of Society for Research in Child Development, Washington, DC.

Belsky, J. (1984). The determinants of parenting: A process model. *Child Development, 55,* 83–96.

Belsky, J., & Cassidy, J. (1994). Attachment: Theory and evidence. In M. Rutter & D. Hay (Eds.), *Development through life* (pp. 373–403). London: Blackwell.

Belsky, J., & Pasco Fearon, R. M. (2002). Early attachment security, subsequent maternal sensitivity, and later child development: Does continuity in development depend upon continuity of caregiving? *Attachment and Human Development, 4*(3), 361–387.

Bowlby, J. (1982). *Attachment and loss. Vol. 1: Attachment.* New York: Basic Books. (Original work published 1969)

Bowlby, J. (1988). *A secure base.* London: Routledge.

Bretherton, I., & Munholland, K. A. (1999). Internal working models in attachment relationships: A construct revisited. In J. Cassidy & P.R. Shaver (Eds.), *Handbook of attachment: Theory, research, and clinical applications* (pp. 89–111). New York: Guilford Press.

Bretherton, I., Ridgeway, D., & Cassidy, J. (1990). Assessing internal working models of attachment relationships: An attachment story completion task for 3-year-olds. In M. T. Greenberg, K. Cicchetti, & E. M. Cummings (Eds.), *Attach-

ment in the preschool years: Theory, research and intervention (pp. 273–308). Chicago: University of Chicago Press.

Cassidy, J. (1988). Child–mother attachment and the self in six-year-olds. *Child Development, 59,* 121–134.

Cassidy, J., & Shaver, P. R. (Eds.). (1999). *Handbook of attachment: Theory, research, and clinical applications.* New York: Guilford Press.

Dazzi, N., De Coro, A., Ortu, F., & Speranza, A. M. (1999). L'intervista sull'attaccamento in preadolescenza: un'analisi della dimensione della coerenza [Attachment Interview for Childhood: Analysis of coherence of transcript]. *Psicologia Clinica dello Sviluppo, 3*(1), 129–153.

De Wolff, M., & van IJzendoorn, M. (1997). Sensitivity and attachment: A meta-analysis on parental antecedents of infant attachment. *Child Development, 68,* 571–591.

Dunn, J. F., Plomin, R., & Daniels, D. (1986). Consistency and change in mothers' behavior towards young siblings. *Child Development, 57,* 348–356.

Dunn, J. F., Plomin, R., & Nettles, M. (1985). Consistency and change in mothers' behavior toward infant siblings. *Developmental Psychology, 21,* 1188–1195.

Erickson, M. F., Sroufe, L. A., & Egeland, B. (1985). The relationship of quality of attachment and behavior problems in preschool in a high risk sample. In I. Bretherton & E. Waters (Eds.), Growing points in attachment theory and research (pp. 147–186). *Monographs of the Society for Research in Child Development, 50*(1–2, Serial No. 209).

George, C., Kaplan, N., & Main, M. (1996). *Adult Attachment Interview Protocol* (3rd ed.). Unpublished manuscript, University of California at Berkeley.

Gloger-Tippelt, G., Gomille, B., Koenig, L., & Vetter, J. (2002). Attachment representations in 6-year-old: Related longitudinally to the quality of attachment in infancy and mothers' attachment representations. *Attachment and Human Development, 4*(3), 318–339.

Greenberg, M. T., Cicchetti, D., & Cummings, E. M. (Eds.). (1990). *Attachment in the preschool years: Theory, research, and intervention.* Chicago: University of Chicago Press.

Greenberg, M. T., Siegel, J. M., & Leitch, C. J. (1983). The nature and importance of attachment relationships to parents and peers during adolescence. *Journal of Youth and Adolescence, 12,* 373–386.

Hamilton, C. E. (2000). Continuity and discontinuity of attachment from infancy through adolescence. *Child Development, 71*(3), 690–694.

Hinde, R., & Stevenson-Hinde, J. (1991). Perspectives on attachment. In C. Parkes, J. Stevenson-Hinde, & P. Morris (Eds.), *Attachment across the life cycle* (pp. 52–65). London: Routledge.

Jacobvitz, D., Curran, M., & Moller, N. (2002). Measurement of adult attachment: The place of self-report and interview methodologies. *Attachment and Human Development, 4*(2), 207–215.

Kerns, K. A., Tomich, P. L., Aspelmeier, J. E., & Contreras, J. M. (2000). Attachment based assessments of parent–child relationships in middle childhood. *Developmental Psychology, 36,* 614–626.

Klagsbrun, M., & Bowlby, J. (1976). Response to separation from parents: A clinical test for young children. *British Journal of Projective Psychology, 21*, 7–21.

Kobak, R. R., & Sceery, A. (1988). Attachment in late adolescence: working models, affect regulation, and representations of self and others. *Child Development, 59*, 135–146.

Kohut, H. (1971). *The analysis of self.* New York: International Universities Press.

Kotler, T., & Omodei, M. (1988). Attachment and emotional health: A life span approach. *Human Relations, 41*, 619–640.

Lamb, M. E., Thompson, R., Gardner, W., & Charnov, E. (1985). *Infant–mother attachment: The origins and developmental significance of individual differences in Strange Situation behavior.* Hillsdale, NJ: Erlbaum.

Lewis, M. (1997). *Altering fate: Why the past does not predict the future.* New York: Guilford Press.

Lewis, M., Feiring, C., & Rosenthal, S. (2000). Attachment over time. *Child Development, 71*(3), 707–720.

Lyons-Ruth, K., Repacholi, B., McLeod, S., & Silva, E. (1991). Disorganized attachment behavior in infancy: Short-term stability, maternal and infant correlates, and risk-related subtypes. *Development and Psychopathology, 3*, 377–396.

Main, M., & Cassidy, J. (1988). Categories of response to reunion with the parent at age 6: Predictable from infant attachment classifications and stable over a 1-month period. *Developmental Psychology, 24*(3), 415–426.

Main, M., & Goldwyn, R. (1998). *Adult attachment scoring and classification system.* Unpublished manuscript, University of California at Berkeley.

Main, M., Kaplan, N., & Cassidy, J. (1985). Security in infancy, childhood and adulthood: A move to the level of representation. In I. Bretherton & E. Waters (Eds.), Growing points of attachment theory and research (pp. 66–104). *Monographs of the Society for Research in Child Development, 50*(1–2, Serial No. 209).

Maslin, C., Bretherton, I., & Morgan, G. A. (1986, April). *Influence of attachment security and maternal scaffolding on mastery motivation.* Paper presented at the International Conference on Infant Studies, Los Angeles.

Muscetta, S., Bovet, A., Candelori, C., Mancone, A., & Speranza, A. M. (1999). Funzione riflessiva materna e stile di attaccamento nei bambini [Maternal reflective function and attachment patterns in children]. *Psicologia Clinica dello Sviluppo, 3*(1), 109–128.

Nelson, K. (1999). Event representations, narrative development, and internal working models. *Attachment and Human Development, 1*, 239–252.

Resnick, G. (1997, April). *The correspondence between the Strange Situation at 12 months and the Separation Anxiety Test at 11 years in an Israeli Kibbutz sample.* Paper presented at the biennal meeting of the Society for Research in Child Development, Washington, DC.

Slough, N. M., Goyette, M., & Greenberg, M. T. (1988). *Scoring indices for the Seattle version of the Separation Anxiety Test.* Unpublished manuscript, University of Washington.

Slough, N. M., & Greenberg, M. T. (1990). Five-year-olds' representations of separation from parents: Responses from the perspective of self and other. *New Direction for Child Development, 48,* 67–84.

Solomon, J., & George, C. (1999). The measurement of attachment security in infancy and childhood. In J. Cassidy & P. R. Shaver (Eds.), *Handbook of attachment: Theory, research, and clinical applications* (pp. 287–316). New York: Guilford Press.

Spangler, G., & Zimmermann, P. (1999). Attachment representation and emotion regulation in adolescents: A psychobiological perspective on internal working models. *Attachment and Human Development, 1*(3), 270–290.

Sroufe, L. A. (1979). The coherence of individual development: Early care, attachment, and subsequent developmental issues. *American Psychologist, 34,* 834–841.

Sroufe, L. A. (1989). Relationships, self, and individual adaptation. In A. J. Sameroff & R. N. Emde (Eds.), *Relationship disturbances in early childhood* (pp. 70–94). New York: Basic Books.

Sroufe, L. A., Carlson, E. A., Levy, A. K., & Egeland, B. (1999). Implications of attachment theory for developmental psychopathology. *Development and Psychopathology, 11,* 1–13.

Stern, D. (1985). *The interpersonal world of the infant.* New York: Basic Books.

Teti, D. M., Sakin, J., Kucera, E., Corns, K. M., & Das Eiden, R. (1996). And baby makes four: Predictors of attachment security among preschool-aged firstborns during the transition to siblinghood. *Child Development, 67,* 579–596.

Touris, M., Kromelow, S., & Harding, C. (1995). Mother–firstborn attachment and the birth of a sibling. *American Journal of Orthopsychiatry, 65*(2), 293–297.

van IJzendoorn, M. H (1995). Adult attachment representations, parental responsiveness, and infant attachment: A meta-analysis on the predictive validity of the Adult Attachment Interview. *Psychological Bulletin, 117*(3), 387–403.

van IJzendoorn, M. H., Moran, G., Belsky, J., Pederson, D., Bakermans-Kranenburg, M. J., & Kneppers, K. (2000). The similarity of siblings' attachments to their mother. *Child Development, 71*(4), 1086–1098.

van IJzendoorn, M. H., Schuengel, C., & Bakermans-Kranenburg, M J. (1999). Disorganized attachment in early childhood: Meta-analysis of precursors, concomitants, and sequelae. *Development and Psychopathology, 11,* 225–249.

Verschueren, K., & Marcoen, A. (1999). Representation of self and socioemotional competence in kindergartners: Differentials and combined effects of attachment to mother and to father. *Child Development, 70,* 183–201.

Verschueren, K., Marcoen, A., & Schoefs, V. (1996). The internal working model of self, attachment, and competence in five-years-olds. *Child Development, 67,* 2493–2511.

Wartner, U. G., Grossmann, K., Fremmer-Bombik, E., & Suess, G. (1994). Attachment patterns at age six in South Germany: Predictability from infancy and implications for preschool behavior. *Child Development, 65,* 1014–1027.

Waters, E., Merrick, S., Treboux, D., Crowell, J., & Albersheim, L. (2000). Attachment security in infancy and early adulthood: A twenty-year longitudinal study. *Child Development, 71*(3), 684–689.

Weinfield, N. S., Sroufe, A. L., & Egeland, B. (2000). Attachment from infancy to early adulthood in a high-risk sample: Continuity, discontinuity, and their correlates. *Child Development, 71*(3), 695–702.

Wright, J. C., Binney, V., & Smith, P. K. (1995). Security of attachment in 8–12-year-olds: A revised version of the Separation Anxiety Test, its psychometric properties and clinical interpretation. *Journal of Child Psychology and Psychiatry, 56*(5), 757–774.

Zimmermann, P., Fremmer-Bombik, E., Spangler, G., & Grossmann, K. E. (1995, March). *Attachment in adolescence: A longitudinal perspective.* Poster presented at the biennal meeting of the Society for Research in Child Development, Indianapolis, IN.

CHAPTER 7

◆ ◆ ◆

The Construct of Coherence as an Indicator of Attachment Security in Middle Childhood

The Friends and Family Interview

HOWARD STEELE
MIRIAM STEELE

This chapter draws on findings obtained in the context of our 11-year follow-up of the London Parent–Child Project, in which we had previously observed the parents of these firstborn children during the prenatal period and later followed up the children during infancy (Steele, Steele, & Fonagy, 1996). Given that attachment during infancy is a relationship-specific construct (Sroufe, 1988), with much evidence that infant–mother attachments are statistically independent from infant–father attachments, further research is needed to elucidate the processes whereby representations of specific relationships to mother and to father during early childhood become, in the course of development, integrated within higher order metarepresentational systems. In this chapter we report on our attempts to observe such evidence of metarepresentations of attachment in 11-year-old children and the extent to which these were related to previously observed attachment characteristics of the children or their parents. Both attachment research and the broader domain of normative developmental research provided the impetus to design the Friends and Family Interview, which, we argue, is appropriate to the aim of assessing representations of attachment in middle childhood.

Middle childhood is the period for which metatheoretical perspectives on one's own and other's cognitions and emotions have been widely documented (Broughton, 1978; Harter, 1998; Selman, 1980), and this topic customarily receives prominent attention in textbooks on child development when the focus is on the late elementary school years or middle childhood (e.g., Dehart, Sroufe, & Cooper, 1999; Hetherington & Parke, 1999). From both the Piagetian and information-processing perspectives, normally developing 11-year-old children have become highly proficient at hierarchical classification or semantic organization, that is, organizing information to be remembered by means of categorization and hierarchic relationships. Against this background, children of this age should be able to recall past interactions that illustrate their higher order views or evaluations of themselves and their relationships to their mothers and their fathers. Such achievement should be fueled by the normatively developing capacities for using others as a source of information to evaluate oneself (e.g., Ruble, 1983). Furthermore, their growing awareness that different situations may require different behavior toward others (Damon & Hart, 1988) should contribute to the likelihood that 11-year-old children would be able to compare and contrast their relationships to their mothers and fathers and to comment on features of these relationships that they would most like to preserve and other features that they would most like to change. We expected that young people who had benefited from security in their early family experiences would be best able to meet this challenge of demonstrating metarepresentational awareness of the positive and negative elements of relationships with family and friends and strategies for how to resolve interpersonal and intrapersonal conflicts.

With respect to children's developing understanding of emotions, it is has been suggested that the capacity to label and understand mixed or blended emotions and diverse emotions arising in the same person toward a target person or situation is normally evident by 11 years of age (Harter & Buddin, 1987). We have previously shown that individual differences in this capacity may be linked to individual differences in early attachment, and when a child benefits from security in the mother–child relationship, an understanding of mixed emotions may be evident as early as 6 years of age (Steele, Steele, Croft, & Fonagy, 1999). Similarly, others have observed that children who benefit from security in their attachment relationships to their mothers have an enhanced understanding of negative emotion in particular (Laible & Thompson, 1998), presumably stemming from more frequent, wide-ranging, and open discussions of emotion in the home. Thus we anticipated that discussions of self and attachment relationships at 11 years of age may be similarly influenced by previously assessed individual differences in attachment because of the varying patterns of emotional communication that are known to underpin and result from differing attachment patterns. Briefly, insecure, especially avoidant, infant–parent attachments are linked to restricted parental responsiveness to negative emotions (Grossmann, Grossmann, & Schwan, 1986), and secure infant–mother attachments are linked to later evidence of open, balanced, and flexible patterns of mother–child conversation concerning emotion (Etzion-Carraso & Oppenheim, 2000).

We conceive of attachment in middle childhood as an emerging property of the individual child that is accessible via a structured interview, informed by but distinct from the Adult Attachment Interview (AAI; Main, Kaplan, & Cassidy, 1985). Since Main and colleagues (1985) first advocated a move to the level of representation beyond attachment behaviors readily observed in the Strange Situation (Ainsworth, Blehar, Waters, & Wall, 1978), numerous narrative tasks, particularly the Attachment Story Completion Task (ASCT), have been proposed or revisited as potential indicators of attachment security in children. Validity of these approaches has depended on making comparisons either with earlier infant–parent or parent measures of attachment security (Gloger-Tippelt, Gomille, Koenig, & Vetter, 2002; Steele et al., 2003) or with concurrent measures of children's well-being (Easterbrooks & Abeles, 2000; Oppenheim, Emde, & Warren, 1997). Suggestive findings have been arrived at by both these approaches, underlining the value of relying on the child's view of self and family relationships as a meaningful indicator of attachment security. Notably, the doll-play literature tends to rely on scoring of the manifest content (e.g., antisocial or prosocial themes) in the child's story completion, as opposed to overall narrative coherence of his or her speech according to the maxims of "good conversation" embraced as central in the most widely used and accepted scoring system applied to the AAI (see Hesse, 1999). This suggests that doll-play tasks are a useful means for demonstrating how interactions with parents are represented in young children's minds, but it is unclear as to whether doll-play tasks can elicit higher order abstract and organized concepts of the positive and negative aspects of relationships with parents, as these are likely to depend on metacognitive abilities and memory skills that are not evident until the end of the primary or elementary school years. The very question, posed early in the AAI, "Tell me about your early relationship with your parents from as far back as you can remember," simply does not seem appropriate until a child is firmly established in, or at the end of, middle childhood. Not surprisingly, then, some researchers have sought to extend the possible use-fulness of doll play for assessing attachment forward, to cover early school age through to the final years of elementary school (i.e., 9- to 11-year-olds), and this strategy no doubt has many applications (see the doll-play task and scoring system suggested by Granot & Mayseless, discussed in Kerns, Schlegelmilch, Morgan, & Abraham, Chapter 3, this volume). Our strategy has been to extend the possible usefulness of questions and scor-ing criteria—especially that of coherence—backward from the AAI litera-ture.

The criterion of coherence is easily applied to speaker's responses to the AAI, in which global evaluations of a relationship are first elicited (e.g., "Give me five adjectives that describe your relationship with your mother during early childhood through the age of about 12. I'll give you a moment to think about it and then I'll ask you about each adjective in turn"). Then specific memories that might illustrate the evaluation are re-quested (e.g., "you said 'loving'; now, when you think about your relation-ship during early childhood with your mother as 'loving,' what comes to mind?"). AAI raters or judges pay close attention to the extent to which recalled memories support or fill out the picture suggested by the adjec-tives provided. High levels of coherence may be demonstrated regardless of the adjective's positive or negative connotations—the crucial elements are correspondence, consistency, and, ultimately, credibility. This is a cen-tral, though not the only, consideration when rating coherence in AAIs. The AAI scoring system (see Hesse, 1999), as concerns coherence, leans heavily on Grice's (1975) maxims of "good conversation"; that is, being truthful, relevant, economical, and conventionally polite. Adherence to these maxims has been shown to be fundamental to an attachment inter-view deemed autonomous-secure and likely to reflect an adult speaker ca-pable of being a good-enough (sensitive and responsive) parent (van IJzendoorn, 1995). Given the developmental evidence that metacognitive abilities and memory skills are vastly improved by 11–12 years of age, as compared with the early school-age years, we anticipated that this age group would be well able to handle the challenge of providing a coherent narrative about self, family, and friends.

Almost as soon as coherence was identified as a central marker of at-tachment security in adulthood, appropriate psychometric queries were raised as to whether coherence in an AAI was distinct from verbal IQ. A number of reports have confirmed that coherence when describing and evaluating attachment relationships (in the context of the AAI) is largely orthogonal to verbal IQ (Bakermans-Kranenburg & van IJzendoorn, 1993; Crowell et al., 1996; Steele, 1991). In other words, a lawyer or doc-tor may be low on coherence in the AAI, whereas an unskilled worker lacking a high school diploma may be high on coherence. This evidence of discriminant validity pertaining to the AAI sets the goalpost for any proposed interview-based measure of attachment security in middle childhood. In other words, to be persuaded that our Friends and Family Interview (FFI) was indeed assessing attachment processes, we proposed to show that a rating of coherence applied to the interview could be reliably achieved without being wholly subsumed by an independent measure of verbal IQ. What we hypothesized was that the overlap between verbal IQ and coherence in the FFI would be limited and no greater in magnitude than the overlap between verbal IQ and coherence in the AAIs obtained many years before from the children's parents.

One further psychometric issue concerns our claim that coherence at age 11 in an attachment narrative is similar to coherence in an AAI. One way of investigating whether coherence at age 11 is a metarepresentational capacity, rooted in but not defined by experience, would be to rate both coherence and evidence of secure–base availability of each parent in the interviews from the 11-year-olds. If these ratings were then found to be completely overlapping, we would be hard pressed to claim that coherence at age 11 is anything like coherence when rated in the context of an AAI. This is so because, in the AAI literature, coherence has been widely shown to be both largely independent from probable past experiences with caregivers *and* a superior predictor of infant–parent attachment quality (Fonagy, Steele, & Steele, 1991; Main et al., 1985; van IJzendoorn, 1995).

We anticipated that coherence in discussing relationships with friends and family at 11 years of age would be significantly related to prior assessments of attachment obtained from the children and their parents. To test for this possibility, we compared ratings of coherence in the interviews provided by the 11-year olds with their earlier observed attachments to mother (at 12 months) and to father (at 18 months) and with the AAIs obtained from their parents in the prenatal period (Steele et al., 1996). In this way, we hoped to explore the extent to which early relationship-specific attachments may be represented and integrated in the mind of the 11-year-old child on the cusp of adolescence. Several questions arise from the fact that our longitudinal design did not include concurrent observations of parent–child interaction at age 11. If coherence at age 11 was related to our previously assessed early-attachment variables, what evidence would we have that it was these early patterns of attachment, as opposed to the continuous and stable nature of parent–child interactions, that have influenced the 11-year outcome? And, if coherence at age 11 was not associated with our early-attachment assessments, should this be taken as evidence that parent–child relations have changed significantly since early childhood? In only one sense could our longitudinal research design explore the possibility that later, as opposed to very early, parent–

child interactions were influencing coherence at age 11. This becomes evident when we consider the four sources of information we have about
early attachments within the family. Two of these are the AAIs provided
by each parent before the child was born. The other two are the infant–
mother attachment at 12 months and the infant–father attachment at 18
months. If we observed that only the AAIs and not the infancy assessments were predicting coherence at age 11, this may suggest that later,
and not early, parent–child interactions were influencing the 11-year outcome. To the extent that the infancy Strange Situation assessment(s) could
be shown to independently predict coherence at age 11, even after taking
account of the parents' AAIs, we would then be on more solid ground in
assuming a long-term influence of early experience with mother, father,
or both attachment figures.

In thinking about what to expect from interviews about self, family,
and friends at age 11, we could not ignore the literature on gender differences. As gender-segregated peer behavior becomes normative in
middle childhood, with all range of activities and judgments being increasingly made in accordance with gender stereotypes (see Ruble &
Martin, 1998), we entertained the possibility that girls would be more
advanced than boys in talking about diverse emotions and relationships
and showing a metarepresentational understanding of attachment. Thus,
in the results reported in this chapter, we explore whether metarepresentations of attachment would be more evident in girls than in boys
and whether the influence of attachment on the narratives provided by
11-year-olds in our sample would be similarly evident in boys as opposed
to girls.

METHOD

Sample

Fifty-seven children were visited in their homes in the year or so following
their 11th birthdays. The mean age of children in the follow-up was 11
years, 6 months; range = 11 years, 1 month through 12 years, 7 months;
SD = 3.8 months. In other words, approximately 70% of the young people
seen at follow-up were between 11 years 2 months and 11 years 10 months
old. In terms of gender, there was an even split, with 28 boys and 29 girls.
AAIs from the parents (obtained during the pregnancy phase of the
study) and infant–parent Strange Situation assessments were available for
all the participants at 11-year follow-up, with the exception of one girl
who had not been observed with her father in the Strange Situation at 18
months. Thus analyses including infant–father attachment data are based
on 56 cases.

Early Attachment Measures

Adult Attachment Interview

The interview administered to all parents who were expecting their first children closely followed the schedule outlined by George, Kaplan, and Main (1985). The AAI is structured entirely around the topic of attachment, principally the individual's relationship to mother and to father (and/or to alternative caregivers) during childhood. Participants are asked both to describe their relationships with their parents during childhood and to provide specific memories to support global evaluations. The interviewer asks directly about childhood experiences of rejection, about being upset, ill, and hurt, as well as about loss, abuse, and separations. In addition, the participants are asked to offer explanations for the parents' behavior and to describe their current relationships with their parents and the influence they consider their childhood experiences to have had on their adult personalities. Ultimate classification of the interview into the secure or one of the insecure (dismissing or preoccupied) groups depends largely on the extent to which the narrative is judged to satisfy four criteria of coherence. These four criteria comprise (1) a good fit between memories and evaluations concerning attachment; (2) a succinct yet complete picture; (3) the provision of relevant details; and (4) clarity and orderliness (see Hesse, 1999). An insecure–dismissing narrative is brief and incomplete, marked by a lack of fit between memories and evaluations, often punctuated or sustained by an unrealistically positive evaluation of parents and/or self. An insecure–preoccupied narrative is neither succinct nor complete and contains many irrelevant details, together with much passive (weak, nonspecific) speech or highly involving anger toward one or both parents. By contrast, the autonomous secure narrative robustly fulfils all or most of the criteria of coherence, whether or not the speaker was well cared for during childhood. Ratings and classifications of the interviews were carried out independently by four trained raters, with highly reliable results (see Steele et al., 1996).

The Results section in this chapter also refers to "probable past experiences" of the parents with their mothers and fathers (how well cared for they were) in terms of the extent of supportive, loving experiences they had, which can be readily identified in an AAI. Here 9-point rating scales were applied to the AAIs by the trained raters, who achieved high levels of interrater agreement, median $r = .76$, range $= .73-.91$ (Steele, 1991).

Strange Situation

The Strange Situation is widely regarded for its reliability and validity and extensively employed as an assessment of the quality of child–parent attachments (Ainsworth et al., 1978). This 20-minute laboratory-based assessment involves two brief separations and two 3-minute reunions with the parent. Focus is on the infant's behavior, especially during the reunions, in which individual differences are measured in terms of the strategies employed to cope with this stressful situation that is within the range of normal infant experience (i.e., introduction to an unfamiliar place and person and two brief separations from the parent).

Of the three originally identified major patterns of response, two reflect an insecure attachment to the parent (either avoidant or resistant), and one indicates a secure attachment to the parent (Ainsworth et al., 1978). Infants whose attachment is classified insecure–avoidant tend to appear undistressed during separation and to avoid proximity to the parent on reunion. Infants whose attachment is classified secure may or may not be distressed by separation, but on reunion they are pleased to see the parent and, if distressed, are easily comforted. Infants whose attachment is classified insecure–resistant tend to be distressed by separation and to seek contact during reunion, but rather than being settled by the parent's return, they appear inconsolable. Some children do not fit easily into one of the traditional three patterns because of their atypical "disorganized" response to the situation, assumed to reflect fear of the attachment figure. When this judgment is made, a best-fitting alternate (avoidant, secure, or resistant) assignment is made. This applied to less than 5 of the cases in the current sample. The videotapes of the Strange Situations were classified by a team of raters who were blind both to the parents' interview data and also to the child's attachment status with the other parent. Two coders independently classified each infant–parent tape. There was 90% agreement on the four-way classifications of infant–parent attachment, with conferencing involving a third trained rater being relied on to settle the disagreements.

Attrition from Earlier Phases of the Study

We examined attrition by computing cross-tabulations of AAI profiles (insecure vs. autonomous–secure) of each parent with children's observed attachment status (insecure vs. secure) with mother (at 12 months) and with father (at 18 months). These cross-tabulations revealed highly similar levels of intergenerational concordance in attachment patterns (75% for mothers and 66% for fathers) to those observed in the larger sample of 90 families from which these 57 come (Steele et al., 1996). In another important respect, the 11-year follow-up sample also resembled the earlier, larger cohort insofar as the proportions of security and insecurity in mothers, fathers, and children were similar at the two time periods, despite the absence of 33 families from the 11-year follow-up. Attrition, it was clear, was not unduly influenced by attachment variables. We were thus persuaded that the sample recruited for the 11-year follow-up was, in terms of attachment security, were very much like the original cohort. Attrition appears to have been much more strongly influenced by migration factors, with a third of the original sample having moved far from their original contact addresses, and most of these we were unable to locate at the time of the 11-year follow-up.

Verbal Intelligence: WISC-III^{UK}

The Vocabulary and Similarities subscales of this widely used and UK-standardized "intelligence" test were administered to control for those aspects of verbal intelligence most likely to be related to the capacity for coherence in discussing relationships (Wechsler, 1992). In the Similarities subtest, the child is asked how stimulus words are similar. The words represent concepts or objects and are presented orally to the child. The child must respond verbally. A maximum raw score of 33 is possible on the Similarities subtest. For the present sample, the mean Similarities score achieved was 23 (SD = 4), range = 14–31. In the Vocabulary subtest, the examiner reads a word, and the child is required to give a spoken definition. A maximum score of 60 is possible. For the present sample, the mean Vocabulary score achieved was 37 (SD = 6), range = 23–49. Remarkably, the mean Similarities score achieved is suggestive of a test age of 15 years, 10 months. The Vocabulary score achieved is suggestive of a test age of 13 years, 2 months. In other words, the sample would appear to be highly verbally intelligent.

Verbal intelligence of the parents had been assessed at the initial pregnancy phase of the study with the short form of the Mill Hill Vocabulary Scales (Raven, Court, & Raven, 1986). The parents were presented with a series of target words of increasing difficulty, and they were asked to define each and use it in a sentence. There are 17 words on the short form. For the parents of the children participating in the 11-year follow-up, the mothers' mean score was 11.1 (SD = 2.3); range = 6–16; the fathers' mean score was 12.3 (SD = 2.6); range = 5–17. These average scores of the parents reflect a level of verbal intelligence that is among the upper third of the British adult population, as Raven and colleagues (1986) report that the 11th word in the list of 17 presents difficulty to approximately 65% of the population.

Friends and Family Interview

Our search for an interview protocol that was appropriate to our aim of assessing coherence concerning attachment relationships and that was also able to elicit the interest of 11-year-old children led us in two directions. First, the mainstream developmental literature and classic theorizing on psychosocial relationships (Erikson, 1951/1963; Sullivan, 1953) led us to consider the domain of friendship as a topic of inquiry. Children's social health by late middle childhood depends very much on forming and maintaining friendships outside the family, beyond long-standing relations to siblings and parents. Thus, to assess coherence concerning relationships, we would have to ask about best friendships and how they are going. At the same time, we were driven by our ongoing interest in close family relationships, as discussed by Bowlby in the 1956 lecture he delivered on the centenary of Sigmund Freud's birth: "In our early years it is the rule and not the exception that towards both our siblings and our parents we are impelled by feelings of anger and hatred as well as those of concern and love" (Bowlby, 1979, p. 4). Bowlby (1979) elaborates in this lecture on the need for children to develop a well-functioning capacity for regulating this conflict of love and hate and, "through this, [a] capacity to experience in a healthy way [both] anxiety and guilt" (p. 3). Thus normal development is depicted in terms of having just the right amount, neither too much nor too little, of anxiety and guilt. How else could we ever seek to change or repair an aspect of ourselves or an important relationship if we did not feel some sense of anxiety or guilt over things not having proceeded as well as they might? This view of the negative emotions owes much to Freud's (1926/1959) account of anxiety being a danger signal that calls the ego (or self) into action aimed at minimizing the threat to internal and social cohesion. Against this background, then, we designed the FFI as a way of systematically inquiring about the young person's view of the complex and often conflicting emotions arising in one's closest relationships.

We not only drew on developmental research and psychoanalytic theories in conceiving of the interview protocol we would assemble, but we were also strongly influenced by our own previous findings concerning young children's understanding of emotion. In particular, we recalled how, at age 6 years, the longitudinal sample we would again be visiting had impressed us with their advanced and precocious skills at understanding mixed emotions, but only if their mothers had provided autonomous–secure and coherent attachment interviews or if they had been securely attached to mothers at 1 year of age (Steele et al., 1999).

We knew that it was perhaps too much to expect 11-year-old children to show themselves to have a coherent developmental perspective on their childhood while they were still in the middle of it. Thus we aimed to prime the 11-year-olds we interviewed to think about diverse aspects of their feelings concerning self, parents, siblings, and friends. We did this by beginning the interview that we would come to call the Friends and Family Interview with the following invitation:

"I want to get an idea about you, what sort of person you are, what you like to do, and most of all how you think and feel about your relationships with friends and family. One thing we sort of take to be true about all people and relationships is that there are things we like best in ourselves and in other people (things we might like to keep the same), and other things that we like least (or not very much at all) in ourselves and other people (things we might like to change). So this might be something we talk about as I ask you the following questions."

The subsequent questions of the interview took as their focus, in turn, self, peers (best friend), siblings, and parents. With regard to each of these domains, the respondents were asked to describe the best and worst bits, most liked and least liked aspects, of how things were. Specific probes included queries about disagreements that arose and how they were negotiated, with requests for supporting memories that could fill out the picture. Indeed, throughout, the respondents were asked to illustrate their stories with examples from daily life. Coming from the attachment tradition, we asked early on, under the heading of questions about the self, "What do you do when you are upset?" We saved those questions that we imagined to be most taxing on these young people's capacity for coherent speech until the end of the interview protocol. These were such questions as, "What kind of person does your mother (or father) think you are?" "How would you describe their relationship to one another (i.e., the marital relationship)?" "Has your relationship to your parents changed since you were younger?" and "What do you think the relationship will be like in 5 years?" (The full FFI protocol and full scoring system are available from the authors by request.) The interviews collected were both tape-recorded (for later transcription) and videotaped.

For the purposes of this chapter, we rely on four-point ratings of coherence and secure-base availability of each parent. These rating scales were applied to the interview transcripts by graduate students working independently and without access to prior attachment-related information about the 11-year-old speakers whose narratives they were rating. Coherence was rated on four subscales, stemming from the AAI literature: Truth, or quality (a good fit between specific memories and general evaluations); Economy, or quantity (a succinct but complete picture); Relation (the provision of relevant detail); and Manner (being conventionally polite, clear, and orderly in presentation). As well, each interview was assigned both a 4-point rating for global or overall coherence and a 4-point rating for evidence of secure-base availability of (1) mother and (2) father. The 4 points for these scales were defined as 0 = no evidence, 1 = a little evidence, 2 = moderate evidence, and 3 = robust marked evidence. The four sets of ratings for coherence were examined for reliability by considering the Cronbach's alpha coefficients when each person's rating was treated as an item. For the alphas computed, each was greater than .74 (range = .74–.88). A single score for Truth, Economy, Relation, Manner, and overall coherence was computed for each interview, based on summing up and averaging the individual four ratings that were assigned.

Importantly, the narratives provided by the 11-year-olds could be scored for evidence of social competence, or "quality of best friendship" and "quality of sibling relationship." However, in this chapter we focus on the global construct of overall coherence in order to consider our hypothesis related to the young person's capacity for providing a cohesive and credible account of his or her attachment experiences, self-construct, and peer relationships. This approach is in line with the widely accepted attachment theory construct of an internal working model of self and others becoming established early in life (a reflection of which is observable on reunion with the caregiver in the Ainsworth Strange Situation). And, further, the internal working model of one's relationship with mother and (often independent) model of one's relationship with father influence one's experiences with peers and eventually become integrated into a higher order representational model that informs one's thoughts and feelings about being or becoming a parent (a reflection of which is evident in the speech provided in response to the AAI).

RESULTS

To test the hypotheses under consideration, we arrange results in two sections. First, we report on bivariate correlations concerning coherence in the narratives from the 11-year-olds and their verbal intelligence, as well as parallel results for the parents, and also correlations between the early attachment assessments and coherence at 11 years of age. Second, we report on regression results examining the extent of influence of independent and overlapping predictor variables from the range of demographic, verbal, and earlier attachment measures obtained on the outcome of coherence and metarepresentational processes observed in the 11-year-olds' responses to the FFI.

Bivariate Comparisons

First, we examined the correlations between verbal intelligence of the parents and children and age of the children in relation to their observed attachment-based coherence. All but one of these correlations yielded nonsignificant results. Children's age in months at the time of the 11-year follow-up was correlated positively and significantly with overall coherence (r = .26, p < .05, one-tailed), allowing for the likelihood that one would have predicted this outcome. This result suggests, as might well be expected, that maturation enhances the child's potential for demonstrating metarepresentational capacities. These preliminary tests revealed one further finding of note—namely, that boys and girls did not differ in the scores they received for coherence and secure–base availability in the FFI.

Our next step was to compare ratings of the secure–base availability or loving supportive experiences with each parent with the speaker's coherence or overall attachment security. For the parents, mothers' and fathers' AAI security correlated positively and highly significantly with the ratings of how supportive, loving, and available their mothers (r = .56, n = 57; r = .34, n = 57), and their fathers (r = .59, n = 57; r = .37, n = 57) had been. When we made a similar comparison for the children based on their FFIs, secure-base availability of mothers correlated positively and highly significantly with each of the five coherence ratings (median r = .46, range = .45–.64), whereas secure-base availability of fathers was similarly correlated with the five coherence ratings (median r = .53, range = .43–.58). These consistent correlations in the .40–.60 range are important because of their modest magnitude given that they are based on comparisons between ratings derived from the same narrative. They highlight how 65–80% of the variance in parents' AAI classifications as insecure or secure and in the children's levels of coherence cannot be attributed directly to their experiences of warmth and support from their parents.

We then proceeded to compare the coherence ratings of the FFIs with the binary measures of attachment security from the parents' AAIs (from the pregnancy phase of the study) and the Strange Situation observations made of the infant–mother relationship (at 12 months) and the infant–father relationship (at 18 months). In Tables 7.1 and 7.2, we show the pattern of correlations that was observed for daughters and sons separately, together with the observed results for the full sample. We followed this strategy in order to consider the question of whether the links with early attachment may depend on the gender of the child, as well as of the parent. Table 7.1 reveals that quality, or truthfulness, in the FFI responses of the 11-year-olds was consistently and significantly higher for both sons and daughters if mother's AAI had been classified autonomous–secure. Uniquely, this is the only coherence correlation in Table 7.1 that is significant for both sons and daughters. Mothers whose AAIs were classified autonomous–secure had sons who at age 11 were impressively well-mannered in the FFI context (r = 40). The remaining significant correlations of coherence variables in Table 7.1 all point to influences of the fathers' AAIs on their sons' FFI responses in terms of every index of coherence: Truth (r = .42), Economy (r = .60), Relation (r = .39), Manner (r = .40), and overall coherence (r = .47).

TABLE 7.1. Ratings of Friends and Family Interview at 11-Year Follow-Up Correlated with Binary Measures of Parents' Security Assessed during Pregnancy with the Adult Attachment Interview

| | AAI Autonomy/Security | | | | | |
| | Mothers (n = 57) | | | Fathers (n = 57) | | |
11-year-olds' FFIs	Daughters	Sons	Full sample	Daughters	Sons	Full sample
Truth	.54**	.42*	.48**	−.09	.42*	.16
Economy	−.18	.25	.03	.03	.60**	.29*
Relation	.13	.22	.18	.06	.39*	.24
Manner	.14	.40*	.27*	−.17	.40*	.12
Overall coherence	.29	.33	.31*	.00	.47*	.23
Secure-base availability of mother	.38*	.39*	.39**	−.02	.47*	.20
Secure-base availability of father	.17	.12	.15	−.02	.38*	.19

Note. Full sample = 29 daughters and 28 sons.
*p < .05, two-tailed; **p < .01, two-tailed.

TABLE 7.2. Ratings of the Friends and Family Interview at 11-Year Follow-Up Correlated with Binary Measures of Infant–Parent Attachment Security

| | Infant–Parent Attachment Security | | | | | |
| | With mother at 12 months | | | With father at 18 months | | |
11-year-olds' FFIs	Daughters	Sons	Full sample	Daughters	Sons	Full sample
Truth	.25	.07	.16	.26	.40*	.31*
Economy	−.09	.13	.02	.02	.52**	.27*
Relation	.02	.01	.01	.19	.41*	.29*
Manner	.10	.06	.08	.06	.52*	.26
Overall Coherence	.09	−.06	.02	.20	.45*	.31*
Secure-base availability of mother	.01	.02	.02	.23	.50**	.38**
Secure-base availability of father	.34^{+}	.12	.22	.20	.17	.16

Note. *p < .05, two-tailed; **p < .01, two-tailed; ^{+}p < .10, two-tailed.

Table 7.1 also indicates that evidence in sons' FFIs of secure-base availability of mother is significantly and positively correlated to both their mothers' AAI security (r = .39) and their fathers' AAI security (r = .47). With daughters, by contrast, availability-of-mother ratings were uniquely and significantly related to mothers' AAI security (r = .38). Table 7.1 also shows that secure-base availability of father, as rated in the FFIs, is significantly correlated to fathers' AAI security, but only for sons.

Table 7.2 looks at the correlations observed between the FFI and the early observations of infant–parent attachment security, with results for sons, daughters, and the full sample presented separately.

Table 7.2 shows a consistent pattern of positive significant correlations between infant–father attachment security and each observed index of coherence in the FFI at age 11, but for sons only. Daughters' speech about relationships, in terms of truthfulness and overall coherence, appears to also be positively influenced by having been securely attached to father at 18 months, but the magnitude of these correlations does not reach significance. Truthfulness of daughters is also correlated positively, but not significantly, with infant–mother attachment at 12 months. Also, with respect to secure-base availability ratings of mother and father in the FFIs, it is for the sons that positive correlations are more evident, one of these highly significantly. This is the correlation in Table 7.2 between secure-base availability of mother (in sons' FFIs) and infant–father attachment security at 18 months (r = .50, p = .007, two-tailed). A parallel correlation, significant at the level of a trend, is observed between secure-base availability of father (in daughters' FFIs) and infant–mother attachment security at 12 months (r = .34, p = .08, two-tailed).

Regression Results

Having established that early attachment variables appear to predict various aspects of our coding of the FFI at 11 years of age, and considering the influence of the child's age and verbal intelligence, we then set out to explore the extent to which these could be said to be overlapping or independent predictive influences.

With regard to the daughters, there was only one robust predictor (mothers' AAI security) of their coherence (the scale concerning truthfulness or credibility) in the FFI, about which we wondered whether the daughter's age or verbal intelligence contributed any independent predictive power. Thus we computed a hierarchical linear regression analysis, entering at the first step the daughter's age as predictor, then her Similarities subtest WISC score (as this was more suggestive of significance than the Vocabulary subtest score), and finally mother's AAI security, in order to see what remaining predictive power mothers' AAI security would have after taking into account these maturational and verbal IQ variables. This regression analysis revealed that age of daughter when entered made a limited (beta = .17) and nonsignificant (p = .35) contribution to the model until, at step 3 (after the AAI of the mother was entered), age dropped out altogether (beta = .03, p = .88). This hierarchical regression also revealed that a daughter's capacity for scoring highly on the verbal intelligence (WISC) subtest of Similarities, entered after age, increased R^2 by 6%, but this was not a significant increase, Fchange (1, 26) = 1.62, p = .21. By contrast, when maternal AAI autonomy/security was added to the model at step 3, there was a substantial and highly significant leap in R^2 by 24%, Fchange (1, 25) = 9.16, p = .006. Overall, 33% of the variance in daughters' coherence (truthfulness) in the FFI was accounted for by the model that included age of daughter, WISC score for Similarities subtest, and maternal AAI security.

With respect to the sons, a range of attachment variables were shown at the bivariate level to be linked with levels of coherence in the FFI. We therefore computed a hierarchical linear regression in order to examine the extent of overlapping, as opposed to independent, influences at work. We concentrated on the sons' speech in terms of truthfulness, both because this was the variable found to be most relevant in the daughter-based analyses and because this variable was variously correlated at the bivariate level with each parent's AAI autonomy/security and with infant–father attachment security. At the first step in the regression analysis, age of son (months over 11 years) was entered as the predictor variable, with sons' truthfulness or credibility in the FFI entered as the dependent variable. This yielded an impressive estimate of variance accounted for of 6%, but, given the small sample size, it was not a significant effect. At the second step, the sons' verbal intelligence scores on the WISC subtest for Similarities were entered, and this added a negligible and nonsignificant increase of 2% to the variance accounted for in the sons' FFI coherence. The contribution to the model at steps 3 and 4 made by sons' verbal intelligence remained trivial and nonsignificant. Statistical significance appeared in the model at step 3, when mothers' AAI security was added, increasing the variance accounted for by 20% to a cumulative total of 28%, Fchange (1, 23) = 6.31, p < .05. Notably, when fathers' AAI security was added at step 4, the variance accounted for increased by a further 12%, to 40%, Fchange (1, 22) = 4.38, p < .05, with mothers' AAI autonomy/security remaining as a significant predictor, independent of the significance contributed by fathers' AAI autonomy/security and of their sons' coherence in the FFI at age 11. Note that infant–father attachment security does not figure in these results, although it did figure in the bivariate correlations. Including this variable in the regression model did not enhance the predictive power of the model, on account of overlapping variance with fathers' AAI security, the more powerful predictor well able to carry the weight of prediction on its own.

DISCUSSION

The results reported herein provide compelling reasons to believe that by 11 years of age boys and girls are capable of telling a coherent and integrated story about their thoughts, feelings, and experiences concerning self, friends, parents, and siblings. The FFI was the method used to elicit these stories, and the discussion accordingly focuses on why this interview method may be particularly useful for studying attachment processes in middle childhood. Observed links between young people's coherence in the FFI and their parents' responses to the AAI, collected more than 11 years previously, merits careful consideration. In particular, we provide an account of the somewhat surprising gender-specific findings that emerged, highlighting the significance for sons' coherence at age 11 of both maternal and paternal AAI security, whereas for daughters the significant influence on their coherence at age 11 appeared to be much more exclusively tied to their mothers' (not their fathers') AAI security.

It is not new to suggest, as we have here, that 11-year-old children can speak about their views of themselves and of their relationships with their parents, siblings, and friends in a thoughtful, reflective, and credibly insightful way. Others have documented this developmental step characteristic of advancing social cognition in the middle childhood and adolescent years (Broughton, 1978; Damon & Hart, 1988; Harter, 1998; Selman, 1980). Nor is it new to suggest that a differentiated self-understanding, including the ability to express positive and negative beliefs about the self, is concurrently linked to attachment security in middle childhood (Easterbrooks & Abeles, 2000). The arguably unique contribution made by the current results stems from the longitudinal research design employed. This allowed us to highlight how individual differences in the capacity to provide a coherent and credible evaluation of the self and important relationships (to parents, siblings, and peers) at age 11 is a reflection of long-standing individual differences in attachment security within the family.

With respect to our approach to scoring the FFIs that we collected, reliance on the construct of coherence (Grice, 1975), as it has been applied to the scoring and classification of AAIs (Hesse, 1999), proved a rewarding investment. Coherence at age 11 in the narratives about self, friends, and family was not shown to be any more influenced by verbal intelligence than is the case with adults or parents who provide their narratives about attachment experiences in the AAI. Furthermore, when we considered whether coherence in the FFI was a dimension distinct from estimates of secure-base availability (supportive parenting), the findings were highly suggestive. The majority of variance in coherence scores in the FFI could not be accounted for in terms of supportive parenting received. Indeed, the proportion of overlap between ratings of coherence and of secure-base availability in the FFI was broadly similar to the observed overlap between ratings of coherence and supportive parenting received in their parents' AAIs. Thus it would seem that coherence is operating in the FFI much like coherence is presumed to operate in the AAI—that is, as an organizer of experience, including reflections, evaluations, and redescriptions of experience at a metarepresentational level within the mind.

Clues as to the only moderate (and not major) influence of early attachment experiences upon coherence at age 11 come from the observed correlations between previously observed infant–parent patterns of attachment and coherence ratings derived from the FFIs. Infant–mother attachment security at 12 months, though positively related to some of the FFI ratings, was not significantly related to any of them. And, with respect to infant–father attachment security observed at 18 months, this variable did relate positively and significantly to every index of coherence in the FFI and also to secure-base availability of the mother, but for sons only. Notably, in the regression analysis predicting boys' coherence (truthfulness), the infant–father attachment variable was occluded by the overlapping and more powerful influences of fathers' and mothers' AAI security/coherence. So early experience, although undeniably contributing to coherence, is perhaps not as important as later attachment experiences, tapped (albeit indirectly) by the AAIs collected from the parents in the pregnancy phase of our longitudinal research. A key assumption here, which remains to be tested, is the long-term stability of parental responses to the AAI. We would assume greater stability for responses to the AAI during adulthood in the parenthood phase than is the case for infant–parent attachment security across childhood. In other words, we understand the AAIs we collected from expectant parents to be a predictor not only of infant–parent attachment but also of later parental availability. This is confirmed by the current results showing a strong and significant correlation between our ratings of secure-base availability of the parent(s) and the 11-year-olds' capacity to provide a credible and coherent attachment narrative, or FFI.

In this respect, we regard the coherent responses we obtained to the FFI as evidence of the representational power of the developing human mind, including the capacity to store and recall details of past and current social interactions and to examine these experiences and the emotional impact they carry. Both daughters and sons in the current study who showed this capacity in the FFI (i.e., to be truthful and coherent) were more likely to have had mothers—and in the case of sons—fathers, too, who, prior to the child's birth, showed this same capacity in the AAI. The discriminant validity findings mentioned here, with respect to verbal intelligence (a well-known heritable characteristic), would seem to rule out a behavior genetic account of these intergenerational findings. More probable is a social transmission model, in which parents' understanding and communication of emotion is a central factor.

The strong influence of mothers' AAIs on both sons and daughters evokes consideration of mothers as primary attachment figures who, for this sample, as in most, spend more time than fathers involved in caregiving to their children. That it was mothers' AAIs and not the early infant–mother relationship that predicted FFI coherence speaks for the *ongoing*, as opposed to early, quality of mother–child interactions. Not having home observations to draw upon, we can only assume that those young people with highly coherent FFIs benefited from many experiences of having their mothers listen well and respond appropriately in the context of conversations about both positive and negative emotions leading to and arising from social experiences. We expect this to have been the case given ample prior research that highlights a relative ease of emotional expression concerning positive and *negative* experiences as a marker of attachment security (Easterbrooks & Abeles, 2000; Laible & Thompson, 1998; Main et al., 1985; Steele et al., 1999). Notably, our rating of coherence in the FFI depended on the young person providing credible evidence to support his or her positive and negative appraisals of self, parents, siblings, and peers.

That levels of coherence in the FFIs from the sons, as opposed to the daughters, should be more influenced by the early father–child relationship and by both parents' (as opposed to only the mothers') AAIs is consistent with diverse developmental theories. Whether we think, for example, in terms of gender schema theory (Martin & Halverson, 1981) or classical psychoanalytic theory (Freud, 1905/1953), there is little surprise in the observation that from earliest childhood on sons—as opposed to daughters—would have been particularly attentive to their fathers in defining their emerging sense of self. To the extent that mothers' AAIs influenced both sons' and daughters' levels of coherence in the FFI, it is appealing to consider that mother is typically the first attachment relationship for both genders, and it is only sons who must later revoke in some measure this primary attachment in order to embrace an identification (or new attachment) with the father (Chodorow, 1978). Thus the challenge of integrating representations of both parents into a singular coherent metarepresentation of attachment may be less straightforward for sons. The attachment history of one 11-year-old boy from our study seems to illustrate this phenomenon well. His responses to the FFI were scored very high for coherence. His parents had each provided AAIs that were judged autonomous–secure/coherent at the initial pregnancy phase of the study. At 12 months he was anxiously resistant in his attachment to his mother, and in a post hoc analysis we identified this type of "mismatch" as a statistically significant group of mothers with a "fragile" form of security (Fonagy, Steele, & Steele, 1991). These mothers' AAIs pointed to a more idealized childhood history (than those of other autonomous–secure mothers with securely attached infants), perhaps making these women especially vulnerable to stress and disappointment, such as can be occasioned by the birth of a first child. At 18 months, the boy was observed to have a secure attachment to his father. In the FFI at 11 years, he described his relationship with his mother as one in which they spent much time together, more than he spent with his father, as she picked him up from school, was able to see his side of an argument (giving as an example a teacher who unfairly gave him a "detention"), and was generally available. He was then prompted for something in the relationship with his mother that was perhaps not as he would like, something he might like to change, or something that he perhaps liked least about his relationship with his mother but could not change. He then commented:

> "Umm, sometimes it's either she doesn't understand me, she doesn't, and sometimes when she doesn't she just physically can't see what I am on about. Umm, this is the least confusing way I can put it. But it's confusing anyway. . . . She either violently agrees with me or violently disagrees. And then she violently agrees. I don't get much in the way of a word, and if I do, then it's kind of discarded which, umm, I don't complain about because, umm, 99.9% of the time everything is fine and she just agrees with me. The thing I don't like that much is, umm, it's either-or."

When asked about his relationship with his father, the tone and content became lighter as he alluded to the positive friendly exchanges they have:

> "Yap. Umm, umm, he always tells rather marvelous stories. They are ones from the paper or ones from his childhood. And, umm, we always laugh about those. And, umm, discuss them. Have a bit of a joke. Umm, most of them involve, umm, doing something he shouldn't have done. And it's quite hard to imagine because I admire him as a grown-up, and I can't imagine him doing all these naughty things he tells me does, he did, rather. And so we have a bit of a laugh about that."

He went on to elaborate in detail on one of the benign stunts his father had engaged in with friends as a child, and overall provided a credible, coherent account of his relationships with each parent, siblings, and friends.

FFIs rated low on coherence often failed to provide experiential details of the "best liked" or especially "least liked" aspects of self, parents, siblings, or friends, and thus "truthfulness" (having evidence for what you say) emerged as the most significant subscale of coherence. This is perhaps typical of the late-middle-childhood–early-adolescent age group, in which dismissal/avoidance (as opposed to preoccupation/rumination) is the more characteristic form of insecurity manifested in a low-risk sample (Ammaniti, van IJzendoorn, Speranza, & Tambelli, 2000).

With respect to the developmental course to be negotiated throughout infancy, early childhood, middle childhood, and beyond, we wish to underscore that the FFI is not the AAI, which no doubt provides a more demanding test of metarepresentational capacities and for which some colleagues have demonstrated the appropriateness for young people age 12 or older (see Ammaniti et al., 2000). Given the evidence we have presented here that a difference of even a few months between ages 11 and 12 can contribute to enhanced coherence, it may be that the FFI is most useful in beginning to engage young people in the task of providing an autobiographical attachment narrative. An AAI may be the next step, appropriate from 12 years on, when middle childhood is widely agreed to have drawn to a close. It may be that what the middle childhood years provide, in attachment terms, is a set of experiences with parents, siblings, and peers that may optimally cohere in such a way as to facilitate the initial integration of diverse mental representations of one's ongoing interactions (and relationship histories) with mother, father, and others.

ACKNOWLEDGMENTS

The research on which this chapter was based was supported by a generous grant from the Köhler Stiftung, Germany, administered by the Anna Freud Centre, London. To the families participating in the research, who kindly give of their time and interest, we owe an enormous debt of gratitude.

REFERENCES

Ainsworth, M. D. S., Blehar, M. C., Waters, E., & Wall, S. (1978). *Patterns of attachment: A psychological study of the Strange Situation*. Hillsdale, NJ: Erlbaum.
Ammaniti, M., van IJzendoorn, M. H., Speranza, A. M., & Tambelli, R. (2000). Internal working models of attachment during late childhood and early adoles-

cence: An exploration of stability and change. *Attachment and Human Development, 2*, 328–346.

Bakermans-Kranenburg, M. J., & van IJzendoorn, M. H. (1993). A psychometric study of the Adult Attachment Interview: Reliability and discriminant validity. *Developmental Psychology, 29*, 870–879.

Bowlby, J. (1979). *The making and breaking of affectional bonds*. London: Routledge.

Broughton, J. (1978). Development of concepts of self, mind, reality, and knowledge. In W. Damon (Ed.), *New directions for child development: Vol. 1. Social cognition* (pp. 75–100). San Francisco: Jossey-Bass.

Chodorow, N. (1978). *The reproduction of motherhood*. Berkeley and Los Angeles: University of California Press.

Crowell, J. A., Waters, E., Treboux, D., O'Connor, E. O., Colon-Downs, C., Feider, O., et al. (1996). Discriminant validity of the Adult Attachment Interview. *Child Development, 67*, 2584–2590.

Damon, W., & Hart, D. (1988). *Self-understanding in childhood and adolescence*. Cambridge, UK: Cambridge University Press.

Dehart, G., Sroufe, A., & Cooper, R. (1999). *Child development: Its nature and course* (4th ed.). Boston: McGraw-Hill.

Easterbrooks, M. A., & Abeles, R. (2000). Windows to the self in 8–year-olds: Bridges to attachment representation and behavioral adjustment. *Attachment and Human Development, 2*, 85–106.

Erikson, E. H. (1963). *Childhood and society*. New York: Norton. (Original work published 1951)

Etzion-Carraso, A., & Oppenheim, D. (2000). Open mother–pre-schooler communication: Relations with early secure attachment. *Attachment and Human Development, 2*, 347–370.

Fonagy, P., Steele, H., & Steele, M. (1991). Maternal representations of attachment during pregnancy predict the organization of infant–mother attachment at one year of age. *Child Development, 62*, 891–905.

Freud, S. (1953). Three essays on the theory of sexuality. In J. Strachey (Ed. & Trans.), *The standard edition of the complete works of Sigmund Freud* (Vol. 7, pp. 125–243). London: Hogarth Press. (Original work published 1905)

Freud, S. (1959). Inhibitions, symptoms and anxiety. In J. Strachey (Ed. & Trans.), *The standard edition of the complete works of Sigmund Freud* (Vol. 20, pp. 77–174). London: Hogarth Press. (Original work published 1926)

George, C., Kaplan, N., & Main, M. (1985). *The Adult Attachment Interview*. Berkeley: University of California, Department of Psychology.

Gloger-Tippelt, G., Gomille, B., Koenig, L., & Vetter, J. (2002). Attachment representations in 6–year-olds: Related longitudinally to the quality of attachment in infancy and other's attachment representations. *Attachment and Human Development, 4*(3), 318–335.

Grice, H. (1975). Logic and conversation. In P. Cole & J. Moran (Eds.), *Syntax and semantics* (Vol. 3., pp. 41–58). New York: Academic Press.

Grossmann, K. E., Grossmann, K., & Schwan, A. (1986). Capturing the wider view of attachment: A reanalysis of Ainsworth's Strange Situation. In C. E. Izard & P. Read (Eds.), *Measuring emotions in infants and children* (Vol. 2, pp. 124–171). Cambridge, UK: Cambridge University Press.

Harter, S. (1998). The development of self representations. In W. Damon (Series Ed.) & N. Eisenberg (Vol. Ed.), *Handbook of child psychology: Vol. 3. Social, emotional, and personality development* (5th ed., pp. 553–617). New York: Wiley.

Harter, S., & Buddin, B. J. (1987). Children's understanding of the simultaneity of two emotions: A five-stage developmental acquisition sequence. *Developmental Psychology, 3*, 388–399.

Hesse, E. (1999). The Adult Attachment Interview: Historical and current perspectives. In J. Cassidy & P. R. Shaver (Eds.), *Handbook of attachment: Theory, research, and clinical applications* (pp. 395–433). New York: Guilford Press.

Hetherington, E., & Parke, R. (1999). *Child psychology: A contemporary viewpoint.* Boston: McGraw-Hill.

Laible, D. J., & Thompson, R. A. (1998). Attachment and emotional understanding in preschool children. *Developmental Psychology, 34*, 1038–1045.

Main, M., Kaplan, N., & Cassidy, J. (1985). Security in infancy, childhood, and adulthood: A move to the level of representation. In I. Bretherton & E. Waters (Eds.), Growing points of attachment theory and research (pp. 66–104). *Monographs of the Society for Research in Child Development, 50*(1–2, Serial No. 209).

Martin, C. L., & Halverson, C. F. (1981). A schematic-processing model of sex typing and stereotyping in children. *Child Development, 52*, 1119–1134.

Oppenheim, D., Emde, R. N., & Warren, S. (1997). Children's narrative representations of mothers: Their development and associations with child and mother adaptation. *Child Development, 68*, 127–138.

Raven, J. C., Court, J. H., & Raven, J. (1986). *Manual for Raven's Progressive Matrices and Vocabulary Scales.* London: Lewis.

Ruble, D. (1983). The development of social-comparison processes and their role in achievement-related self-socialization. In E. T. Higgins, D. N. Ruble, & W. W. Hartup (Eds.), *Social cognition and social development: A socio-cultural perspective* (pp. 134–157). Cambridge, UK: Cambridge University Press.

Ruble, D., & Martin, C. (1998). Gender development. In W. Damon (Series Ed.) & N. Eisenberg (Vol. Ed.). *Handbook of child psychology: Vol. 3. Social, emotional, and personality development* (5th ed., pp. 933–1016). New York: Wiley.

Selman, R. (1980). *The growth of interpersonal understanding: Developmental and clinical analyses.* New York: Academic Press.

Sroufe, L. A. (1988). The role of infant–caregiver attachment in development. In J. Belsky & T. Nezworski (Eds.), *Clinical implications of attachment* (pp. 18–38). Hillsdale, NJ: Erlbaum.

Steele, H. (1991). *Adult personality characteristics and family functioning: The development and validation of an interview-based technique.* Unpublished doctoral dissertation, University of London.

Steele, H., Steele, M., Croft, C., & Fonagy, P. (1999). Infant–mother attachment at one year predicts children's understanding of mixed emotions at six years. *Social Development, 8*, 161–177.

Steele, H., Steele, M., & Fonagy, P. (1996). Associations among attachment classifications of mothers, fathers, and their infants. *Child Development, 67*, 541–555.

Steele, M., Steele, H., Woolgar, M., Yabsley, S., Johnson, D., Fonagy, P., & Croft, C. (2003). An attachment perspective on children's emotion narratives: Links across generations: The MacArthur story stem battery and parent–child narrative. In R. Emde, D. Wolf, & D. Oppenheim (Eds.), *Revealing the inner worlds of young children* (pp. 163–181). Oxford, UK: Oxford University Press.

Sullivan, H. S. (1953). *The interpersonal theory of psychiatry.* New York: Norton.

van IJzendoorn, M. H. (1995). Adult attachment representations, parental responsiveness and infant attachment: A meta-analysis on the predictive validity of the Adult Attachment Interview. *Psychological Bulletin, 117,* 387–403.

Wechsler, D. (1992). *Wechsler Intelligence Scale for Children–3rd (1) WISC-III UK.* London: Psychological Corporation.

CHAPTER 8

◆ ◆ ◆

Attachment and Friendship Predictors of Psychosocial Functioning in Middle Childhood and the Mediating Roles of Social Support and Self-Worth

CATHRYN BOOTH-LaFORCE
KENNETH H. RUBIN
LINDA ROSE-KRASNOR
KIM B. BURGESS

Links between children's relationships with their parents and with their peers have received significant theoretical and empirical attention in the past 15 years. This focus has grown, in part, from peer researchers seeking out meaningful answers about why some children are socially competent and engaged with their peer group in positive ways, whereas others display maladaptive behaviors and have significant difficulties with their peers. At the same time, researchers identifying individual differences in early parent–child relationships have searched for meaningful developmental sequelae of these differences beyond the social world of the family. These merging interests have resulted in considerable attention to the links between the child–parent and child–peer systems (Ladd, 1992).

Author Note: Cathryn Booth-LaForce was formerly Cathryn L. Booth.

ATTACHMENT, PEER RELATIONS, AND FRIENDSHIP

Although relationships with parents may influence relations with peers in numerous ways, our focus in this chapter is based on premises drawn from attachment theory. According to attachment theory, the child who receives responsive and sensitive parenting from the primary caregiver forms an internal working model of that caregiver as a trustworthy and dependable source of care when it is needed, as well as a model of the self as someone who is worthy of such care (Bowlby, 1973, 1982). Through experience with a responsive and sensitive caregiver, the child also learns reciprocity in social interactions (Elicker, Englund, & Sroufe, 1992), a prosocial/empathic orientation (Clark & Ladd, 2000), and a set of specific social skills that can be used in relationships that extend beyond the boundaries of the family. Also, the securely attached child is able to use the caregiver as a secure base for exploration (Ainsworth, Blehar, Waters, & Wall, 1978), including the exploration of relationships with peers. Such exploration leads the child to develop the ability to interact and play competently with peers. Moreover, through play experiences, the child learns about normative roles, rules, and how to negotiate his or her way through interpersonal dilemmas (e.g., Rubin, Fein, & Vandenberg, 1983). Thus the child who has trusting and supportive caregivers is able to form positive expectations regarding relationships and has opportunities to learn the necessary social skills for negotiating the social world (Sroufe, 1988). In contrast, children who are insecurely attached are at risk for developing problematic relationships with peers, which may be based, in part, on negative attributions about peer behavior (Cassidy, Kirsh, Scolton, & Parke, 1996; Dodge & Newman, 1981) and emotion-regulation difficulties (Cassidy, 1994), as well as poor social skills and negative expectations about relationships.

In support of attachment theory, a substantial number of studies have linked child–parent attachment security with peer-group functioning and relationships. In a recent meta-analysis of 63 studies, Schneider, Atkinson, and Tardiff (2001) found a small to moderate effect size linking these two domains (see also Cassidy, Aikins, & Chernoff, 2003; Finnegan, Hodges, & Perry, 1996; Verschueren & Marcoen, 1999, 2002). Although connections between attachment security and social competence are theoretically meaningful, there is an even more compelling rationale for the link between attachment security and friendship. Specifically, the trust and intimacy that characterizes secure child–parent relationships would be expected to engender a set of internalized relationship expectations that would affect the nature and quality of relationships with friends (Belsky & Cassidy, 1994; Sroufe & Fleeson, 1986; Youngblade & Belsky,

1992). In fact, Schneider and colleagues (2001) found a larger effect size linking attachment security with friendship than with peer relationships more generally (see also Chipuer, 2001; Hodges, Finnegan, & Perry, 1999; Lieberman, Doyle, & Markiewicz, 1999).

Attachment and Psychosocial Functioning

In addition to considering links between child–parent attachment security and social competence/relationships with peers, it is important to consider, in middle childhood, the influence of attachment security on psychosocial functioning more broadly. In fact, a number of researchers have found that the quality of the child–parent attachment relationship predicts indices of well-being and of externalizing and internalizing problems in school-age children and young adolescents. For example, Kerns, Klepac, and Cole (1996) found that children who felt secure and supported by their primary caregivers had higher levels of perceived competence in multiple domains and felt less lonely. Additionally, insecurity has been associated with both internalizing and externalizing problems in middle childhood (Easterbrooks & Abeles, 2000; Granot & Mayseless, 2001; Simons, Paternite, & Shore, 2001). *less lonely*

Friendship and Psychosocial Functioning

Given that attachment security and friendship quality have been linked both theoretically and empirically, it is useful to consider what is known about the effects of friendship quality on psychosocial functioning in middle childhood. Friendship quality has been associated negatively with loneliness (Parker & Asher, 1993). Having high-quality friendships also is related positively to indices of peer-assessed sociability and leadership (Berndt, Hawkins, & Jiao, 1999). Among a sample of shy children, Fordham and Stevenson-Hinde (1999) found that friendship quality was correlated with lower trait anxiety. The long-term influence of friendship quality also has been demonstrated in a 12-year longitudinal study by Bagwell, Newcomb, and Bukowski (1998), who found that fifth-graders without friends, compared with those with friends, had lower self-esteem and more psychopathological symptoms in adulthood. More recently, we have shown that fifth-grade children without friends were rated by their peers as more aggressive, less popular and prosocial, and more rejected and victimized than those children who possessed mutual best friendships (Rubin, Wojslawowicz, Burgess, Booth-LaForce, & Rose-Krasnor, 2003); similarly, Hodges, Boivin, Vitaro, and Bukowski (1999) demonstrated that having a best friend decreased peer victimization.

Interaction of Attachment and Friendship

Given the importance of both parent–child relationships and friendships in middle childhood, it is likely that the nature and quality of these relationships may interact in meaningful ways to predict psychosocial functioning. First, it is possible that attachment security and friendship each contributes uniquely to the prediction of outcomes. Second, attachment security may be the primary predictor of outcomes, with friendship characteristics serving as mediating variables. Finally, friendship characteristics may moderate the relation between attachment security and psychosocial functioning. That is, relationships with friends may serve a compensatory function when family relationships are inadequate (see Cooper & Cooper, 1992) by providing the intimacy and support that is lacking in the family. This compensatory model typically refers to relationships in adolescence, but it may apply to middle childhood as well. According to this model, the presence of an emotionally supportive friend might be viewed as a protective factor in the sense that the potentially negative effects of insecurity or lack of mother's support on psychosocial functioning would be reduced.

Most studies investigating these compensatory processes have not assessed child–parent attachment security per se but have measured conceptually related aspects of the parent–child relationship and the family environment. For example, Stocker (1994) found that in a sample of 8-year-olds, high friendship warmth compensated for low maternal warmth in terms of the children's adjustment scores. However, van Aken and Asendorpf (1997) did not find such compensatory effects among 12-year-olds.

In another study, Gauze, Bukowski, Aquan-Assee, and Sippola (1996) found that quality of friendship in grades 4–6 predicted perceived social competence and general self-worth more strongly for children from families with low adaptability and cohesion than for children from higher functioning families. That is, high-quality friendships appeared to buffer children whose family experiences were less than optimal. Furthermore, family experiences of cohesion and adaptability were stronger predictors of adjustment for those children without a best friend than for those whose best friendship was qualitatively poor.

Schwartz, Dodge, Pettit, and Bates (2000) examined whether early harsh home environment and number of children's friendships predicted peer victimization. They found that children who experienced harsh home environments in the preschool years were more likely to be victimized by peers in the third and fourth grades; however, this correlation was stronger for those who had a lower number of friendships. Overall, early harsh environment was not predictive of victimization for children who reported having many friendships. More recently, Criss, Pettit, Bates, Dodge, and Lapp (2002) examined the role of children's peer relationships in the link between family adversity and child externalizing behavioral problems. They found that family adversity and child externalizing behaviors were not related for children who had a large friendship network.

Possible Mediators

So far, we have provided evidence of links between attachment security and friendship quality, as well as links (and interactions) between these constructs and psychosocial functioning in middle childhood. However, a significant question concerns the *process* whereby attachment security and friendship quality are linked with outcomes. That is, what are the mediating variables connecting these constructs? Very few researchers have evaluated these mediating variables, even though potential candidates have been suggested in the literature. These include social information processing (Dodge & Newman, 1981; Simons et al., 2001), emotion regulation (Cassidy, 1994; Thompson, 1994), communication skills (Bretherton, 1990), and self-esteem (Granot & Mayseless, 2001; Simons et al., 2001; Verschueren & Marcoen, 2002). In the present report, we consider the child's perceptions of *self-worth*, as well as the child's perceptions of the availability of *social support* from others, as potential mediators.

Self-Worth

A central tenet of attachment theory is that on the basis of primary attachment relationships, children develop an internal working model of the self as worthy and lovable. This view of the self is carried into other relationships, and thereby affects their nature and quality (see Bretherton, 1985; Cassidy, 1988, 1990; Ladd, 1992). Evidence for the link between attachment security and feelings of self-worth in middle childhood is relatively scarce. However, in our own work, we found that perceptions of self-worth were predicted by attachment security in relation to both mother and father in fifth grade (Rubin et al., in press). Among kindergarten children, Verschueren and Marcoen (1999) and Verschueren, Marcoen, and Schoefs (1996) found that security of attachment to mother was related to self-esteem. Similar links were demonstrated in early adolescence (Engels, Finkenauer, Meeus, & Dekovic, 2001; Simons et al., 2001), and adolescent attachment to parents predicted adult self-esteem (Giordano, Cernkovich, Groat, Pugh, & Swinford, 1998).

Perceptions of self-worth also have been linked with psychosocial functioning in middle childhood. For example, Verschueren, Buyck, and

Marcoen (2001) found that positive self-perceptions at age 5 were related to school adjustment/independence as rated by teachers at age 8. Also among 8-year-olds, Easterbrooks and Abeles (2000) found that self-worth was related to peer competence, to school adjustment, and (negatively) to behavior problems. Fordham and Stevenson-Hinde (1999) found that self-worth was negatively related to loneliness and anxiety and positively related to perceptions of social acceptance and classmate support in a sample of shy children in middle childhood. Additionally, perceptions of self-worth have been linked to friendship quality in middle childhood (Franco & Levitt, 1998), and the presence of a close friendship in the preadolescent years predicted self-esteem in adulthood (Bagwell et al., 1998).

Perceptions of Emotional Support

Another candidate for the role of mediating variable in the association between attachment security, friendship, and psychosocial functioning is the child's *perceptions of emotional support* (see also Yunger, Corby, & Perry, Chapter 5, this volume). We reasoned that children who were securely attached to their mothers would have a history of experiencing their mothers as responsive and emotionally available when needed. Therefore, these children would be more likely than insecurely attached children to view their mothers as primary, effective sources of support in middle childhood. As Bowlby (1973) indicated, "On the structure of these complementary models [of self and attachment figures] are based that person's forecasts of how accessible and responsive his attachment figures are likely to be should he turn to them for support. And . . . it is on the structure of those models that depends, also, whether he feels confident that his attachment figures are in general readily available or whether he is more or less afraid that they will not be available . . ." (p. 203).

Although we are not taking a large conceptual leap in linking attachment security with children's perceptions of support, there are very few data-based publications connecting these constructs. In one such study of 4-year-olds (Bost, Vaughn, Washington, Cielinski, & Bradbard, 1998), attachment security predicted social-support networks, which served as a mediating variable linking security with social competence. Also, among 6-year-old children, earlier attachment security predicted social support, which mediated links between attachment and adjustment (Anan & Barnett, 1999). There are other indications in the child development literature that perceptions of support are linked with children's positive adaptational outcomes (e.g., Bost, 1995; Bost et al., 1998; Bryant, 1985; Dubow & Tisak, 1990; Dubow, Tisak, Causey, Hryshko, & Reid, 1991; see also Belle, 1989).

A Conceptual Model

In thinking about the links between attachment, friendship, and psychosocial functioning in middle childhood, as well as the possible mediating roles of perceptions of self-worth and social support, we have found it useful to consider a conceptual model developed by Sarason, Pierce, and Sarason (1990). We adapted this model in an earlier paper (Booth, Rubin, & Rose-Krasnor, 1998) and have slightly modified it again for this chapter, as shown in Figure 8.1. According to the Sarason model, self-worth, or a *sense of acceptance*, is viewed as a stable personality characteristic that derives from the quality of the primary attachment relationship and that is sustained via the development of internal working models of the self in relation to others. That is, feelings of being lovable and worthy that evolve from sensitive and responsive parental care develop into more codified cognitive representations of the self that are reinforced by stability in parental behavior, as well as subsequent social experiences and interpretation of those experiences. Thus thoughts and feelings of being accepted influence the quality of social relationships in the sense that expectations of acceptance and support from others and interpretation of others' behavior as supportive affect how people interact with others in social relationships. Families provide emotional security so that children feel comfortable developing personal relationships with others (Antonucci & Akiyama, 1994).

Sarason and colleagues (1990) also posited that perceptions of the availability of social support, as well as perceptions of support received, are actually manifestations of the sense of acceptance. That is, they pro-

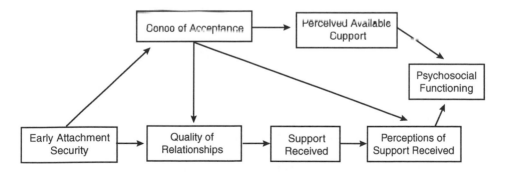

FIGURE 8.1. Conceptual model linking attachment security, quality of relationships, sense of acceptance, and perceived social support to psychosocial functioning, based on Sarason et al. (1990). From Booth, Rubin, and Rose-Krasnor (1998, p. 428). Copyright 1998 by the Society for Research in Child Development. Adapted by permission.

vided evidence (see Sarason, Shearin, Pierce, & Sarason, 1987) that a common theme linking various assessments of social support is that they measure the degree to which individuals feel "accepted, loved, and involved in relationships with open communication" (Sarason et al., 1990, pp. 109–110). It is the *perception* of available support, rather than actual support received, that is most directly linked with attachment security and is most predictive of positive adjustment outcomes (Komproe, Rijken, Ros, Winnubst, & 't Hart, 1997; Sarason et al., 1990).

In this chapter, we use our version of the Sarason model to test a number of hypotheses about predicted relations among relevant variables. Specifically, we present data from two studies (the Seattle Study and the Maryland Study) in which we investigated attachment and friendship variables as predictors of psychosocial functioning, evaluated the role of perceived social support and sense of acceptance as mediators of these relations, and evaluated the moderating role of friendship characteristics in the links between attachment and psychosocial functioning in middle childhood.

THE SEATTLE STUDY

The Seattle Study was a longitudinal investigation of the concurrent and predictive links between the quality of the mother–child relationship and the child's social competence with peers at ages 4 and 8 years (see Booth, Rose-Krasnor, McKinnon, & Rubin, 1994; Booth, Rose-Krasnor, & Rubin, 1991; Booth et al., 1998; Rose-Krasnor, Rubin, Booth, & Coplan, 1996; Rubin, Lynch, Coplan, Rose-Krasnor, & Booth, 1994). Of particular relevance in the present context is an article we published in 1998 (Booth et al., 1998) in which we introduced the Sarason model and tested propositions arising from it. A condensed description of the study and our results follows.

The participants in the study were 65 children (89% European American) and their mothers. During the first phase of this longitudinal research project, mothers and their 4-year-old children participated in a videotaped mother–child–peer interaction session in our laboratory. The segment most relevant to the present analyses involved a reunion between the focal child and his or her mother that occurred after a 15-minute separation. Each focal child's *security of attachment to mother* was rated using a 5-point version of the 9-point security rating scale developed by Cassidy and Marvin with the MacArthur Working Group (1989).

Social support and child adjustment were measured at age 8. One of the most central measures was *My Family and Friends* (Reid, Landesman, Treder, & Jaccard, 1989), an interview designed to assess 6- to 12-year-old children's perceptions of the availability of social support from individuals in their network and their satisfaction with the support they receive. After the members of a child's social network were identified, the child was asked a series of five emotional support questions and, for each, asked to indicate the order in which he or she would turn to network members. Ranks for each person were averaged across the five emotional support items, with scores converted so that higher scores indicated lower, that is, more favorable, ranks. *Ratings* of the effectiveness of emotional support were also averaged across items for each network member. In addition, mothers' interactive style was rated from a mother–child interaction session that included free play and structured activities. The *maternal warmth summary score* comprised the summed z-scores for ratings of proximity, positive affect, responsivity, and positive control.

Finally, at age 8, each focal child returned to the laboratory for a videotaped peer-play session with a new set of three unacquainted, same-sex, same age (± 6 months) control peers. Each child also provided ratings of the other members of the quartet. The observational measures, peer ratings of acceptance and aggression, and the mothers' ratings of behavior problems on the Child Behavior Checklist (CBCL; Achenbach, 1991) comprised the adjustment measures at age 8. The measures were factored (see Booth et al., 1998) to yield scores for (1) *social engagement/acceptance,* (2) *internalizing problems,* and (3) *externalizing problems.*

Back to Our Model

Going back to our conceptual model, the hypothesized interrelations among the variables and measures are shown in Figure 8.2. We hypothesized that (1) attachment security at age 4 would predict perceptions of emotional support from mother at age 8; (2) security would predict inclusion of the best friend in the emotional support network, as well as perceptions of support from the best friend; (3) psychosocial functioning at age 8 would be predicted by perceptions of emotional support from mother and from best friend, as well as early attachment security; and (4) perceived best-friend support would serve a compensatory role in enhancing psychosocial functioning among insecurely attached children.

Attachment Security, Maternal Warmth, and Maternal Support

Our first hypothesis received partial support: We found that security at age 4 was significantly related to the child's ranking of mother's perceived availability for support ($r = .29$, $p < .05$ for boys; $r = .61$, $p < .001$ for girls), but not to the rating of how much better the child would feel after receiving support from the mother. We also found that in a hierarchical multiple-regression analysis, regardless of order of entry, preschool at-

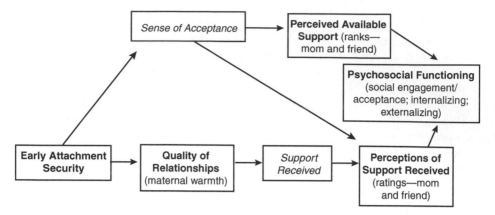

FIGURE 8.2. The Seattle Study: Conceptual links between early attachment security, maternal warmth, perceptions of support from mother and best friend, and psychosocial functioning. Constructs in **bold type** were assessed in the study.

tachment security was a significant predictor of the child's ranking at age 8 of the mother's perceived availability for support and that maternal warmth was not. Thus this analysis suggested that the internal working model of the attachment relationship was a more salient factor than the mother's contemporaneous behavior in influencing the child's perceptions of support.

Security and Friend Support

Next, we tested the hypothesis that security would be positively related to perceptions of support from the best friend. We found that 60% of the secure children and 39% of the insecure children included their best friend as a source of emotional support on at least four of the five emotional support items. However, this difference was not significant by a chi-square test. Also, we found that attachment security among the boys was not related to the best friend's rank or rating. However, among the girls, the greater the attachment security, the *less* perceived satisfaction with support from the best friend ($r = -.52$, $p < .05$).

Psychosocial Functioning, Support, and Attachment

Our third hypothesis was that psychosocial functioning at age 8 would be positively linked with perceptions of maternal and best-friend support and with early attachment security. As expected, we found that attachment security was a significant predictor of social engagement/acceptance ($r =$

.49, $p < .001$) and a negative predictor of internalizing problems ($r = -.30$, $p < .01$) but not externalizing problems.

Contrary to our predictions, we found that perceptions of maternal support (both ranks and ratings) were not significantly related to any of the psychosocial functioning variables. In terms of friend support, we found that children who included their best friend in their support network, compared with those who did not, scored significantly higher on the social engagement/acceptance factor ($M = .24$, $SD = .81$, vs. $M = -.33$, $SD = 1.01$), $t (56) = 2.37$, $p < .05$, but did not differ on the internalizing and externalizing factors. Bivariate correlations between the best friend's rank and the dependent variables indicated that, contrary to our hypothesis, the greater the perceived reliance on the best friend for emotional support, the greater the externalizing problems, for boys only, $r (21) = .41$, $p < .05$. None of the other correlations between friendship variables and outcomes was significant.

Moderating Role of Friendship

Our final hypothesis was that best-friend support would serve a compensatory role in the sense of enhancing psychosocial functioning among children with insecure attachment relationships with their mothers. We performed a series of hierarchical multiple-regression analyses in which the predictors were (in order) attachment security at age 4, the best friend's rank at age 8, and the interaction between these two variables.

For the social engagement/acceptance analyses, neither the best friend's rank nor the interaction term made a significant contribution to the prediction of this outcome. A similar pattern was obtained for internalizing problems; for externalizing problems, both the best friend's rank and the interaction term were significant. Specifically, the *higher* the best friend's rank, the higher the externalizing score. When we probed this interaction, we found that among the securely attached children, the best friend's rank was not related to externalizing problems; but among the insecures, this relation was significant. These data suggest that when a child is insecurely attached, reliance on a friend for emotional support may potentiate rather than reduce externalizing problems, which is the opposite of the effect we expected.

Summary and Discussion

To summarize, we found that:

1. Preschool attachment security predicted observed maternal warmth, perceptions of availability of support from mother (but not per-

ceptions of satisfaction with support received), peer social engagement/ acceptance, and low internalizing problems in middle childhood. Preschool attachment security was a better predictor than 8-year maternal warmth of 8-year perceptions of availability of support from mother.

2. Perceptions of support from mother were not related to any of the measures of psychosocial functioning.

3. Including a best friend in one's support network was related to peer social engagement/acceptance but was not predicted by preschool attachment security. Reliance on the best friend for support did not compensate for the effects of insecurity on psychosocial functioning but appeared to potentiate them.

In relation to our conceptual model, the results were mixed. On the positive side, the results provide support for hypothesized links between attachment security and psychosocial functioning and are congruent with previous middle-childhood studies (e.g., Easterbrooks & Abeles, 2000; Granot & Mayseless, 2001; Kerns et al., 1996; Simons et al., 2001). They also suggest a degree of continuity in the child's internal working model of the self in relation to mother from the preschool period to middle childhood, and link attachment security with perceptions of emotional support from mother and with the quality of the mother's interactive behavior.

On the negative side, we were surprised to find that perceptions of support from mother were not related at all to psychosocial functioning (and—obviously—did not serve as mediating variables linking attachment with outcomes). Based on prior research and premises from attachment theory, we expected to find these links (Anan & Barnett, 1999; Bost, 1995; Bost et al., 1998; Bryant, 1985; Dubow & Tisak, 1990; Dubow et al., 1991; van Aken & Asendorpf, 1997). Thus a central part of our model was not supported.

Additionally, the friendship variables did not perform as expected. Attachment theory and research led us to expect that children who were securely attached to their mothers would be more likely to have emotionally supportive friendships (see Belsky & Cassidy, 1994; Schneider et al, 2001). However, attachment security was not related to friendship, except in a primarily negative way. Specifically, insecure attachment among the girls was related to perceptions of *lower* effectiveness of support received from the best friend. Also, among insecurely attached children, the more they relied on the best friend for emotional support, the greater were their externalizing problems. These results suggest to us that perceiving one's best friend as a potential source of emotional support may have negative consequences at this age when coupled with insecurity in the child–

parent relationship. That is, the best friendships of insecurely attached children might arise from less healthy (and early) intimacy and support needs that are not being met in the home environment.

It is relevant in this context to think about the goals of friendship at different developmental stages. According to Sullivan (1953), companionship and validation are two of the most salient functions of friendship in middle childhood, and the intimacy and support functions of friendship become more important in adolescence (see Buhrmester & Furman, 1987; Furman & Buhrmester, 1992; Kerns et al., 1996). Thus it is possible that reliance on the best friend as a source of emotional support at age 8 is developmentally inappropriate and perhaps maladaptive.

THE MARYLAND STUDY

The second study to be described in this chapter, the Maryland Study, is currently in progress. The Maryland Study is a longitudinal investigation of the role of children's friendships and family relationships in predicting psychosocial functioning in the transition from elementary school (fifth grade) to middle school (sixth grade). In the present context, we were interested in the relations among these variables in fifth grade. Whereas we used the data from the Seattle Study in part to focus on perceived social support as a mediating factor in the relation between attachment security, friendship, and psychosocial functioning, we are using data from the Maryland Study in part to evaluate the mediating role of the children's perceptions of self-worth.

Participants

The participants in the study were drawn from a sample of 828 fifth-grade students (407 boys, 421 girls) from 39 classrooms in eight public elementary schools in the Washington, D.C., metropolitan area, for whom parental permission was received (consent rate = 84%). The mean age of the sample was 10.33 years (SD = .52). Approximately 58% of the children were European American, 13% African American, 17% Asian, and 9% Hispanic.

Classroom Procedures

Research assistants administered two questionnaires in group format in the classrooms. The first questionnaire involved friendship nominations (Bukowski, Hoza, & Boivin, 1994). Participants were asked to write the names of their "very best friend" and their "second best friend" at their school. Only *mutual* (reciprocated) same-sex best friendships were considered for a subsequent laboratory visit (see the next section). The second questionnaire was an extension of the *Revised Class Play* (RCP; Masten, Morison, & Pellegrini, 1985)—the *Extended Class Play* (ECP; Burgess, Rubin, Wojslawowicz, Rose-Krasnor, & Booth, 2003). The children were instructed to pretend to be the directors of an imaginary class play and to nominate their classmates for various positive and negative roles, with one boy and one girl for each role. The same person could be selected for more than one role. Ten items were added to the original *RCP*, including two aggression items; five items descriptive of social reticence, shyness, and social disinterest; and three items descriptive of victimization. All item scores were standardized within sex and within classroom to adjust for the number of nominations received and also the number of nominators. A principal-components factor analysis with varimax rotation yielded five orthogonal factors: Aggression, Shyness/Withdrawal, Rejection/Victimization, Leadership/Prosocial, and Popularity/Sociability. The standardized item scores were summed to yield five different total scores for each participant.

Laboratory Visit

From the original group of class participants, 162 children visited our laboratory (81 pairs of mutual best friends). Thirty-nine of the children were classified as aggressive (14 boys, 25 girls), 34 as withdrawn (15 boys, 19 girls), 13 as both aggressive and withdrawn (5 boys, 8 girls) and 76 as nonaggressive and nonwithdrawn (35 boys, 41 girls). Data from all of these children ($n = 162$) were used in the analyses reported here.

During the lab visit, mothers completed the CBCL (Achenbach, 1991), and the children ($n = 162$) completed several questionnaires. One was the *Network of Relationships Inventory* (NRI; Furman & Buhrmester, 1985), which was used as a proxy measure of the children's internal working models of the child–mother and child–father attachment relationship. The 30-item NRI comprises 10 conceptually distinct subscales that load onto two factors (e.g., Furman, 1996): (1) *support* (affection, admiration, instrumental aid, companionship, intimacy, nurturance, and reliable alliance); and (2) *negativity* (antagonism, conflict). The support subscale, which was the score of primary interest, was highly correlated with the Security Scale (Kerns et al., 1996) for a subsample of the children, r (73) = .65, $p < .001$ (for mother) and r (68) = .66, $p < .001$ (for father). Thus, given the magnitude of these correlations, as well as the nature of the NRI items, and precedents in the literature (e.g., Karavasilis, Doyle, & Markiewicz, 2003), we concluded that it was reasonable to use the NRI support score as an indicator of attachment security with mother and with father.

The children (n = 162) also completed the *Friendship Quality Questionnaire–Revised* (FQQ; Parker & Asher, 1989), which assessed their self-perceived quality of friendship with the best friend. The FQQ yields six subscales in the areas of companionship/recreation, validation/caring, help/guidance, intimate disclosure, conflict/betrayal, and conflict resolution; and a total score, which is used in this chapter. Finally, the *Self-Perception Profile for Children* (Harter, 1985) was administered. This measure yields six subscales in the areas of scholastic competence, social acceptance, athletic competence, physical appearance, behavioral conduct, and global self-worth. The latter score is used in this chapter.

Child Adjustment Measures

An index of *externalizing difficulties and aggression* was formed by standardizing and aggregating the scores of the mother-rated externalizing difficulties (CBCL) and peer-nominated aggression (ECP) measures. Similarly, an index of *internalizing difficulties and shyness/withdrawal* was formed by standardizing and aggregating the scores of mother-rated internalizing difficulties (CBCL) and peer-nominated shyness/withdrawal (ECP) measures. We also used the peer-nominated *rejection/victimization* and *popularity/sociability* scores.

Back to Our Model, Again

Going back to our conceptual model, the constructs and specific variables we measured in the Maryland Study are shown in Figure 8.3. Although we did not use a measure of early attachment security in the study, we used the NRI support scores as measures of concurrent security with mother and father. The Harter Global Self-Worth score was the measure of sense of acceptance, and the FQQ total positive score was a measure of the quality of the relationship with the best friend. Finally, the adjustment outcomes were peer-nominated popularity/sociability and rejection/victimization, and the aggregated scores for internalizing and externalizing problems.

In this version of the model, we hypothesized that (1) attachment security, perceptions of self-worth, and friendship quality would all be associated positively with popularity/sociability and negatively with rejection/victimization, internalizing, and externalizing problems; (2) attachment security and friendship quality would be positively related; (3) self-worth would be a significant mediator between attachment security and friendship quality, and between attachment security and outcomes; and (4)

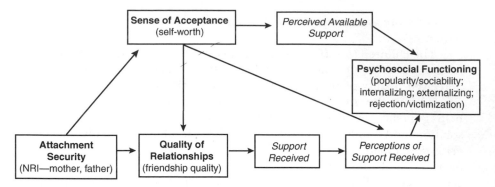

FIGURE 8.3. The Maryland Study: Conceptual links between attachment security, friendship quality, self-worth, and psychosocial functioning. Constructs in **bold type** were assessed in the study.

friendship quality would serve as a moderating factor in protecting children with relatively poor parent–child relationships from negative outcomes.

Security, Friendship, Self-Worth, and Outcomes

To test our first hypothesis about the links between psychosocial functioning and attachment security, self-worth, and friendship quality, we computed bivariate correlations, presented in Table 8.1. We found that popularity/sociability was significantly and positively related to friendship quality and self-worth, but not to attachment security with either parent. As expected, internalizing problems were significantly and negatively associated with all of the predictor variables. Externalizing problems were significantly and negatively related to attachment security with both parents but were not significantly related to friendship quality or self-worth. Finally, rejection/victimization was significantly and negatively related to all predictors except security with mother. These correlations provided partial support for our first hypothesis.

Security and Friendship Quality

Our second hypothesis, that attachment security and friendship quality would be positively related, was tested via bivariate correlations. The significant positive correlations between friendship quality and attachment security with mother and father, shown in Table 8.1, confirmed this hypothesis.

TABLE 8.1. Correlations among Predictors, and between Predictors and Outcomes

	n	Security with mother	Security with father	Friendship quality	Global self-worth
Security with father	162	.45**			
Friendship quality	162	.35**	.33**		
Global self-worth	162	.23**	.34**	.34**	
Popularity/sociability	162	.10	.06	.15*	.17*
Internalizing problems	144	−.24**	−.20*	−.24**	−.24**
Externalizing problems	144	−.22**	−.33**	−.15	−.16
Rejection/victimization	162	−.08	−.20*	−.28**	−.31**

Note. *p < .05; **p < .01.

Self-Worth as a Mediator

Our third hypothesis was that self-worth would serve as a mediator between attachment security and friendship quality and between attachment security and outcomes. For the first part of this hypothesis, we performed a series of regression analyses in accordance with the Baron and Kenny procedures for testing mediation. However, rather than using the Baron and Kenny criterion for mediation—that the effect of the independent variable on the dependent variable decreases when the mediator is in the model—we used the Sobel (1982) test to formally evaluate whether statistically significant mediation had occurred. The Sobel test indicated that self-worth was a significant mediator of the relation between attachment security with mother and friendship quality, z = 2.38, p = .02, and between attachment security with father and friendship quality, z = 2.74, p = .01.

For the second part of this hypothesis, we tested whether self-worth mediated the link between attachment security and outcomes. Once again, we used the Baron and Kenny (1986) procedures and the Sobel (1982) test. Several outcomes were not included in the mediation tests because they were not related significantly to attachment security with mother (popularity/ sociability, rejection/victimization), attachment security with father (popularity/sociability), or self-worth (externalizing problems). For those outcomes that we did test, our mediation hypothesis was supported. Specifically, in terms of security with mother, we found that self-worth was a nearly significant mediator of the relation between attachment and internalizing problems, z = −1.88, p = .06. For security with father, we found that self-worth was a significant mediator of the relation between attachment and internalizing problems, z = −2.18, p = .03, and between attachment and rejection/victimization, z = −2.71, p = .01.

Moderating Role of Friendship

Our fourth hypothesis was that friendship quality would serve as a moderating factor in protecting children with relatively poor parent–child relationships from negative outcomes. To test this hypothesis, we performed hierarchical multiple regression analyses to predict (separately) popularity/sociability, internalizing problems, externalizing problems, and peer rejection/victimization from the following variables (each entered on a separate step): child sex, attachment security in relation to mother (NRI), positive friendship quality (FQQ), the two-way interaction of attachment and friendship quality, and the three-way interaction of child sex with attachment and friendship quality. In a second set of regressions, attachment security with father replaced attachment security with mother.

In searching for moderating effects, we were particularly interested in any significant interactions involving attachment and friendship quality. The results for the main effects of attachment security (with both parents) and friendship quality reiterated the results of the bivariate correlations linking these variables with psychosocial functioning. We did not find significant Security × Friendship Quality interactions for popularity/sociability, externalizing problems, or rejection/victimization. However, for internalizing problems, we found that after controlling for security with *mother* and friendship quality, the Security × Friendship Quality and the Sex × Security × Friendship Quality interactions yielded significant changes in R^2 (beta = .14, p = .04 and beta = .51, p = .04, respectively).

The three-way interaction was probed separately for girls and boys by restructuring the equation to express the regression of internalizing problems on friendship quality for children in the lowest third, middle third, and highest third in terms of attachment scores. For boys with low attachment scores, internalizing problems decreased significantly as friendship quality increased (beta = –.44, p = .03). But for boys with medium and high attachment scores, internalizing problems did not change significantly as friendship quality increased (beta = –.30, p = .17 and beta = –.09, p = .73, respectively).

For girls with low attachment scores, internalizing problems also decreased significantly as friendship quality increased (beta = –.50, p = .02). For girls with medium attachment scores, there was a trend for internalizing problems to decrease as friendship quality increased (beta = –.31, p = .08), but for girls with high attachment scores, internalizing problems did not change in relation to values of friendship quality (beta = –.09, p = .67).

Thus these results indicate that friendship quality may have a buffering effect on internalizing problems under conditions of low felt security with mother.

Summary and Discussion

To summarize, we found that:

1. Psychosocial functioning measures varied in the extent to which they were related to our predictor variables of attachment security, self-worth, and friendship quality. Both internalizing problems and rejection/victimization were significantly related to most of the predictors, but externalizing problems were related only to attachment security, and popularity/sociability was related only to friendship quality and self-worth.

2. Self-worth was a significant mediator of the relation between attachment security with father and both internalizing problems and rejection/victimization, and a near-significant mediator of the relation between attachment security with mother and internalizing problems.

3. Attachment security to both parents was related to friendship quality, and self-worth was a significant mediator of this relation, in both cases.

4. Friendship quality served as a compensatory factor in relation to internalizing problems under conditions of low felt security with mother, but this effect was not observed for other outcome variables.

Referring again to our model, it is clear that most of the hypothesized relations among the study variables were supported. As expected, the children's felt security with both parents was associated with their feelings of self-worth. Also, greater security was associated with fewer internalizing and externalizing problems and with less rejection/victimization (in relation to security with father only). These findings are consistent with a growing body of research indicating that school-age children and young adolescents are better adapted when they feel secure and supported by a primary caregiver (Granot & Mayseless, 2001; Kerns et al., 1996; Simons et al., 2001). In the present study, we expanded on previous work in that perceived *paternal* support also predicted psychosocial functioning.

The children's perceptions of friendship quality also were associated with their perceptions of self-worth, attachment security in relation to both parents, popularity/sociability, internalizing problems, and rejection/victimization—all in the expected direction. These findings are consistent with studies indicating that children who are in high-quality friendships, characterized by warmth and validation, are better adjusted than children who do not have a friend or who are in low-quality friendships (e.g., Berndt et al., 1999; Fordham & Stevenson-Hinde, 1999; Ladd, Kochenderfer, & Coleman, 1996; Parker & Asher, 1993; Stocker, 1994).

We also found that self-worth was related to attachment security, which is consistent with the results of previous research (Engels et al., 2001; Rubin et al., in press; Simons et al., 2001; Verschueren & Marcoen, 1999; Verschueren et al., 1996). Additionally, other investigators have found that self-worth is a significant predictor of both friendship and psychosocial functioning in middle childhood (Easterbrooks & Abeles, 2000; Fordham & Stevenson-Hinde, 1999; Franco & Levitt, 1998), and we obtained these results as well. More significantly, perceptions of self-worth mediated relations between attachment security and both friendship quality and psychosocial functioning in the present study. These findings support the idea that children develop an internal working model of the self as worthy and lovable on the basis of primary attachment relationships, and this view of the self is carried into other relationships and other contexts. These findings also are congruent with those of Verschueren and Marcoen (Chapter 10, this volume), who reported that perceptions of self-worth mediated the link between security with father and peer acceptance.

There was some evidence that quality of attachment with parents and quality of best friendship interacted in their effects on outcomes in relation to internalizing problems. That is, friendship quality appeared to compensate for the effects of insecure attachment. However, moderating effects of friendship quality were not found for other outcomes. Other researchers have found that having reciprocated friendships may moderate the effects of family adversity, including harsh parenting (Criss et al., 2002; Schwartz et al., 2000; Stocker, 1994), and that experiences in high-quality friendships may buffer the effects of poor family functioning (Gauze et al., 1996). However, van Aken and Asendorpf (1997) did not find such effects. It is clear that additional investigation is needed to shed more light on the ways in which friendship characteristics may interact with parent–child relationship qualities in affecting psychosocial functioning.

BACK TO OUR MODEL ONE MORE TIME

We began this chapter with a model relating attachment, self-worth, friendship, and social support to psychosocial functioning; and we tested the model using data from two different studies. In testing the model, we learned a number of things. First, we learned that in both studies, attachment security operated (mostly) as predicted from attachment theory and from prior research. It is important to note that links between attachment security and other measures varied somewhat according to the gender of the parent, suggesting that this is an important factor to consider in future research. Second, we provided some evidence that characteristics of the children's best friendships were related in expected ways to outcomes and that these relations were more apparent among the fifth-graders in the Maryland Study than among the 8-year-olds in the Seattle Study.

Third, we learned that at age 8, social support did not function in the way that we supposed it would. Although perceived support was related to preschool attachment security, it did not predict outcomes. It is not clear why this would be the case, but it is possible that measurement issues or developmental issues were responsible. The paucity of research in the area of social support in middle childhood suggests the need for further investigation of these issues.

The fourth thing we learned is that perceptions of self-worth did, in fact, serve a mediating role in linking attachment security with both friendship quality and psychosocial functioning. These results are consistent with attachment theory and also provide much-needed evidence about the processes linking security with outcomes.

Finally, when looking at the interaction between attachment security and friendship, we learned that at age 8, reliance on the best friend for emotional support appeared to exacerbate the negative effects of insecure attachment. Among the fifth graders, we did find that friendship quality buffered the effects of low felt security on internalizing problems, but not on externalizing problems or rejection/victimization. Thus we were not able to determine conclusively whether friendship serves a compensatory role when parent–child relationships are less than optimal. Once again, measurement issues (e.g., assessing perceived best friend support vs. quality of best friendship) and developmental issues (i.e., the functions of friendship at different age periods) need to be considered in this context.

LIMITATIONS

In thinking about our conceptual model, it is useful to note some limitations inherent in this chapter. First, the results of the two studies cannot be compared directly because different measures were used for similar constructs and the ages of the participants varied. Second, we did not test the full model with either set of data. Ideally, we would have a larger number of participants and multiple indicators of each construct so that the model could be tested fully, with sufficient power to detect meaningful associations among variables. Third, in the Seattle Study, the attachment assessment occurred at age 4, and the other measures were obtained at age 8; but in the Maryland Study, the predictor and outcome variables were assessed relatively contemporaneously. Ideally, it would be better to predict outcomes longitudinally. Fourth, some of the relations specified in our model may function in a bidirectional way. For example, self-worth may be affected by friendship quality, as well as influencing it.

Finally, it is clear that, particularly in the Maryland Study, we could have made other choices about which measures index which constructs in the model. For example, one could argue that the NRI is a measure of perceptions of support, rather than a substitute variable for attachment security; or one could view perceptions of self-worth as an indicator of psychosocial functioning rather than as a mediator between attachment security and outcomes. With respect to the attachment issue, and with due respect to researchers who have developed middle-childhood attachment measures (see Kerns, Schlegelmilch, Morgan, & Abraham, Chapter 3, this volume), it is clear that more work is needed to delineate what secure and insecure attachments "look like" in the middle-childhood years.

CONCLUSIONS

The results of both studies provided support for some of the basic tenets of attachment theory and partial support for the Sarason model. Further investigation of the utility of the latter model in explaining links between attachment security and psychosocial functioning would benefit from a broader longitudinal investigation, with more intensive measurement and particular attention to the varying relations among variables from early to late middle childhood (see Mayseless, Chapter 1, this volume). Additionally, further development and refinement of methods for assessing attachment security would provide much-needed answers about the ways in which felt security or insecurity are expressed during the middle-childhood years. Finally, continued investigation into the links between child–parent and child–peer systems in middle childhood holds promise for providing more evidence about the shift in adolescence from primary orientation toward parents to primary orientation toward peers (Fraley & Davis, 1997; Hazan & Shaver, 1994; Mayseless, Chapter 1, this volume) and the role of best friendship in this process.

ACKNOWLEDGMENTS

The research included in this chapter was supported by grants from the National Center for Nursing Research (NR01635), the National Institute of Child Health and Human Development (HD27806), and the National Institute of Mental Health (MH58116).

REFERENCES

Achenbach, T. M. (1991). *Manual for the Child Behavior Checklist: 4–18*. Burlington, VT: Associates in Psychiatry.

Ainsworth, M. D., Blehar, M. C., Waters, E., & Wall, S. (1978). *Patterns of attachment: A psychological study of the Strange Situation*. Hillsdale, NJ: Erlbaum.

Anan, R. M., & Barnett, D. (1999). Perceived social support mediates between prior attachment and subsequent adjustment: A study of urban African American children. *Developmental Psychology, 35,* 1210–1222.

Antonucci, T. C., & Akiyama, H. (1994). Convoys of attachment and social relations in children, adolescents, and adults. In F. Nestmann & K. Hurrelmann (Eds.), *Social networks and social support in childhood and adolescence. Prevention and intervention in childhood and adolescence* (Vol. 16, pp. 37–52). New York: de Gruyter.

Bagwell, C. L., Newcomb, A. F., & Bukowski, W. M. (1998). Preadolescent friendship and peer rejection as predictors of adult adjustment. *Child Development, 69,* 140–153.

Baron, R. M., & Kenny, D. A. (1986). The moderator–mediator variable distinction in social psychological research: Conceptual, strategic, and statistical considerations. *Journal of Personality and Social Psychology, 51,* 1173–1182.

Belle, D. (1989). *Children's social networks and social supports*. New York: Wiley.

Belsky, J., & Cassidy, J. (1994). Attachment: Theory and evidence. In M. L. Rutter, D. F. Hay, & S. Baron-Cohen (Eds.), *Development through life: A handbook for clinicians* (pp. 373–402). Oxford, UK: Blackwell.

Berndt, T. J., Hawkins, J. A., & Jiao, Z. (1999). Influences of friends and friendships on adjustment to junior high school. *Merrill-Palmer Quarterly, 45,* 13–41.

Booth, C. L., Rose-Krasnor, L., & Rubin, K. H. (1991). Relating preschoolers' social competence and their mothers' parenting behaviors to early attachment security and high-risk status. *Journal of Social and Personal Relationships, 8,* 363–382.

Booth, C. L., Rose-Krasnor, L., McKinnon, J., & Rubin, K. H. (1994). Predicting social adjustment in middle childhood: The role of preschool attachment security and maternal style. *Social Development, 3,* 189–204.

Booth, C. L., Rubin, K. H., & Rose-Krasnor, L. (1998). Perceptions of emotional support from mother and friend in middle childhood: Links with social-emotional adaptation and preschool attachment security. *Child Development, 69,* 427–442.

Bost, K. K. (1995). Mother and child reports of preschool children's social support networks: Network correlates of peer acceptance. *Social Development, 4,* 149–164.

Bost, K. K., Vaughn, B. E., Washington, W. N., Cielinski, K., & Bradbard, M. R. (1998). Social competence, social support, and attachment: Demarcation of construct domains, measurement, and paths of influence for preschool children attending Head Start. *Child Development, 69,* 192–218.

Bowlby, J. (1973). *Attachment and loss: Vol. 2. Separation, anxiety, and anger*. London: Penguin Books.

Bowlby, J. (1982). *Attachment and loss: Vol. 1. Attachment* (2nd ed.). New York: Basic Books. (Original work published 1969)

Bretherton, I. (1985). Attachment theory: Retrospect and prospect. In I. Bretherton & E. Waters (Eds.), Growing points of attachment theory and research (pp. 3–35). *Monographs of the Society for Research in Child Development, 50*(1–2, Serial No. 209).

Bretherton, I. (1990). Open communication and internal working models: Their role in the development of attachment relationships. In R. A. Thompson (Ed.), *Nebraska Symposium on Motivation, 1988: Vol. 36. Socioemotional development: Current theory and research in motivation* (pp. 57–113). Lincoln: University of Nebraska Press.

Bryant, B. (1985). The Neighborhood Walk: Sources of support in middle childhood. *Monographs of the Society for Research in Child Development, 50*(3, Serial No. 210).

Buhrmester, D., & Furman, W. (1987). The development of companionship and intimacy. *Child Development, 58,* 1387–1398.

Bukowski, W. M., Hoza, B., & Boivin, M. (1994). Measuring friendship quality during pre- and early adolescence: The development and psychometric properties of the Friendship Qualities Scale. *Journal of Social and Personal Relationships, 11*(3), 472–484.

Burgess, K. B., Rubin, K. H., Wojslawowicz, J., Rose-Krasnor, L., & Booth, C. (2003, April). *The Extended Class Play: A longitudinal study of its factor structure, reliability, and validity.* Poster presented at the biennial meeting of the Society for Research in Child Development, Tampa, FL.

Cassidy, J. (1988). Child–mother attachment and the self in six-year-olds. *Child Development, 59,* 121–134.

Cassidy, J. (1990). Theoretical and methodological considerations in the study of attachment and the self in young children. In M. T. Greenberg, D. Cicchetti, & E. M. Cummings (Eds.), *Attachment in the preschool years: Theory, research, and intervention* (pp. 87–119). Chicago: University of Chicago Press.

Cassidy, J. (1994). Emotional regulation: Influences of attachment relationships. In N. A. Fox (Ed.), The development of emotion regulation: Biological and behavioral considerations. *Monographs of the Society for Research in Child Development, 59*(2–3, Serial No. 240), 228–249.

Cassidy, J., Aikins, J. W., & Chernoff, J. J. (2003). Children's peer selection: Experimental examination of the role of self-perceptions. *Developmental Psychology, 39,* 495–508.

Cassidy, J., Kirsh, S. J., Scolton, K. L., & Parke, R. D. (1996). Attachment and representations of peer relationships. *Developmental Psychology, 32,* 892–904.

Cassidy, J., Marvin, R., & the MacArthur Working Group. (1989). *Attachment organization in three- and four-year-olds: Coding guidelines.* Unpublished manuscript, University of Virginia, Charlottesville.

Chipuer, H. M. (2001). Dyadic attachments and community connectedness: Links with youths' loneliness experiences. *Journal of Community Psychology, 29,* 429–446.

Clark, K. E., & Ladd, G. W. (2000). Connectedness and autonomy support in parent–child relationships: Links to children's socioemotional orientation and peer relationships. *Developmental Psychology, 36,* 485–498.

Cooper, C. R., & Cooper, R. G., Jr. (1992). Links between adolescents' relationships with their parents and peers: Models, evidence, and mechanisms. In R. D. Parke & G. W. Ladd (Eds.), *Family–peer relationships: Modes of linkage* (pp. 135–158). Hillsdale, NJ: Erlbaum.

Criss, M. M., Pettit, G. S., Bates, J. E., Dodge, K. A. & Lapp, A. L. (2002). Family adversity, positive peer relationships, and children's externalizing behavior: A longitudinal perspective on risk and resilience. *Child Development, 74,* 1220–1237.

Dodge, K. A., & Newman, J. P. (1981). Biased decision-making processes in aggressive boys. *Journal of Abnormal Psychology, 90,* 375–379.

Dubow, E. F., & Tisak, J. (1990). The relation between stressful life events and adjustment in elementary school children: The role of social support and social problem-solving skills. *Child Development, 66,* 1412–1423.

Dubow, E. F., Tisak, J., Causey, D., Hryshko, A., & Reid, G. (1991). A two-year longitudinal study of stressful life events, social support, and social problem-solving skills: Contributions to children's behavioral and academic adjustment. *Child Development, 63,* 583–599.

Easterbrooks, M. A., & Abeles, R. (2000). Windows to the self in 8–year-olds: Bridges to attachment representation and behavioral adjustment. *Attachment and Human Development, 2,* 85–106.

Elicker, J., Englund, M., & Sroufe, L. A. (1992). Predicting peer competence and peer relationships in childhood from early parent–child relationships. In R. D. Parke & G. W. Ladd (Eds.), *Family–peer relationships: Modes of linkage* (pp. 77–107). Hillsdale, NJ: Erlbaum.

Engels, R. C. M. E., Finkenauer, C, Meeus, W., & Dekovic, M. (2001). Parental attachment and adolescents' emotional adjustment: The associations with social skills and relational competence. *Journal of Counseling Psychology, 48,* 428–439.

Finnegan, R. A., Hodges, E. V. E., & Perry, D. G. (1996). Preoccupied and avoidant coping during middle childhood. *Child Development, 67,* 1318–1328.

Fordham, K., & Stevenson-Hinde, J. (1999). Shyness, friendship quality, and adjustment during middle childhood. *Journal of Child Psychology and Psychiatry and Allied Disciplines, 40,* 757–768.

Fraley, R. C., & Davis, K. E. (1997). Attachment formation and transfer in young adults' close friendships and romantic relationships. *Personal Relationships, 4,* 131–144.

Franco, N., & Levitt, M. J. (1998). The social ecology of middle childhood: Family support, friendship quality, and self-esteem. *Family Relations: Journal of Applied Family and Child Studies, 47,* 315–321.

Furman, W. (1996). The measurement of friendship perceptions: Conceptual and methodological issues. In W. M. Bukowski, A. F. Newcomb, & W. W. Hartup (Eds.), *The company they keep: Friendships in childhood and adolescence* (pp. 41–65). Cambridge, UK: Cambridge University Press.

Furman, W., & Buhrmester, D. (1985). Children's perceptions of the personal relationships in their social networks. *Developmental Psychology, 21,* 1016–1024.

Furman, W., & Buhrmester, D. (1992). Age and sex differences in perceptions of networks and personal relationships. *Child Development, 63,* 103–115.

Gauze, C., Bukowski, W. M., Aquan-Assee, J., & Sippola, L. K. (1996). Interactions between family environment and friendship and associations with self-perceived well-being during adolescence. *Child Development, 67,* 2201–2216.

Giordano, P. C., Cernkovich, S. A., Groat, H. T., Pugh, M. D., & Swinford, S. P. (1998). The quality of adolescent friendships: Long term effects? *Journal of Health and Social Behavior, 39,* 55–71.

Granot, D., & Mayseless, O. (2001). Attachment security and adjustment to school in middle childhood. *International Journal of Behavioral Development, 25,* 530–541.

Harter, S. (1985). *Manual for the Self-Perception Profile for Children.* Denver, CO: University of Denver.

Hazan, C., & Shaver, P. R. (1994). Attachment as an organizational framework for research on close relationships. *Psychological Inquiry, 5,* 1–22.

Hodges, E. V. E., Boivin, M., Vitaro, F., & Bukowski, W. M. (1999). The power of friendship: Protection against an escalating cycle of peer victimization. *Developmental Psychology, 35,* 94–101.

Hodges, E. V. E., Finnegan, R. A., & Perry, D. G. (1999). Skewed autonomy-relatedness in preadolescents' conceptions of their relationships with mother, father, and best friend. *Developmental Psychology, 35,* 737–748.

Karavasilis, L., Doyle, A. B., & Markiewicz, D. (2003). Associations between parenting style and attachment to mother in middle childhood and adolescence. *International Journal of Behavioral Development, 27,* 153–164.

Kerns, K. A., Klepac, L., & Cole, A. (1996). Peer relationships and preadolescents' perceptions of security in the child–mother relationship. *Developmental Psychology, 32,* 457–466.

Komproe, I. H., Rijken, M., Ros, W. J. G., Winnubst, J. A. M., & 't Hart, H. (1997). Available support and received support: Different effects under stressful circumstances. *Journal of Social and Personal Relationships, 14,* 59–77.

Ladd, G. W. (1992). Themes and theories: Perspectives on processes in family-peer relationships. In R. D. Parke & G. W. Ladd (Eds.), *Family–peer relationships: Modes of linkage* (pp. 3–34). Hillsdale, NJ: Erlbaum.

Ladd, G. W., Kochenderfer, B. J., & Coleman, C. C. (1996). Friendship quality as a predictor of young children's early school adjustment. *Child Development, 67,* 1103–1118.

Lieberman, M., Doyle, A., & Markiewicz, D. (1999). Developmental patterns in security of attachment to mother and father in late childhood and early adolescence: Associations with peer relations. *Child Development, 70,* 202–213.

Masten, A. S., Morison, P., & Pellegrini, D. S. (1985). A revised class play method of peer assessment. *Developmental Psychology, 21*(3), 523–533.

Parker, J. G., & Asher, S. R. (1989). *Friendship Quality Questionnaire–Revised: Instrument and administrative manual.* (Available from the first author, Department of Psychology, Pennsylvania State University, University Park, PA 16802-1503)

Reid, M., Landesman, S., Treder, R., & Jaccard, J. (1989). "My family and friends": Six- to twelve-year-old children's perceptions of social support. *Child Development, 60,* 896–910.

Rose-Krasnor, L., Rubin, K. H., Booth, C. L., & Coplan, R. (1996). The relation of maternal directiveness and child attachment security to social competence in preschoolers. *International Journal of Behavioral Development, 19,* 309–325.

Rubin, K. H., Dwyer, K. M., Booth-LaForce, C., Kim, A. H., Burgess, K. B., & Rose-Krasnor, L. (in press). Attachment, friendship, and psychosocial functioning in early adolescence. *Journal of Early Adolescence.*

Rubin, K. H., Fein, G., & Vandenberg, B. (1983). Play. In P. H. Mussen (Series Ed.) & E. M. Hetherington (Vol. Ed.), *Handbook of child psychology: Vol. 4. Socialization, personality, and social development* (4th ed., pp. 693–774). New York: Wiley.

Rubin, K. H., Lynch, D., Coplan, R., Rose-Krasnor, L., & Booth, C. L. (1994). "Birds of a feather..": Behavioral concordances and preferential personal attraction in children. *Child Development, 65,* 1778–1785.

Rubin, K. H., Wojslawowicz, J. C., Burgess, K. B., Booth-LaForce, C., & Rose-Krasnor, L. (2003). *The best friendships of aggressive children and shy/withdrawn children: Prevalence, stability, and relationship quality.* Manuscript submitted for publication.

Sarason, B. R., Pierce, G. R., & Sarason, I. G. (1990). Social support: The sense of acceptance and the role of relationships. In B. R. Sarason, I. G. Sarason, & G. R. Pierce (Eds.), *Social support: An interactional view* (pp. 97–128). New York: Wiley.

Sarason, B. R., Shearin, E. N., Pierce, G. R., & Sarason, I. G. (1987). Interrelations of social support measures: Theoretical and practical implications. *Journal of Personality and Social Psychology, 52,* 813–832.

Schneider, B. H., Atkinson, L., & Tardiff, C. (2001). Child–parent attachment and children's peer relations: A quantitative review. *Developmental Psychology, 37,* 86–100.

Schwartz, D., Dodge, K. A., Pettit, G. S., & Bates, J. E. (2000). Friendship as a moderating factor in the pathway between early harsh home environment and later victimization in the peer group. *Developmental Psychology, 36,* 646–662.

Simons, K. J., Paternite, C. E., & Shore, C. (2001). Quality of parent/adolescent attachment and aggression in young adolescents. *Journal of Early Adolescence, 21,* 182–203.

Sobel, M. E. (1982). Asymptotic intervals for indirect effects in structural equations models. In S. Leinhart (Ed.), *Sociological methodology 1982* (pp. 290–312). San Francisco: Jossey-Bass.

Sroufe, L. A. (1988). The role of infant–caregiver attachment in development. In J. Belsky & T. Nezworski (Eds.), *Clinical implication of attachment* (pp. 18–38). Hillsdale, NJ: Erlbaum.

Sroufe, L. A., & Fleeson, J. (1986). Attachment and the construction of relationships. In W. W. Hartup & Z. Rubin (Eds.), *Relationships and development* (pp. 57–71). Hillsdale, NJ: Erlbaum.

Stocker, C. M. (1994). Children's perceptions of relationships with siblings, friends, and mothers: Compensatory processes and links with adjustment. *Journal of Child Psychology and Psychiatry and Allied Disciplines, 35,* 1447–1459.

Sullivan, H. S. (1953). *The interpersonal theory of psychiatry.* New York: Norton.

Thompson, R. A. (1994). Emotion regulation: A theme in search of definition. In N. A. Fox (Ed.), The development of emotion regulation: Biological and behavioral considerations. *Monographs of the Society for Research in Child Development, 59*(2–3, Serial No. 240), 25–52.

van Aken, M. A. G., & Asendorpf, J. B. (1997). Support by parents, classmates, friends, and siblings in preadolescence: Covariation and compensation across relationships. *Journal of Social and Personal Relationships, 14,* 79–93.

Verschueren, K., Buyck, P., & Marcoen, A. (2001). Self-representations and socioemotional competence in young children: A 3-year longitudinal study. *Developmental Psychology, 37,* 126–134.

Verschueren, K., & Marcoen, A. (1999). Representation of self and socioemotional competence in kindergartners: Differential and combined effects of attachment to mother and to father. *Child Development, 70,* 183–201.

Verschueren, K., & Marcoen, A. (2002). Perceptions of self and relationship with parents in aggressive and nonaggressive rejected children. *Journal of School Psychology, 40,* 501–522.

Verschueren, K., Marcoen, A., & Schoefs, V. (1996). The internal working model of the self, attachment, and competence in five-year-olds. *Child Development, 67,* 2493–2511.

Youngblade, L. M., & Belsky, J. (1992). Parent–child antecedents of 5-year-olds' close friendships: A longitudinal analysis. *Developmental Psychology, 28,* 700–713.

CHAPTER 9

◆ ◆ ◆

Quality of Attachment at School Age

Relations between Child Attachment Behavior,
Psychosocial Functioning, and School Performance

ELLEN MOSS
DIANE ST-LAURENT
KARINE DUBOIS-COMTOIS
CHANTAL CYR

Secure Base

Study of the relation between attachment and development during middle childhood is a relatively new field requiring both theoretical and empirical clarification. According to attachment theory, parents continue to serve as a secure base throughout childhood, and the child's internal working model of the interactional history with caregivers influences perceptions of social events and expectations regarding relationships (Bowlby, 1969/1982). Parent–child interactions continue to be important mediators between the quality of child attachment in middle childhood and further socioemotional and academic adjustment. The secure child is not only able to use the parent as a secure base in stressful circumstances but also—because of the greater openness of emotional expression and problem resolution that characterizes the secure parent–child relationship in childhood—continues to learn more complex coping skills, which are scaffolded by the parent (Laible & Thompson, 2000). In essence, the attachment relationship during the preschool period and beyond is increasingly reflected in the integration of child goals, plans, and behavior with those of the attachment figure in a goal-corrected partnership (Bowlby, 1953; Marvin, 1977). Although children may have qualitatively distinct attachment relationships with different caregivers, the child's behavior in extrafamilial settings, such as the peer group, and representations of family and caregiving relationships reflect a developing individual attachment internal working model. How children integrate their various attachment relationships and evolve an individual internal working model of attachment, which can be measured using instruments such as the Adult Attachment Interview (AAI), is one of the current cutting-edge questions in attachment research. Clearly, greater understanding of the development of attachment during the middle-childhood period is critical to furthering our understanding of this issue.

In this chapter, we explore the relation between family ecology, quality of parent–child relationships, and child attachment as predictors of child socioemotional and academic development during the early school-age period. Our reflections are based on results of an 8-year (two-cohort) longitudinal study of approximately 240 Canadian children and their families who were followed from ages 3 to 9 (cohort 1) and 3 to 6 (cohort 2). As part of the study, quality of parent–child attachment was observed at preschool and school age using modified separation–reunion procedures for older children (Cassidy & Marvin, 1992; Main & Cassidy, 1988). In addition, stressful life events, maternal psychosocial measures, mother–child interactive patterns, and child behavior problems were evaluated during both the preschool and early-school-age periods.

MEASUREMENT OF ATTACHMENT USING SEPARATION–REUNION AT EARLY SCHOOL AGE

The major source of information concerning links between quality of attachment, mother–child interaction, and adaptation in extrafamilial contexts has been longitudinal studies linking infant or toddler Strange Situation classifications with later outcomes (Erickson, Sroufe, & Egeland, 1985; Lyons-Ruth, Alpern, & Repacholi, 1993). With the development of measures for assessing reunion behavior in children ages 3 to 7 (Cassidy & Marvin, 1992; Main & Cassidy, 1988), it became possible to examine concurrent and later correlates of attachment during the preschool and school-age years. The Cassidy–Marvin procedure is more flexible than the infant separation–reunion procedure. It essentially consists of two consecutive separation–reunion episodes lasting 3–5 minutes each between the child and the caregiver. Although the child is always left alone during the second separation, in some lab protocols a stranger remains with the child during the first separation, whereas in others the child is left alone during both separations. The procedure developed by Main and Cassidy for early-school-age children involves longer separations than the infant or preschool procedures do (approximately 45 minutes), during which the child often completes tasks with an assistant while the mother completes questionnaires in another room. Just prior to the 5-minute reunion period, there is usually a free-play session during which a research assistant is available to the child. In order to permit the observation of consistency in reunion patterns, it is recommended that a second 45-minute separation and 5-minute reunion period (structured like the first) take place. The child's attachment classification is given on the basis of behavior observed during both reunion periods.

There is considerable conceptual similarity between the Main and Cassidy (1988) school-age coding system and both infancy and preschool (Cassidy & Marvin, 1992) systems. All systems use a four-classification coding scheme (A, avoidant; B, secure; C, ambivalent; D, disorganized, controlling, and insecure–other), with coding decisions based on observer evaluations of child's physical proximity to mother, affective expression, and verbal exchanges. Beyond infancy, conversational exchanges assume increasing importance as a function of child age. In the Main and Cassidy classification system, the *secure* (B) pattern is manifested when the child responds to the mother's return in a confident, relaxed, and open manner. The child seems relaxed throughout the reunion and shows some pleasure being with the parent. The *insecure–avoidant* (A) pattern is characterized by the child's neutral coolness toward the parent, including minimizing physical or verbal contact. Generally, these children avoid intimacy rather than avoid their attachment figures in a more global manner. In the *insecure–ambivalent/dependent* (C) attachment pattern, the child shows exaggerated intimacy and dependency with the attachment figure through cute, babyish, or angry behavior. Ambivalence is shown through moderate avoidance displayed when the child seeks proximity. Like their infancy and preschool counterparts, the A, B, and C patterns can be considered to be organized, both representationally and behaviorally, in terms of accessing the attachment figure in times of stress.

At early school age, there are three subcategories of disorganization (D): controlling–punitive, controlling–caregiving, and insecure–other. Although children showing any of these patterns are considered to be disorganized at the level of representation, important behavioral differences exist between the subgroups at the level of behavioral organization. Children are considered to be insecure–controlling if they show punitive or caregiving strategies that are organized compensatory responses to parental insufficiency (Teti, 1999). As identified by Main and Cassidy (1988), *controlling–caregiving* behavior is manifested when the child focuses on helpfully guiding, orienting, or cheering up the parent. A *controlling–punitive* child uses hostile, directive behavior with the caregiver, which may include verbal threats or harsh commands. Certain children include both caregiving and punitive elements in a general controlling style, with the child directing the parent's activities and conversational exchanges. Children are classified *behaviorally disorganized or insecure–other* if they seem unable to use the caregiver as a secure base for exploration but do not clearly show either the A or C pattern. Children may display disordered, incomplete, or undirected sequencing of movements; some confusion or apprehension or other anomalous behavior similar to that described in the Main and Solomon (1990) infant disorganized pattern; or a combination of other insecure patterns (A and C).

Although studies using postinfancy separation–reunion measures have been ongoing for more than 10 years, some still question their validity. In fact, a substantial number of studies have established the predictive validity of the Main and Cassidy (1988) and Cassidy and Marvin (1992) attachment measures for both high-risk and normative samples of 3- to 7-year-old children with respect to socioemotional and academic adaptation (Cassidy, 1988; Cohn, 1990; Easterbrooks, Davidson, & Chazan, 1993; Main, Kaplan, & Cassidy, 1985; Moss, Bureau, Cyr, Mongeau, & St-Laurent, 2004; Moss, Cyr, Bureau, Tarabulsy, & Dubois-Comtois, 2004; Moss, Cyr, & Dubois-Comtois, 2004; Moss, Parent, Gosselin, Rousseau, & St-Laurent, 1996; Moss, Rousseau, Parent, St-Laurent, & Saintonge, 1998; Moss, Smolla, & Mazzarello, 2004; Moss & St-Laurent, 2001; Solomon, George, & De Jong, 1995; Speltz, Greenberg, & De Klyen, 1990). In addition—although in comparison with the infant literature there are still only a few stability studies that include separation–reunion measures for older children—these have found high stability (over 80%) between infancy and age 6 (Main & Cassidy, 1988; Wartner, Grossmann, Fremmer-Bombik, & Suess, 1994), further supporting the validity of both the Preschool Attachment Classification System (Cassidy & Marvin, 1992) and the Main and Cassidy systems as measures of attachment during the preschool/early-school-age years.

CONTINUITY/DISCONTINUITY IN ATTACHMENT BETWEEN PRESCHOOL AND SCHOOL AGE

According to Bowlby (1969/1982), early experiences with attachment figures lead to more generalized representations of self and others through the mediation of internal working models. Although internal working models develop in infancy, they continue to evolve throughout childhood and adolescence as a function of attachment-relevant experiences. Because internal working models are flexible, they may be revised in light of changing experiences occurring beyond infancy. However, persistence of a representational model will render it increasingly less likely that new attachment-related events will result in a changed attachment pattern. These theoretical ideas raise interesting issues concerning the relative impact of earlier and later experiences on the stability of attachment and how children's life circumstances will affect the evolution of their attachment patterns.

A few recently published studies have examined stability between infancy and adolescence or adulthood (Hamilton, 2000; Lewis, Feiring, & Rosenthal, 2000; Waters, Merrick, Treboux, Crowell, & Albersheim, 2000; Weinfeld, Sroufe, & Egeland, 2000). Results of these studies indicate that stability is higher in middle-class samples, in which children are likely to experience more stable, lower risk environments, and is lower in high-risk samples, in which families have experienced difficult life experiences. These studies have shown that particular events or circumstances that affect the quality of caregiving are related to discontinuity in child attachment patterns.

In our own mixed-socioeconomic-status (SES) sample, we examined the extent to which changes in parent–child interactive patterns, level of family risk, marital difficulties, and experience of potentially traumatic events such as death of family members or prolonged parental hospitalization would be related to stability and change in child attachment between preschool and school age. In a recent study of stability of attachment in our mixed-SES sample, we examined the extent to which changes in parent–child interactive patterns, level of family risk, marital difficulties, and experience of potentially traumatic events such as death of family members or prolonged parental hospitalization would be related to stability and change in child attachment between preschool and school age (Moss, Cyr, Bureau, et al., 2004). Our results indicated continuity of both secure and insecure patterns (two-way classification analysis: 77%, kappa = .53; four-way classification analysis: 68%, kappa = .45). Consistent with other studies (Cicchetti & Barnett, 1991; Main & Cassidy, 1988; Wartner et al., 1994), we found that the secure (72%) and disorganized (77%) classifications showed high stability. The ambivalent classification also showed continuity (62%). As for the avoidant classification, our findings on stability are in line with the findings of Egeland and Farber (1984) and Howes and Hamilton (1992), with 44% of this group showing continuity between Time 1 and Time 2.

These results are consistent with Bowlby's idea (1958) that security and insecurity represent two diverging pathways that become increasingly resistant to convergence given continuity in life circumstances. In the case of the secure preschool child, the basic structures for effective communication and negotiation, not only with the caregiver but also with other social partners, are in place (Moss et al., 1998; Stevenson-Hinde & Shouldice, 1995). The secure preschool child's ability to participate in goal-corrected partnerships may facilitate the maintenance of a secure relationship with the caregiver. In the case of the disorganized child, the lack of flexibility and openness in the relationship structure may contribute to a downward spiral in which the child's defenses become stronger with time and in which transitioning to security becomes less likely with development. The state of fear that characterizes the internal working model of the disorganized child may overwhelm the child's cognitive capacity, further impeding affect regulation and integration of attachment-related information (Solomon & George, 1999). Children in the D group not only use defensive processes to exclude threatening information—as do ambivalent and avoidant children—but they also do so in an extreme way by segregating attachment-related information from consciousness. This extreme defensive process renders change in internal working models more difficult (Bowlby, 1980). Given that children who show ambivalent and avoidant attachment strategies with the caregiver have less distorted attachment-related representational processes, changes in attachment consequent to changes in caregiving quality or family circumstances is more likely to occur. Consistent with these ideas was our disturbing finding that not a single disorganized child in our study changed toward security between preschool and school age, whereas 27% of ambivalent children and 14% of avoidant children did.

Our findings also supported the theoretical prediction that parent–child communication patterns are closely linked to continuity and change in child attachment (Thompson, 2000). Children who changed from secure to insecure patterns by school age experienced accompanying decreases in quality of communication with their mothers, in contrast to the stable secure group, who maintained dyadic relationships characterized by emotional openness, appropriate role structure, and reciprocity. Similarly, children who changed from insecurity to security had a more affectively supportive communication pattern with the caregiver than did those children who stayed insecure.

Our findings further indicated that difficult family circumstances occurring during the preschool period were associated with change from security to insecurity. Those secure preschoolers who became insecure had mothers who reported less satisfaction in their couple relationship and families in which level of overall risk and likelihood of hospitalization of an attachment figure was higher than in the stable secure group. At least two possible processes may explain these associations. Mothers who are coping with financial or personal difficulties are less accessible as emotional support to the preschool or school-age child who is still in need of an attachment figure. Difficult events that occur in the larger family system may also more directly influence the child's representational model of attachment relations. Exposure to parental destructive conflict in the course of marital disagreements may cause considerable discordance with a secure view of relationships (Davies, Harold, Goeke-Morey, & Cummings, 2002; Frosch, Manglesdorf, & McHale, 2000). Such exposure may interrupt consolidation of newly evolved attachment representations involved in maintaining goal-corrected partnerships, such as open expression of emotions, reciprocal modes of communication, negotiation, and compromise. In a similar fashion, the absence of a parent due to hospitalization is likely to compromise the child's confidence in and representation of parents as a source of security.

Our data on stressful life events in families were less informative in explaining changes from insecurity to security. However, it is possible that child characteristics not measured in our study (e.g., temperament) or positive peer experiences may also play a role in transitioning toward security in middle childhood (Kerns, Klepac, & Cole, 1996). In addition, it is also likely that attachment relationships with other caregivers, such as fathers or preschool teachers (Howes & Hamilton, 1992), may positively influence the child's attachment representations or interactions with the caregiver.

In summary, these results support the idea that attachment representations remain open to revision during the preschool and early-school-age period. The ability to engage in goal-corrected partnership is a new developmental acquisition that characterizes security in preschoolers (Marvin, 1977). Considerable scaffolding of these skills between ages 3 and 6, in the course of parent–child interactions, is still necessary for their integration in the child's behavioral repertoire and representational models of socioemotional relationships. Our findings that changes in attachment were predictably associated with changes in quality of parent–child communication and attachment-related family variables support the idea that early working models based on children's representations of the sensitivity of parental care may be modified by family events that significantly change the caregiving climate (Thompson, 2000).

ATTACHMENT AND CHILD ADAPTATION
DURING MIDDLE CHILDHOOD

In middle childhood, effective performance and integration in the school setting is an important marker of real-world success. Successful adaptation in the school environment involves socioemotional maturity, as well as application of both cognitive and metacognitive skills. According to attachment theory, the quality of parent–child relationships has a continuing effect on adaptation both within and outside of the family context (Bowlby, 1982). Acceptance or rejection in the peer group and performance in the school setting is related to motivational, self-regulatory, and behavioral patterns that, in part, stem from and are maintained through family processes. In the course of our longitudinal study of the associations between attachment at school age and child developmental outcomes, we have extensively investigated links between particular child attachment patterns and both socioemotional and cognitive markers of adaptation in the school setting (Moss et al., 1996, 1998; Moss, Bureau, et al., 2004; Moss & St-Laurent, 2001; Moss, St-Laurent, & Parent, 1999). Measures have included teacher reports and child self-reports of behavior problems, measures of joint and individual problem-solving ability, and academic records. Because our study includes measures of attachment at early school age, we have been able to test models concerning the salience of concurrent patterns of parent–child interaction as mediators of child school-age outcomes, in contrast to the bulk of the attachment literature that has emphasized the salience of early internalized patterns of attachment with the caregiver in predicting long-term adaptive outcomes.

The Role of Attachment in the Development of Behavior Problems

Past research supports the view that the secure child's capacity to be appropriately self-reliant while openly communicating emotions and needs, to negotiate interpersonal difficulties, and to coconstruct joint plans should engender a higher level of adaptation in the school setting in comparison with insecure peers (Easterbrooks et al., 1993; Greenberg, Speltz, De Klyen, & Endriga, 1991; Moss et al., 1998; Wartner et al., 1994). However, considerable evidence indicates that the particular type of insecurity is critical in predicting level of behavior problems, with the most consistent associations between attachment and behavior problems found for insecure behaviorally disorganized or controlling children. In several longitudinal studies with high-risk and more normative samples, children classified D in infancy showed a higher rate of externalizing problems at preschool and school age than any other attachment group (Lyons-Ruth et al., 1993; Lyons-Ruth, Easterbrooks, & Cibelli, 1997; Shaw, Owens, Vondra, & Keenan, 1996). Similarly, children with insecure–controlling attachment patterns at preschool and school age are significantly more likely to be rated as externalizing or aggressive (Moss et al., 1996, 1998; Solomon et al., 1995). A few studies have established associations between behaviorally disorganized or controlling attachment and internalizing symptoms (Carlson, 1998; Moss et al., 1998; Shaw, Keenan, Vondra, Delliquadri, & Giovanelli, 1997). In general, studies have been inconclusive with respect to the degree and type of behavior-problem risk associated with the avoidant and ambivalent attachment groups (Greenberg, 1999). This ambiguity may be partially due to the fact that the D classification was not included in studies published prior to 1985.

Consistent with these studies, our longitudinal data have shown that school-age attachment classifications significantly predict teacher-reported behavior problems at the transition to school and 2 years later (Moss et al., 1996, 1998). When compared with the secure group, insecure attachment groups were more likely to manifest behavior problems. However, the D group was the only attachment group that presented clinical cutoff levels of problem behaviors at both 5–7 and 7–9 years of age. There was also some indication of behavior problem risk for other insecure groups. Ambivalent children had higher externalizing scores at ages 5–7, which appeared to attenuate by ages 7–9, whereas avoidant boys manifested higher internalizing scores at ages 7–9 only. A subsequent study of a second cohort of children from a similar mixed–SES sample supported these results in showing that, by age 3, teacher ratings of both externalizing and internalizing symptoms for the disorganized group were significantly higher than those of their secure peers (Moss, Bureau, et al., 2004).

The peer behavior of disorganized children has been described as shifting between social withdrawal and extremely aggressive episodes (Jacobvitz & Hazen, 1999). As interpreted by these authors, because disorganized children may not believe that they can master the challenges of engaging competently with peers and see them as a potential threat, they may demonstrate fight-or-flight behaviors (i.e., aggression accompanied by fearful affect, in which children aggress against peers in order to ward off perceived threats). Studies of the preschool peer behavior of ambivalent children indicate that their immature social behavior elicits exploitation or reciprocal immaturity from other insecure peers and nurturance from secure peers, resulting in conflictual relationships with some group members (Troy & Sroufe, 1987). However, the more intense and bizarre aggressive behavior patterns associated with disorganization are likely to result in more general alienation from the peer group. Concerning avoidant children, our results are consistent with findings from other studies that have generally not indicated associations between psychopathology or aggressive problems and avoidant attachment when the disorganized or controlling classifications are included (Fagot & Kavanagh, 1990; Fagot & Pears, 1996; Lewis, Feiring, McGuffog, & Jaskir, 1984; Lyons-Ruth et al., 1993; Solomon et al., 1995). However, in line with previous studies, there were indications that avoidant children, particularly boys, showed an inhibited level of social participation (Bates & Bayles, 1988; Erickson et al., 1985; Lyons-Ruth et al., 1997; Suess, Grossmann, & Sroufe, 1992; Wartner et al., 1994). The denial of negative affect and expectations of rejection that dominate the internal working models of avoidant children may lead to passive withdrawal from conflictual situations, involving the internalization of negative affective expressions such as anger and sadness.

Further mediational analyses of processes that might explain the association between attachment and behavior problems in middle childhood indicated that the tense, poorly coordinated mother–child interactive patterns of both the ambivalent and disorganized groups contributed to the manifestation of behavior problems in the early-school-age years. However, by 7–9 years, these intrafamilial processes, which played a key role at earlier developmental periods in defining the nature of both attachment relations and extrafamilial relational styles, had diminished in importance as mediators of the association between attachment and maladaptation. Children's own internalized anxieties and fears related to performance, abilities, and self-worth were, however, important mediators of these associations at this age (Moss et al., 1999). Analyses of doll play of early-school-age disorganized children support these ideas in providing evidence of dysregulated representational processes (Solomon & George, 1999). This dysregulation is reflected in the disorganized child's representations of the self as helpless or vulnerable in the face of frightening events and of attachment figures as failing to provide protection. In accordance with George and Solomon's and our own teacher-report findings, our analyses of 8-year-old children's perceptions of their own behavior problems using a self-report measure showed that disorganized children were more likely than their peers to perceive themselves as aggressive or highly anxious in diverse parent–child and peer contexts (Moss, Smolla, & Mazzarello, 2004). Ambivalent children also showed greater likelihood of self-perceived externalizing behavior problems. Thus both internal representational and external behavioral correlates of insecure attachment interact in interfering with the child's ability to explore on both a cognitive and social level in the school setting.

The Role of Attachment in Predicting School Performance

The idea that, by middle childhood, the internalized attachment strategy of the child serves as a marker for the more salient contribution of the current patterns of interaction and engagement in which it is embedded was also supported by our findings concerning attachment and children's academic performance (Moss & St-Laurent, 2001). In attachment theory, caregiver–child relationships, which allow the child to balance attachment and exploration needs, lead to the early development of internal working models that promote self-efficacy and self-esteem (Bretherton, 1985; Cassidy, 1988). These self-regulatory mechanisms govern key areas of schoolage adaptation that include persistence, resourcefulness, and cognitive flexibility. Jacobsen and her colleagues found that attachment was related to differences in children's and adolescents' (ages 7–15) cognitive regulatory activity and academic competence through the mediation of selfconcept (Jacobsen, Edelstein, & Hofmann, 1994; Jacobsen & Hofmann, 1997). In the Jacobsen studies, the disorganized classification was most strongly associated with negative selfregulatory and/or self-concept outcomes.

Deficient evaluations of oneself and others' views of oneself may influence school achievement by having an impact on the goals children set for themselves, on difficulties in maintaining stable levels of reasoning, and on expectations for support from parents, peers, and teachers (Jacobsen et al., 1994; Saxe, Guberman, & Gearhart, 1987). Parent–child communication patterns, characterized by autonomy support, involvement, and reciprocal control, have been shown to predict child selfperceived competence and academic achievement (Grolnick & Ryan, 1989). Better communication processes in dyads that include a secure child may allow parents to support achievement, either directly through providing constructive feedback and being generally supportive about school-relevant activities or indirectly through encouraging development of child motivation and academic self-esteem. Conversely, concerning insecure children, communicative difficulties may interfere with child school performance either directly or through their negative impact on child sense of selfefficacy.

Recent studies conducted by our research group and others in the preschool and early-school-age period support these ideas in showing that secure children are significantly more likely to engage in collaborative regulation of joint problem-solving and reading activities with their caregivers than are their insecure peers (Bus & van IJzendoorn, 1988; Meins, 1997; Moss, Gosselin, Parent, Rousseau, & Dumont, 1997; Moss, Parent, Gosselin, & Dumont, 1993; Moss et al., 1999). In an unstructured interactive context, Moss et al. (1998) found that the levels of attunement, reciprocity, and balanced emotional expression in secure dyads surpassed those of insecure dyads, with the controlling group showing particularly poor coordination and role reversal in comparison with other groups.

Only a few studies have investigated links between insecurity and related psychosocial variables measured in early childhood and later school achievement (Aviezer, Sagi, Resnick, & Gini, 2002; Pianta & Harbers, 1996; Moss et al., 1999; Moss & St-Laurent, 2001; Teo, Carlson, Mathieu, Egeland, & Sroufe, 1996). These studies show that attachment relationships and quality of early caregiving are powerful predictors of school performance in both elementary and high school. Results of one study we conducted indicated that children classified D at age 6 showed deficits in math performance 2 years later (Moss et al., 1999). In that study, children's low perceived competence, metacognitive difficulties, and dysfunctional collaborative problem-solving styles with their mothers predicted poor math performance. We interpreted these results as evidence that disorganization at the level of representation interferes not only with the child's affect regulation and socioempathic skills but also with the activation of high-level self-regulated thought processes involved in planning or other executive functions (Moss et al., 1999).

In a more extensive study (Moss & St-Laurent, 2001), we examined the extent to which children with different attachment classifications showed competence in meeting the demands of the academic setting. We also attempted to identify processes that might explain any demonstrated attachment-risk relations at school age by testing alternative mediational models involving the role of attachment patterns and concurrent measures related to parent–child interaction in explaining school performance. The strong continuity between attachment classifications at infancy or preschool and at age 6 in our own sample (Moss, Cyr, Bureau, et al., 2004) and those of others (Main & Cassidy, 1988; Wartner et al., 1994) supports the view that school-age measures of attachment (particularly in more stable, normative samples) reflect the child's internalized model of the attachment relationship based on the history of experiences with attachment figures. Attachment patterns may be directly related to school performance outcomes, as these internalized patterns may place constraints on child learning and exploration. An alternative model suggests that associations between internalized attachment patterns and school performance are mediated by concurrent school-age experiences in interactive and exploratory contexts. This model is supported by studies that indicate that parent–child communication patterns characterized by autonomy support, involvement, and reciprocal control predict child self-perceived competence and academic performance (Grolnick & Ryan, 1989).

In order to test these models, the affective quality of mother–child interaction patterns and quality of child attachment to mother were evaluated during a lab visit, which included a separation–reunion procedure, that occurred when the children were approximately 6 years of age. Children's academic performance was assessed 2 years later (age 8). Analyses indicated that secure children had higher scores than their insecure peers on communication, cognitive engagement, and mastery motivation. Both avoidant and ambivalent children showed significantly lower levels of cognitive engagement in the joint mother–child problem-solving task and lower levels of mastery motivation than secure children.

However, only children with disorganized–controlling attachment were at risk for school underachievement. Children in the D group, despite their similarity in IQ to other attachment groups, were at greatest risk for poor school performance and showed the most pervasive deficits in other variables related to academic functioning. At age 6, children in the D group showed more inconsistent and incongruent communication patterns involving either highly restricted or exaggerated emotional expression. A negative, tense mood was more likely to prevail, with both mother and child using either ignoring or interfering response styles. Most characteristic of the controlling group was the role-reversed relationship structure.

As described previously, in order to better understand mechanisms that might explain identified links between disorganized attachment and school underachievement, we tested alternative mediational models. In the first model, following the idea that parent–child interaction patterns at school age serve as a setting condition for attachment strategies in facilitating or interfering with adaptation (Moss et al., 1998), we tested the mediational role of mother–child interaction in explaining the demonstrated relation between disorganization and academic performance. An alternative model, which tested the role of attachment as mediator of the relation between parent–child communication and academic performance, was not supported. We interpret this to mean that the evolution in the child of a disorganized–controlling attachment pattern does not place constraints on the child's academic performance above and beyond the constraints placed by current noncollaborative interaction patterns with the caregiver. By school age, the dysfunctional affective interaction patterns that are associated with controlling attachment behavior are directly related to academic risk for this group.

In summary, it is likely that early patterns of infant responding to various styles of parental sensitivity lay at least some of the groundwork for the development of both different attachment patterns and skills relevant to successful school performance. However, these results demonstrate that parent–child interactions during middle childhood still play an important role in explaining associations between attachment and school performance, at least in the case of the disorganized–controlling group. The adoption of a parentified role vis-à-vis the caregiver implies an abdicated caregiving style (Solomon & George, 1996) that may be incompatible with the careful monitoring of and adjustment to the child's state that is required not only for adequate development of child affective-self functions but also to facilitate the development of cognitive regulatory functions during the school-age period (Main, 1991; Vygotsky, 1978). Role reversal in the caregiver–child dyad may interfere with the acquisition and consolidation of higher level cognitive skills important for school success. Results of these mediational analyses suggest that, in the case of children with controlling attachment patterns, interventions related to school underachievement that focus on the role of the child in the family context are likely to be more successful than those focusing only on the individual child's cognitive deficits.

NEW DIRECTIONS FOR ATTACHMENT RESEARCH IN MIDDLE CHILDHOOD: EXAMINING SEPARATE DEVELOPMENTAL TRAJECTORIES OF D SUBGROUPS

One of the main objectives of our research program has been to examine trajectories of children (and their families) who show different types of insecure attachment at early school age. Our results and those of others have indicated that children who show disorganized attachment are the most at-risk attachment group (Lyons-Ruth & Jacobvitz, 1999; Moss, Cyr, & Dubois-Comtois, 2004). However, a few recent studies suggest that there may be differences in the family and child risk profiles associated with different forms of disorganization at early school age (George & Solomon, 1999). In order to further examine this question, we recently examined the preschool to school-age trajectories of children (and their families) who show different types of organized and disorganized attachment at early school age (Moss, Cyr, & Dubois-Comtois, 2004). In order to overcome the obstacle of low frequency of occurrence of these subgroups in normal populations, we combined two cohorts of participants in our longitudinal studies (Moss et al., 1998; Moss, Bureau, et al., 2004; Moss, Cyr, & Dubois-Comtois, 2004).

Results of this study provided the first findings concerning prevalence of subtypes of disorganized attachment at early school age in a normative sample. Our breakdown of the disorganized group, which was possible because of the unusually large sample size, revealed that 68% of the D group (10% of the sample) had developed controlling attachment behaviors with mothers at early school age. As described earlier, this controlling profile was equally distributed between two forms: (1) controlling–punitive or (2) controlling–caregiving. Whereas the controlling–punitive child's interactions with the caregiver seemed designed to humiliate the parent into submission through initiation of hostile and aggressive interactions, the controlling–caregiving child seemed motivated to orient or protect the parent by being excessively cheery, polite, or helpful. Thirty-two percent of the D sample, classified insecure–other, were behaviorally disorganized, showing disordered, incomplete, or undirected sequences of behavior and confusion or apprehension in the presence of the attachment figure. These results support other studies with middle-income low-risk samples that have shown that the majority of disorganized attachments at early school age are of the controlling type (Main & Cassidy,

1988; Moss & St-Laurent, 2001; Wartner et al., 1994). However, they also indicate that, even in normative samples, some children still show behavioral disorganization with the caregiver at early school age. The ratio of insecure–other children to controlling children may be considerably higher in samples of psychiatrically at-risk (Speltz et al., 1990) or maltreated children (Cicchetti & Barnett, 1991), and further research is needed with these populations.

These results also provided the first longitudinal data concerning family precursors and concurrent correlates of school age subtypes of disorganization. Our analyses of the developmental trajectories (preschool to school age) of these different D subgroups revealed considerable heterogeneity in family correlates, maternal psychosocial functioning, and child behavior problem profiles. Our comparisons of maternal reports of stress revealed that, as the controlling–punitive behavior became more evident over the preschool period, mothers of these children felt increasingly unable to cope with the children. However, as the controlling–caregiving behavior developed over the same period, mothers of these children felt increasingly better about their relationships with the children. Thus, despite the similar role-reversal inherent in these patterns and the resulting child feelings of being unprotected and vulnerable, different maternal feelings clearly appear, perhaps because of the negative, humiliating characteristics of the punitive behavior and the therapeutic, empathic nature of the caregiving behavior.

Although the behaviorally disorganized group was less distinguishable from the controlling–punitive or controlling–caregiving groups on maternal stress, results related to marital quality indicated that the former group experienced the most difficult family environment of all attachment groups. Families of these children were characterized by higher levels of severe marital conflict and traumatic life events. The unpredictability and overwhelming nature of the family environment that is disrupted by a conflictual marital relationship, as is the case for the behaviorally disorganized group, may compromise the possibility of the child forming any organized strategy for accessing the caregiver, even of a role-reversed controlling nature.

In line with theoretical ideas that link nonresolution of traumatic life events with child disorganization (Main & Hesse, 1990), we further compared disorganized attachment subgroups with respect to the likelihood of occurrence of several attachment-related events: loss of a close family member through death, parental hospitalization, and parental separation or divorce. Results indicated that behaviorally disorganized children were more likely to have experienced the trauma of parental hospitalization over the course of early childhood than were secure children. Our results further indicated that families of children who showed a controlling–

caregiving profile at early school age were more likely to have experienced the death of a close family member than were those of controlling-punitive, organized–insecure, or secure children. The serious disruption in the family that is occasioned by parental hospitalization or loss of a close family member may be associated with an increase in child fears related to lack of protection for himself or the caregiver, leading to disorganization of attachment-related mental processes (Bowlby, 1980; Robertson, 1962; van IJzendoorn, 1995). Our results did not indicate a greater likelihood of traumatic events for the controlling–punitive group. However, our measure did not include questions concerning exposure to violence or abuse—traumatic events that may have differentiated this group.

Finally, we tested the hypothesis that differences in dyadic emotion regulation styles and internal working models of punitive and caregiving children are associated with different forms of child maladaptation (Lyons-Ruth, Bronfman, & Atwood, 1999; Teti, 1999). We found that all the disorganized subgroups had elevated behavior problem scores relative to the secure group. However, punitive and insecure–other children were rated higher on externalizing problems, and the controlling–caregiving group was higher on internalizing problems. These results concerning differences in emotion regulation styles of children in D subgroups are supported by findings of Solomon and George (1999). These authors noted that the representational models of controlling–punitive children, as revealed in their doll-play themes, were dominated by themes of chaos and destruction, whereas extreme inhibition and portrayals of frightened behavior were evident in the doll-play narratives of controlling–caregiving children.

In summary, this study provides new evidence that the disorganized and controlling classifications should no longer be considered to be a single group with similar family and child behavior problem profiles. Given the emerging nature of this research domain, further studies are needed to clarify the precursors and further trace the trajectories of disorganized and controlling children in the school-age period.

CONCLUSION

In the last decade, the construct validity, stability, and reliability of separation–reunion measures appropriate for older children (3–7 years of age) have been demonstrated. Thompson (1999) has recently pointed to the development of postinfancy separation–reunion measures as one of the main innovations making possible the study of attachment relationships across the lifespan, their role in risk and protection, and the processes that contribute to the relation between qualities of attachment and outcomes. Results of our studies support the view that advances in attachment research require exploration of potential mediating influences between attachment and outcomes, rather than simple antecedent–consequent designs. Of particular importance is the continued role of children's interactions with their caregivers and experience of attachment-related family life events such as parental separation or divorce and loss of close family members in contributing to change or continuity of attachment patterns during the middle childhood period. On the one hand, to what extent do earlier patterns of security buffer children against changes in caregiving or traumatic family events that occur during middle childhood? On the other hand, can positive changes in quality of interactions with parents or family climate that occur in the middle-childhood period reorient children's insecure attachment patterns in a more positive direction? These are important cutting-edge questions for attachment research.

In addition, the dilemma of how to capture different patterns of insecurity in the middle-childhood period still remains. We strongly feel that use of both representational and behavioral measures of attachment will provide the most comprehensive and reliable evaluation of attachment during this age period. The excellent work presented by the authors in this volume has provided some important research tools. In this respect, it will be important to test whether self-report measures such as the Security Scale (Kerns et al., 1996), which assesses children's confidence in caregivers' availability and responsiveness, and the Preoccupied and Avoidant Coping Styles Questionnaire (Finnegan, Hodges, & Perry, 1996), which measures children's style of using the caregiver as a base for exploration, are longitudinally associated with observed attachment patterns of the preschool and early-school-age period. To achieve this end, it will be necessary to develop additional representational measures that capture the range of attachment strategies children use to cope with their caregivers. One of the biggest challenges will be to capture the diversity in the internal working models associated with disorganized attachment. We agree with Yunger, Corby, and Perry (Chapter 5, this volume) that it is insufficient to measure only avoidant and preoccupied styles of insecure coping in middle childhood. It will be interesting to see whether the caregiving–controlling and punitive–controlling behaviors described in this chapter can also be reliably measured using self-report methods and whether such measures can be validated using observed parent–child interactions.

Our own work, described in this chapter, has relied extensively on behaviorally based separation–reunion measures of attachment for research in the early-middle-childhood years. However, the dilemma of how to capture different patterns of insecurity in the later-middle-childhood period still remains. Because there is continued behavioral differentiation throughout childhood and adolescence in the strategies that children use to seek support from caregivers, it would be unwise to rely exclusively on representational measures to study attachment patterns. In order to capture aspects of parent–child relationships that are related to differences in attachment, it might be interesting to consider methodologies similar to those used in couples research to study parent–child communication patterns. In these protocols, the caregiver and child would be asked to separately identify issues that are problematic for the relationship (e.g., homework, friends, household chores) and then to try to make progress in resolving these issues. Secure (balanced affective and reciprocal communication), avoidant (minimization of involvement and affect), ambivalent (enmeshed, negative affective) and controlling (dysregulated affect and role-reversal) communication patterns could be coded from videotape. In addition, further studies that explore generalization of these attachment communication styles in the peer context are likely to enhance our understanding of both stability of attachment patterns between childhood and adulthood and the link between attachment patterns and children's psychosocial functioning in extrafamilial contexts.

REFERENCES

Aviezer, O., Sagi, A., Resnick, G., & Gini, M. (2002). School competence in young adolescence: Links to early attachment relationships beyond concurrent self-perceived competence and representations of relationships. *International Journal of Behavioral Development, 26*, 397–409.

Bates, J. E., & Bayles, K. (1988). The role of attachment in the development of behavior problems. In J. Belsky & T. Nezworski (Eds.), *Clinical implications of attachment* (pp. 253–299). Hillsdale, NJ: Erlbaum.

Bowlby, J. (1953). *Child care and the growth of love*. Harmondsworth, UK: Penguin.

Bowlby, J. (1958). The nature of the child's tie to his mother. *International Journal of Psycho-Analysis, 39*, 350–373.

Bowlby, J. (1980). *Attachment and loss: Vol.3. Loss*. New York: Basic Books.

Bowlby, J. (1982). *Attachment and loss: Vol. 1. Attachment*. New York: Basic Books. (Original work published 1969)

Bowlby, J. (1982). Attachment and loss: Retrospect and prospect. *American Journal of Orthopsychiatry, 52*, 664–678.

Bretherton, I. (1985). Attachment theory: Retrospect and prospect. In I. Bretherton & E. Waters (Eds.), Growing points of attachment theory and research. *Monographs of the Society for Research in Child Development, 50*(1–2, Serial No. 209).

Bus, A. G., & van IJzendoorn, M. H. (1988). Mother–child interactions, attachment, and emergent literacy: A cross-sectional study. *Child Development, 59*, 1262–1272.

Carlson, E. A. (1998). A prospective longitudinal study of disorganized/disoriented attachment. *Child Development, 69*, 1970–1979.

Cassidy, J. (1988). Child–mother attachment and the self in six-year-olds. *Child Development, 59,* 121–135.

Cassidy, J., & Marvin, R. S. (with the MacArthur Working Group on Attachment). (1992). *Attachment organization in 2½ to 4½ year olds: Coding manual.* Unpublished manuscript, University of Virginia, Charlottesville.

Cichetti, D., & Barnett, D. (1991). Attachment organization in maltreated preschoolers. *Development and Psychopathology, 3,* 397–411.

Cohn, D. A. (1990). Child–mother attachment of six-year-olds and social competence at school. *Child Development, 61,* 152–162.

Davies, P. T., Harold, G. T., Goeke-Morey, M. C., & Cummings, E. M. (2002). Child emotional security and interparental conflict. *Monographs of the Society for Research in Child Development, 67*(3, Serial No. 270).

Easterbrooks, M. A., Davidson, C. E., & Chazan, R. (1993). Psychosocial risk, attachment, and behavior problems among school-aged children. *Development and Psychopathology, 5,* 389–402.

Egeland, B., & Farber, E. (1984). Infant–mother attachment: Factors related to its development and changes over time. *Child Development, 55,* 753–771.

Erickson, E., Sroufe, A., & Egeland, B. (1985). The relationship between quality of attachment and behavior problems in a preschool high-risk sample. In I. Bretherton & E. Waters (Eds.), Growing points of attachment theory and research. *Monographs of the Society for Research in Child Development, 50*(1–2, Serial No. 209).

Fagot, B. I., & Kavanagh, K. (1990). The prediction of antisocial behavior from avoidant attachment classifications. *Child Development, 61,* 864–873.

Fagot, B. I., & Pears, K. C. (1996). Changes in attachment during the third year: Consequences and predictions. *Development and Psychopathology, 1,* 15–30.

Finnegan, R. A., Hodges, V. E., & Perry, D. G. (1996). Preoccupied and avoidant coping during middle childhood. *Child Development, 67,* 1318–1328.

Frosch, C. A., Manglesdorf, S. C., & McHale, J. L. (2000). Marital behavior and the security of the preschooler–parent attachment relationships. *Journal of Family Psychology, 14,* 365–379.

George, C., & Solomon, J. (1999). Attachment and caregiving: The caregiving behavioral system. In J. Cassidy & P. R. Shaver (Eds.), *Handbook of attachment: Theory, research and clinical applications* (pp. 649–670). New York: Guilford Press.

Greenberg, M. T. (1999). Attachment and psychopathology in childhood. In J. Cassidy & P. R. Shaver (Eds.), *Handbook of attachment: Theory, research, and clinical applications* (pp. 469–496). New York: Guilford Press.

Greenberg, M. T., Speltz, M. L., De Klyen, M., & Endriga, M. C. (1991). Attachment security in preschoolers with and without externalizing behavior problems: A replication. *Development and Psychopathology, 3,* 413–430.

Grolnick, W. S., & Ryan, R. M. (1989). Parent styles associated with children's self-regulation and competence in school. *Journal of Educational Psychology, 81,* 143–154.

Hamilton, C. (2000). Continuity and discontinuity of attachment from infancy through adolescence. *Child Development, 71*(3), 690–694.

Howes, C., & Hamilton, C. (1992). Children's relationships with child care teachers: Stability and concordance with parental attachments. *Child Development,* *63,* 867–878.

Jacobsen, T., Edelstein, W., & Hofmann, V. (1994). A longitudinal study of the relation between representations of attachment in childhood and cognitive functioning in childhood and adolescence. *Developmental Psychology, 30,* 112–124.

Jacobsen, T., & Hofmann, V. (1997). Children's attachment representations: Longitudinal relations to school behavior and academic competency in middle childhood and adolescence. *Developmental Psychology, 33,* 703–710.

Jacobvitz, D., & Hazen, N. (1999). Developmental pathways from infant disorganization to childhood peer relationships. In J. Solomon & C. C. George (Eds.), *Attachment disorganization* (pp. 127–159). New York: Guilford Press.

Kerns, K., Klepac, L., & Cole, A. (1996). Peer relationships and preadolescents' perceptions of security in the child–mother relationship. *Developmental Psychology, 32,* 457–466.

Laible, D. J., & Thompson, R. A. (2000). Mother–toddler conflict in the toddler years: Lessons in emotion, morality and relationships. *Child Development,* *73*(4), 1187–1203.

Lewis, M., Feiring, C., McGuffog, C., & Jaskir, J. (1984). Predicting psychopathology in six-year-olds from early social relations. *Child Development, 55,* 123–136.

Lewis, M., Feiring, C., & Rosenthal, S. (2000). Attachment over time. *Child Development, 71,* 707–720.

Lyons-Ruth, K., Alpern, L., & Repacholi, L. (1993). Disorganized infant attachment classification and maternal psychosocial problems as predictors of hostile-aggressive behavior in the preschool classroom. *Child Development, 64,* 572–585.

Lyons-Ruth, K., Bronfman, E., & Atwood, G. (1999) A relational diathesis model of hostile–helpless states of mind: Expressions in mother–infant interaction. In J. Solomon & C. C. George (Eds.), *Attachment disorganization* (pp. 33–70). New York: Guilford Press.

Lyons-Ruth, K., Easterbrooks, M. A., & Cibelli, C. D. (1997). Infant attachment strategies, infant mental lag, and maternal depressive symptoms: Predictors of internalizing and externalizing problems at age 7. *Developmental Psychology, 33,* 681–692.

Lyons-Ruth, K., & Jacobvitz, D. (1999). Attachment disorganization: Unresolved loss, relational violence, and lapses in behavioral and attentional strategies. In J. Cassidy & P. R. Shaver (Eds.), *Handbook of attachment: Theory, research, and clinical applications* (pp. 520–554). New York: Guilford Press.

Main, M. (1991). Metacognitive knowledge, metacognitive monitoring, and singular (coherent) vs. multiple (incoherent) models of attachment: Findings and directions for future research. In C. M. Parkes, J. Stevenson-Hinde, & P. Marris (Eds.), *Attachment across the life cycle* (pp. 127–159). New York: Tavistock/Routledge.

Main, M., & Cassidy, J. (1988). Categories of response to reunion with the parent at age six: Predictable from infant attachment classifications and stable over a 1–month period. *Developmental Psychology, 24*(3), 415–526.

Main, M., & Hesse, E. (1990). Parents' unresolved traumatic experiences are related to infant disorganized attachment status: Is frightened and/or frightening parental behavior the linking mechanism? In M. T. Greenberg, D. Cichetti, & M. Cummings (Eds.), *Attachment in the preschool years* (pp. 161–182). Chicago: University of Chicago Press.

Main, M., Kaplan, N., & Cassidy, J. (1985). Security in infancy, childhood, and adulthood: A move to the level of representation. In I. Bretherton & E. Waters (Eds.), Growing points of attachment theory and research. *Monographs of the Society for Research in Child Development, 50*(1–2, Serial No. 209).

Main, M., & Solomon, J. (1990). Procedure for identifying infants as disorganized/disoriented during the Ainsworth Strange Situation. In M. Greenberg, D. Cicchetti, & M. Cummings (Eds.). *Attachment in the preschool years: Theory, research, and intervention* (pp. 121–160). Chicago: University of Chicago Press.

Marvin, R. S. (1977). An ethological-cognitive model of the attenuation of mother–child attachment behavior. In T. Alloway, L. Krames, & P. Pilner (Eds.), *Advances in the study of communication and affect: Vol. 3. Attachment behavior* (pp. 25–60). New York: Plenum Press.

Meins, E. (1997). Security of attachment and maternal tutoring strategies: Interaction within the zone of proximal development. *British Journal of Developmental Psychology, 15*, 129–144.

Moss, E., Bureau, J.-F., Cyr, C., Mongeau, C., & St-Laurent, D. (2004). Correlates of attachment at age 3: Construct validity of the Preschool Attachment Classification System. *Developmental Psychology, 40*, 323–334.

Moss, E., Cyr, C., Bureau, J.-F., Tarabulsy, G. M., & Dubois-Comtois, K. (2004). *Stability of attachment between preschool and early school age and factors contributing to continuity/discontinuity*. Manuscript submitted for publication.

Moss, E., Cyr, C., & Dubois-Comtois, K. (2004). Attachment at early school age and developmental risk: Examining trajectories of controlling-caregiving, controlling-punitive and behaviorally-disorganized children. *Developmental Psychology, 40*, 519–532.

Moss, E., Gosselin, C., Parent, S., Rousseau, D., & Dumont, M. (1997). Attachment and joint problem-solving experiences during the preschool period. *Social Development, 6*, 1–17.

Moss, E., Parent, S., Gosselin, C., & Dumont, M. (1993). Attachment and the development of metacognitive and collaborative strategies. *International Journal of Educational Research, 16*, 555–571.

Moss, E., Parent, S., Gosselin, C., Rousseau, D., & St-Laurent, D. (1996). Attachment and teacher-reported behavior problems during the preschool and early school-age period. *Development and Psychopathology, 8*, 511–525.

Moss, E., Rousseau, D., Parent, S., St-Laurent, D., & Saintonge, J. (1998). Correlates of attachment at school age: Maternal reported stress, mother–child interaction, and behavior problems. *Child Development, 69*, 1390–1405.

Moss, E., Smolla, N., & Mazzarello, T. (2004). *School-age attachment and behavior problems: Concordance between mother, teacher and self-reports*. Manuscript submitted for publication.

Moss, E., & St-Laurent, D. (2001). Attachment at school age and academic performance. *Developmental Psychology, 37*, 863–874.

Moss, E., St-Laurent, D., & Parent, S. (1999). Disorganized attachment and developmental risk at school age. In J. Solomon & C. C. George (Eds.), *Attachment disoganization* (pp. 160–186). New York: Guilford Press.

Pianta, R. C., & Harbers, K. L. (1996). Observing mother and child behavior in a problem-solving situation at school entry: Relations with academic achievement. *Journal of School Psychology, 34,* 307–322.

Robertson, J. (1962). *Hospitals and children: A parents' eye view.* New York: Gollanz.

Saxe, G. B., Guberman, S. R., & Gearhart, M. (1987). Social processes in early number development. *Monographs of the Society for Research in Child Development, 52*(2, Serial No. 162).

Shaw, D., Owens, E., Vondra, J., & Keenan, K. (1996). Early risk factors and pathways in the development of early disruptive behavior problems. *Development and Psychopathology, 8,* 679–699.

Shaw, D. S., Keenan, K., Vondra, J. I., Delliquadri, E., & Giovanelli, J. (1997). Antecedents of preschool children's internalizing problems: A longitudinal study of low-income families. *Journal of the American Academy of Child and Adolescent Psychiatry, 36,* 1760–1767.

Solomon, J., & George, C. C. (1996). Defining the caregiving system: Toward a theory of caregiving. *Infant Mental Health Journal, 17,* 183–197.

Solomon, J., & George, C. C. (1999). The place of disorganization in attachment theory: Linking classic observations with contemporary findings. In J. Solomon & C. C. George (Eds.), *Attachment disorganization* (pp. 3–32). New York: Guilford Press.

Solomon, J., George, C. C., & De Jong, A. (1995). Children classified as controlling at age six: Evidence of disorganized representational strategies and aggression at home and at school. *Development and Psychopathology, 7*(3), 447–464.

Speltz, M. L., Greenberg, M. T., & De Klyen, M. (1990). Attachment in preschoolers with disruptive behavior: A comparison of clinic-referred and nonproblem children. *Development and Psychopathology, 2,* 31–46.

Stevenson-Hinde, J., & Shouldice, A. (1995). Maternal interactions and self-reports related to attachment classifications at 4.5 years. *Child Development, 66*(3), 583–596.

Suess, G., Grossmann, K. E., & Sroufe, L. A. (1992). Effects of infant attachment to mother and father on quality of adaptation in preschool: From dyadic to individual organization of self. *International Journal of Behavioral Development, 15*(1), 43–65.

Teo, A., Carlson, E., Mathieu, P. J., Egeland, B., & Sroufe, L. A. (1996). A prospective longitudinal study of psychosocial predictors of achievement. *Journal of School Psychology, 34,* 285–306.

Teti, D. M. (1999). Conceptualizations of disorganization in the preschool years: An integration. In J. Solomon & C. C. George (Eds.), *Attachment disorganization* (pp. 213–242). New York: Guilford Press.

Thompson, R. A. (1999). Early attachment and later development. In J. Cassidy & P. R. Shaver (Eds.), *Handbook of attachment: Theory, research, and clinical applications* (pp. 265–286). New York: Guilford Press.

Thompson, R. A. (2000). The legacy of early attachments. *Child Development, 71,* 145–152.

Troy, M., & Sroufe, L. A. (1987). Victimization among preschoolers: The role of attachment relationship history. *Journal of the American Academy of Child Psychiatry, 26,* 166–172.

van IJzendoorn, M. (1995). Adult attachment representations, parental responsiveness, and infant attachment: A meta-analysis on the predictive validity of the Adult Attachment Interview. *Psychological Bulletin, 117,* 387–403.

Vygotsky, L. (1978). *Mind in society.* Cambridge, MA: Harvard University Press.

Wartner, U. G., Grossman, K., Fremmer-Bombik, E., & Suess, G. (1994). Attachment patterns at age six in South Germany: Predictability from infancy and implications for preschool behavior. *Child Development, 65,* 1014–1027.

Waters, E., Merrick, S., Treboux, D., Crowell, J., & Albersheim, L. (2000). Attachment security in infancy and early adulthood: A twenty-year longitudinal study. *Child Development, 71,* 684–689.

Weinfeld, N. S., Sroufe, L. A., & Egeland, B. (2000). Attachment from infancy to early adulthood in a high-risk sample: Continuity, discontinuity, and their correlates. *Child Development, 71*(3), 695–702.

CHAPTER 10

◆ ◆ ◆

Perceived Security of Attachment to Mother and Father

Developmental Differences and Relations to Self-Worth and Peer Relationships at School

KARINE VERSCHUEREN
ALFONS MARCOEN

Research has suggested that in middle childhood, children retain a need for parental attachment figures (see Kerns, Tomich, Aspelmeier, & Contreras, 2000; Kobak, Rosenthal, & Serwick, Chapter 4, this volume). However, because of the lack of adequate and age-appropriate assessments of attachment, the nature and the correlates of parent–child attachment during these middle-childhood years have only recently been the subject of empirical investigation. In the past decade, some promising assessments have been developed, including the Security Scale constructed by Kerns, Klepac, and Cole (1996). This measure is based on Bowlby's hypothesis that the set goal of the attachment system in older children becomes psychological availability rather than physical proximity (Ainsworth, 1990; Kerns et al., 2000). In line with this hypothesis, attachment security is operationally defined as the degree to which the child perceives the attachment figure as responsive, available, and open to communication. In contrast to some other measures, the Security Scale is designed to assess children's perceptions of *specific* attachment relations. This allows for a test of the connection between children's perceived attachment to mother and to father, as well as of the differential effects of both.

In several studies, evidence for the reliability and the validity of the Security Scale as a measure of perceived attachment security has been gathered. These studies show that—despite the justified concern that children's self-reports of their attachment relationships may be subject to conscious or unconscious distortion—children's security scores are related in the predicted way to their self-esteem and their functioning in peer relationships (Kerns et al., 1996, 2000; Lieberman, Doyle, & Markiewicz, 1999; Verschueren & Marcoen, 2002). Relations with observed and parent-reported responsiveness have also been reported but appear to be less consistent (Kerns et al., 2000). Finally, some evidence suggesting a connection between security scores based on the Security Scale and children's overall security of attachment assessed by a picture-response procedure has been found (Granot & Mayseless, 2001; Kerns et al., 2000). The shared variance of both attachment-based assessments is, however, only modest to low. This suggests that both methods may tap somewhat different constructs (consciously available and reported perceptions vs. inferred representations of attachment relations; see later in the chapter).

The recent availability of attachment measures such as the Security Scale makes it possible to take further steps into the testing and refinement of attachment theoretic assumptions, especially as they apply to the middle-childhood period. In the longitudinal study presented in this chapter, some of these theoretically relevant questions were addressed. The questions can be grouped into two sections: The first pertain to the developmental changes in attachment security, and the second to the connections with self-perceptions and peer relationships at school.

DEVELOPMENTAL CHANGES IN ATTACHMENT SECURITY ACROSS THE MIDDLE CHILDHOOD YEARS

As stated by Lieberman and colleagues (1999), there are relatively little empirical data on developmental changes in attachment security beyond the early childhood years. The issue of stability and change covers several different interesting questions.

First, does the perceived security of attachment (at the group level) decrease, increase, or remain the same over the middle-childhood years? Lieberman and colleagues (1999) found that, in general, perceptions of parental availability (six items of the Security Scale) did not differ as a function of age, whereas perceptions of dependency on parents (nine remaining items of the Security Scale) declined with increasing age. However, this study was cross-sectional and involved a somewhat older group of children (ages 9–14 years). In our study, a younger sample of children in the middle-childhood years was investigated, and age differences were studied using a longitudinal instead of a cross-sectional design. This rules out any alternative explanations in terms of cohort or sample differences. As in the study of Lieberman and colleagues, potential interactions between genders of parent and child on the development of perceived security were explored.

A second question regarding the developmental changes in attachment security across the middle-childhood years refers to the stability of individual differences in perceived attachment security: Do individual differences in the perceived security of attachment to mother and to father remain relatively stable during the middle-childhood period? In other words, despite a possible decrease or increase of feelings of security at the group level, do children retain their position relative to other children on a continuum of perceived attachment security? Because of its cross-sectional design, this stability of individual differences could not be investigated in the study by Lieberman and colleagues (1999). In a 2-year longitudinal study using a sample of 77 children (followed from grade 3 to grade 5), Kerns and colleagues (2000) found significant stability in perceived security of attachment to father ($r = .31$, $p < .05$), but not to mother ($r = .15$, n.s.). In the study presented here, we reexamined this issue using a 3-year interval and a larger sample of children. This way, we could rule out the possibility that the nonsignificant stability Kerns and colleagues found for mother was merely due to a lack of power.

A third relevant question related to the developmental changes in attachment security is whether the representations of attachment to mother and to father become more integrated or more differentiated during middle childhood. On the one hand, it may be hypothesized that the association between the representation of attachment to mother and to father becomes stronger during the middle-childhood years because of the development of cognitive abilities necessary for the construction of a generalized representation of attachment relationships (Kerns, Schlegelmilch, Morgan, & Abraham, Chapter 3, this volume; Mayseless, Chapter 1, this volume). On the other hand, it may be suggested that older children are more likely to develop differentiated perceptions of their relationships, including their relationships with their parents. In the study reported here, the evidence for both hypotheses was compared.

With regard to this latter question, we need to be make two remarks. First, the juxtaposition of these two hypotheses may obscure the fact that, in our opinion, both may be true. While growing older and developing more advanced cognitive abilities, children may develop more differentiated perceptions of the quality of their specific attachment relationships and the differences between them while also developing a more overall, integrated view of how attachment relationships work in general. In other words, the development of attachment representations may be comparable to the development of self-representations. Here, too, it has been proposed that children's perceptions of self become more differentiated with increasing age, while at the same time a better integration of specific features into a general model of self becomes possible (Harter, 1990, 1998). Hence, it is possible that in our study (using the Security Scale), we can see only part of the picture and that we can test only whether or not perceptions of attachment to mother and father become more differentiated over time. To test the hypothesis of increasing integration between different representations, other assessments probing the degree of integration more directly may be needed.

Second, we must remark on the difference between the terms "representation" and "perception." Although both can be seen as cognitive–affective structures comprising both thoughts and feelings regarding attachment relations, the concept of representation also covers organizational features, such as ease of accessibility, coherence of propositions about the attachment relationship, and so forth. In our opinion, self-report measures such as the Security Scale do not take into account such organizational features (in contrast to narrative, doll-play measures, or the Adult Attachment Interview). Hence, it is most correct to say that this study tests the hypothesis that children's *perceptions* of their attachment relationships become more differentiated with increasing age.

CONNECTIONS BETWEEN ATTACHMENT SECURITY, SELF-PERCEPTIONS, AND PEER RELATIONSHIPS AT SCHOOL DURING MIDDLE CHILDHOOD

The second set of questions addressed in this chapter refers to the connections between attachment security, self-perceptions, and peer relationships during the middle-childhood years.

Without claiming any determinism, attachment theory predicts links between the quality of children's attachment to their primary attachment figures and their competence in relationships with peers. In several studies, the predicted associations have been found, using both observational and representational assessments of attachment (for an overview, see Stevenson-Hinde & Verschueren, 2002; Thompson, 1999). However, most research has focused on the (longer term) correlates of attachment quality in early childhood. Evidence for concurrent or longitudinal connections with attachment quality in middle childhood is far more scarce (Kerns et al., 1996; Ladd, 1992). Kerns and colleagues (1996) found a modest but significant association between children's liking ratings received from their peers and their perceptions of security of attachment to mother as measured by the Security Scale. In a second relevant study, Granot and Mayseless (2001) reported similar findings: Higher felt security in the relationship with mother (measured by the Security Scale) was related to a lower number of negative peer nominations. However, both studies focused only on the attachment to mother. As concluded by Schneider, Atkinson, and Tardif (2001) from a quantitative review of studies, "the implications of paternal attachment for children's peer relations remain largely unexplored" (p. 96; see Granot & Mayseless, 2001, for a similar conclusion for middle childhood). The study presented here was aimed at filling this gap by examining the connections between children's perceptions of attachment to mother and to father and their peer acceptance. Because both the perceived security with mother and the perceived security with father were assessed, we were able to test potential differential associations of attachment to mother and to father with children's peer relationships. In a study with 5-year-olds, Verschueren and Marcoen (1999) found that relations between attachment representations and peer social competence as rated by the kindergarten teacher were more robust for the attachment to father than for the attachment to mother. In a follow-up of this study, the same finding was found using peer sociometric ratings (Verschueren & Marcoen, 2003). Replicating these differential effects using a different age group (middle instead of early childhood) and a different assessment of attachment (direct self-report questionnaire instead of narrative, doll-play assessment) would definitely add to the robustness of the findings.

In trying to explain the connection between attachment to parents and competence in peer relationships, several possible mediating mechanisms have been suggested. In general, explanations refer to differences between secure and insecure children in social (behavioral) skills, in affect regulation, and in views of self and others (e.g., Lieberman et al., 1999). With regard to self-perceptions, attachment theory suggests that children, through their attachment relationships, form a representational model of self that includes expectations about their worthiness and lovableness (Cassidy, 1988; Ladd, 1992). Once internalized, these expectations about the self (in relation to others) are assumed to affect children's behavior and success in other relationships, including their relationships with peers. In other words, "the self provides a mechanism through which the relationship with the attachment figure can continue its influence across many years and in situations where the attachment figure is not present" (Cassidy, 1988, p. 133; see also Booth-LaForce, Rubin, Rose-Krasnor, & Burgess, Chapter 8, this volume; Bretherton, 1985; Hamilton & Howes, 1992; Ladd, 1992; Rose-Krasnor, Rubin, Booth, & Coplan, 1996). Although linkages between attachment security and self-perceptions have been established in samples of kindergartners (Cassidy, 1988; Verschueren & Marcoen, 1999; Verschueren, Marcoen, & Schoefs, 1996), the mediational model explained previously has not yet been tested (but see Booth-LaForge, et al., Chapter 8, this volume). Nevertheless, empirical evaluation of the mediational processes that explain the link between attachment security and social functioning is regarded as a high priority in the current research on attachment (Belsky & Cassidy, 1994; Granot & Mayseless, 2001; Schneider et al., 2001). In the study presented here, we tested this mediational model in a sample of 8- to 11-year-olds.

The preceding discussion has identified a number of questions regarding the developmental changes of attachment security and connections with self-perceptions and peer relationships. As explained previously, these questions refer to: (1) developmental changes in attachment security at the group level, (2) stability of individual differences in attachment security over time, (3) the interrelation over time of the representations of attachment to mother and to father, (4) the connection between security of attachment to mother and father and peer relationships at school, and (5) the mediational role of children's global self-worth in explaining this link. These five questions were addressed in a longitudinal study. The remainder of the chapter describes the methods and results of this study, considering each of these main research questions in turn.

A LONGITUDINAL STUDY ON ATTACHMENT, SELF-WORTH, AND PEER RELATIONSHIPS IN MIDDLE CHILDHOOD

Description of the Method

Longitudinal Sample

Participants were 265 children (129 girls and 136 boys) who were followed from grade 3 to grade 6. At the first measurement, their mean age was 8 years and 10 months (SD = 5 months). The children were recruited from 17 elementary school classes in seven schools in the neighborhoods of Mechelen and Leuven (Flanders, Belgium). Approximately 3 years after the first measurement, the seven schools were contacted again, and a follow-up measurement took place. Children from 15 classes participated. At the time of this second measurement, the children were age 11 years and 9 months on average (*SD* = 5 months). All participating children had received parental permission for participation.

Measures

All instruments were administered in the classroom during normal school hours. After an introductory explanation, the children completed a set of questionnaires, including the ones reported here. At both measurement times, the same set of questionnaires was completed. In the third-grade classes, two research assistants were available for explanations if necessary; in the sixth-grade classes, at least one research assistant was present during the administration of the measures. The entire testing session lasted about 1 hour in each classroom. At the end of the session, all children received a small gift.

The perceived security of the attachment to mother and to father was assessed using the Security Scale of Kerns and colleagues (1996), completed once for mother and once for father (in counterbalanced order). The children's self-perceptions were assessed with Harter's Self-Perception Profile for Children (SPPC; Harter, 1985; Veerman, Straathof, Treffers, Van den Bergh, & ten Brink, 1997). For the analyses reported here, only the scores for the SPPC subscale Global Self-Worth were considered. Items of this scale refer to "liking oneself," "thinking that one is a good person," and so forth. The alpha coefficients of internal consistency for this subscale were .82 and .81, at Time 1 and Time 2, respectively. To assess peer acceptance, a sociometric rating assessment (Singleton & Asher, 1977) was done. All children were asked to indicate on a 5-point "smiley scale" how much they liked to play with all other children in their classroom. A child's score was computed as the average rating received from his or her peers. These mean rating scores were converted into standard scores per classroom.

Main Results and Conclusions

Before reporting on the results for the five main research questions, we discuss the conclusions from preliminary analyses of the psychometric properties of the Security Scale. Specifically, the factor structure of the scale was investigated using exploratory and confirmatory factor analysis. These analyses were performed on the data gathered at Time 1. The final measurement models were also evaluated for the data gathered at Time 2.

Factor Structure of the Security Scale

The Security Scale has most often been used as a unidimensional scale, measuring the child's perceived security of attachment to a specific figure (Kerns et al., 1996). Although the high levels of internal consistency support the assumption of a unidimensional model, Lieberman and colleagues (1999) have suggested that two "somewhat distinct dimensions of attachment" (p. 205) may be probed, labeled *availability* (perceiving parents as available) and *dependency* (seeking or valuing parental help). Up to now, however, no strong evidence for either of these two models has been given. In support of their assumption, Lieberman and colleagues point to the modest correlations between the two subscales they defined a priori (.51 for mother and .64 for father).

An exploratory factor analysis on the 15 Security Scale items in our study revealed that, for mother as well as for father, a one- and a two-factor solution were both appropriate (based on scree plot of eigenvalues). An inspection of the two-factor solution revealed that the factor that accounted for the split of the items was a method factor: Items in which a positive description (description of a secure relationship) was presented first loaded on a different factor than items in which a negative description (description of an insecure relationship) was presented first. In other words, responses to items with a similar format appeared to share more variance in common than could be explained by the common content of the security items. As shown by an inspection of the item means, children tended to agree more with the description of a secure relationship when it was presented first. For the two-dimensional model proposed by Lieberman and colleagues, no evidence was found.

The same results were found using confirmatory factor analysis (LISREL). The 15 items were found to load on a single latent factor, but the fit was satisfying only when the aforementioned method factor was included (chi-square/df = 1.69, RMSEA = .051, p-value test of close fit = .43, GFI = .93, AGFI = .89, CFI = .88 for mother; and chi-square/df = 1.62, RMSEA = .055, p-value test of close fit = .31, GFI = .92, AGFI = .89, CFI = .91 for father). When comparing this model to the two-dimensional model proposed by Lieberman and colleagues (using the AIC and CAIC indices as criteria), the first was found to show better fit to the data. The resulting two-dimensional model (including the method factor) at Time 1 was also evaluated at Time 2. A good fit was found for mother (chi-square/df = 1.87, RMSEA = .057, p-value test of close fit = .22, GFI = .93, AGFI = .89, CFI = .91) and a somewhat lower but still adequate fit was found for father (chi-square/df = 2.48, RMSEA = .078, p-value test of close fit = .00, GFI = .90, AGFI = .86, CFI = .90).

In sum, no evidence was found for the presence of two sub-dimensions labeled *dependency* and *availability*. All items appeared to measure one dimension that was interpretable as "perceived security of an attachment relationship." There was, however, evidence for an effect of the order of presentation of positive and negative descriptions of the parent–child relationship. Despite this, all 15 items were used in the following analyses to derive a total security score for mother and for father. This decision was made not only for the sake of comparability with other studies but also because the preceding analyses showed that all items did probe the same latent construct of perceived attachment security. The alpha-coefficients for the total scale were .73 and .77 for mother and father at Time 1 and .83 and .89 at Time 2. Nevertheless, the results we found show that, when using self-report measures and especially when interpreting the interrelations of several self-report measures, the possibility of (shared) response biases needs to be taken into account.

Developmental Changes in Attachment Security at the Group Level

To address the first research question, a repeated-measures ANOVA, with gender of the child as between-subjects independent variable and age group as within-subjects variable, was performed on the security scores for mother and for father. With regard to the attachment to mother, results showed a significant main effect of child gender, $F (1, 249) = 5.32$, $p < .05$. Girls reported higher levels of perceived security with mother than boys did. Moreover, a significant main effect of age group was found, $F (1, 249) = 6.85$, $p < .01$. As can be seen in Figure 10.1, 11-year-olds reported higher levels of perceived security with mother than 8-year-olds. This finding was unexpected and is certainly not in line with an assump-

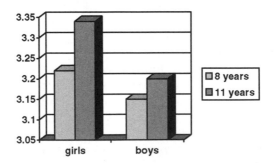

FIGURE 10.1. Security scores for mother as a function of gender and age of the child.

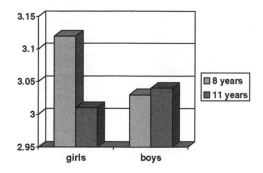

FIGURE 10.2. Security scores for father as a function of gender and age of the child.

tion of disengagement from parental attachment figures during middle childhood (Mayseless, Chapter 1, this volume).

With regard to the attachment to father, no significant main or interaction effect was found. Only a marginally significant interaction between age group and gender emerged (p = .09). As can be seen in Figure 10.2, girls' perceptions of their attachment to father became more negative over the middle-childhood years (3.12 at age 8 vs. 3.00 at age 11), whereas boys' perceptions of security remained the same (3.03 vs. 3.04, respectively). This is in accordance with the finding that, when reaching puberty, girls' relationships with fathers tend to become more distant (Lieberman et al., 1999).

When comparing the mean level of reported security with mother and father (using repeated-measures ANOVAs with gender of the child as the between-subjects and gender of the parent as the within-subjects variable), we found that self-reported security with mother was higher than self-reported security with father. This was true both at age 8, F (1, 253) = 16.66, p < .0001, and at age 11, F (1, 263) = 59.06, p < .0001. In line with results from the previous analyses, a significant interaction between gender of the parent and gender of the child was found at age 11, F (1, 263) = 5.96, p < .05, indicating that the aforementioned difference between the perceived security with mother and father was larger for girls than for boys.

In sum, although studies on the development of parent–child relationships during early adolescence have shown a decrease in self-reported attachment security to both parents with increasing age (Papini, Roggman, & Anderson, 1991), our longitudinal findings suggest that this decrease probably does not take place before the adolescent years. The mean level of security with father remained stable over time, and the mean level of perceived security with mother even increased from age 8 to age 11. Although the latter finding was unexpected, a closer look at the coping literature shows that a similar developmental difference has been found for children's strategies for coping with stress. As concluded by Fields and Prinz (1997), children in the later elementary school years were found to prefer adult support, whereas children in the lower elementary school grades preferred peer support. The authors explain this finding by pointing to the greater awareness of older children of how peers view them, causing them to be less willing to reveal their weaknesses to peers. In line with findings from other studies, feelings of global self-worth (SPPC) did show a decline with increasing age in the present study (mean scores of 3.28 and 3.09, respectively). Maybe the greater vulnerability to peer reactions, combined with an increase in internal stresses (such as an increase of worries about one's worthiness), temporarily lead to more reliance on parental attachment figures, and specifically more reliance on mothers.

Our findings also show that, in middle childhood, children report feeling more secure with their mothers than with their fathers. This means that, on average, they rely more on their mothers when seeking comfort and support and find it easier to communicate openly with their mothers. This is in line with results of Kobak's study (Kobak et al., Chapter 4, this volume) showing that, when probed for the preferred attachment figure, children in middle childhood generally prefer their mothers over their fathers. Our findings suggest that for girls this relative "preference" for mother over father becomes even more pronounced with increasing age.

Stability of Individual Differences in Attachment Security

The correlation between children's perceived security scores at age 8 and at age 11 was .28 ($p < .0001$) for mother and .37 ($p < .0001$) for father. In line with findings from Kerns and colleagues (2000), the stability coefficient was higher for father than for mother. This difference was, however, not significant (indicated by overlapping confidence intervals).

In sum, during the course of middle childhood, children tend to retain their relative positions among others on a continuum of attachment security. Children who are relatively more secure at age 8 are likely to remain relatively more secure at age 11. The stability we found was statistically significant, both for mother and for father. However, as shown by the magnitude of the coefficients, there is a lot of room for interindividual change over time (shared variance is only 8–14%). This modest stability may in part be due to the somewhat lower reliability of the 8-year-olds' responses to the measure. As reported previously, the internal consistency coefficients indeed increased with increasing age (from .73–.77 at age 8 to .83–.89 at age 11). On the other hand, it is possible that different children really show different developmental trajectories over time. In other words, some children may show decreasing and others increasing or stable perceptions of security over time, thus leading to low stability of interindividual differences. In further longitudinal research, involving more than two measurement times, it would be interesting to study the correlates of such differences in developmental trajectories.

Representations of Attachment to Mother and Father: Interrelation over Time

Results from confirmatory factor analyses reveal that, although the representations of attachment to mother and to father were moderately to highly related, a two-dimensional model in which the representation of attachment to mother and to father were treated as two separate dimensions appeared to fit the data better than a unidimensional model in which only one generalized attachment representation was assumed. (The fit of the model was, however, only adequate when a method factor and correlated measurement errors between similar items of the mother and father scales were included.) This provides evidence for the assumption that, in middle childhood, children have built separate representations of their attachment relationships with mother and with father. The correlation between the two latent constructs was higher at Time 1 as opposed to Time 2 (phi = .80 vs. 51). Correlations between the observed security scores for mother and for father were lower but lay in the same direction: Correlations were .60 and .47 at Time 1 and Time 2, respectively. Given that the Security Scale probes relationship-specific perceptions of attachment security, this seems to suggest that older children are better capable of differentiating between the qualities of the specific relationship they have with their mothers and with their fathers.

In sum, using the Security Scale, no evidence was found for the development of one overall, generalized representation of attachment during middle childhood. Instead, we found that older children are better able to differentially respond to the security items for mother and for father than younger children. This points to the development of more differentiated perceptions of the quality of the relationships with mother and father over the middle-childhood years. Hence, it definitely makes sense to separate the perceptions of attachment to mother and to father and to study their differential effects. Although these findings do not lend support to the hypothesis that more generalized attachment representations are developed across middle childhood, they do not contradict it either. As stated before, the Security Scale may not be suitable for testing this latter hypothesis. Other (interview-based) measures that probe the level of integration more directly may be more suitable.

Attachment to Mother and Father and Peer Relationships at School

As explained previously, the connection between attachment to father and peer relationships in middle childhood has been largely unexplored up to now. In this longitudinal study, we examined the association between perceived security of attachment to father and peer acceptance at age 8 and age 11. An examination of the bivariate correlations showed that, at both measurement times, children's perceived security of attachment to father was related significantly to the degree of acceptance by peers, r (255) = .13, p < .05, at age 8 and r (263) = .13, p < .05, at age 11. The correlations between perceived security of attachment to mother and the degree of peer acceptance was not significant in this study, r (254) = .01, $n.s.$ at age 8 and r (261) = −.08, $n.s.$ at age 11. In a longitudinal study in which children were followed from kindergarten to third grade, Verschueren and Marcoen (2003) also found that peer acceptance was predicted significantly by the earlier representation of attachment to father and not by the earlier representation of attachment to mother. These results add to the conclusion from Schneider and colleagues (2001) that felt security with mother may be especially predictive of children's functioning in more intimate small group or dyadic interactions, rather than of their popularity in the larger peer group. The reverse may be true for fathers (Verschueren & Marcoen, 2003).

Although the findings in this study support the differential effects found by Verschueren and Marcoen (2003), caution needs to be paid. First, the association of peer acceptance with the attachment to father was significant but only weak. Second, other studies (Granot & Mayseless, 2001; Kerns et al., 1996) did reveal a significant association between security of attachment to mother and acceptance within the larger peer group, indicating that the present findings call for further replication. Third, when the predictive value of security scores for mother and for father was compared directly by entering both as predictors into one multiple regression equation, we found that, at age 8, the predictive value of child–father attachment was not significantly higher than the predictive value of child–mother attachment (beta = .19, p < .05, for father vs. beta = −.11, $n.s.$ for mother). Only at age 11 was a significant difference between both regression coefficients obtained (beta = .21, p < .01, for father vs. beta = −.18, p < .05, for mother). Unexpectedly, we found that, when the effect of child–father attachment was controlled for, higher security scores for mother predicted lower acceptance in the peer group. In other words, in a group of children reporting equal levels of security with the father, 11-year-olds who reported feeling more secure with their mothers were (somewhat) less well liked in the peer group than age mates who reported feeling less secure.

In sum, both multivariate regression analyses and bivariate correlational analyses reveal that higher felt security with father (assessed by the Security Scale) was related to better social acceptance in school. This connection was found in third grade as well as in sixth grade. Given the lack of empirical research on the connection between child–father attachment and social functioning, especially in middle childhood, this finding is important in itself. The present study is less clear when it comes to evaluating the effects of child–mother attachment (as measured by the Security Scale) on children's acceptance in the peer group. Bivariate correlations were not significant, and—when controlling for effects of child–father attachment—a negative association even emerged. Although these findings need further replication, they point to the importance of (1) including both the attachment to mother and the attachment to father in future research on the correlates of attachment security and (2) taking into account the age of the children (or their developmental status) when formulating hypotheses concerning family–peer linkages: What may be beneficial for children's peer relations in one developmental period may turn out to be a risk factor later on.

Mediational Model: Does Global Self-Worth Mediate the Link between Attachment to Parents and Peer Acceptance?

Attachment theory not only predicts a link between the quality of attachment to parents and children's functioning in peer relationships but also offers an explanation for this relation. In this study, we tested whether the children's feelings of global self-worth could be considered a plausible mediating mechanism in explaining the link between attachment to parents and peer acceptance.

According to Baron and Kenny (1986), three conditions must hold in order to establish mediation. First, regression analysis must show that variations in the mediator (global self-worth) are significantly predicted by variations in the predictor (security of attachment). Second, when regressing the criterion variable (peer acceptance) on the predictor (attachment security), significant regression coefficients must be obtained. And third, when regressing the criterion variable on both the predictor and the mediator, the mediator must significantly affect the criterion. Given that these conditions are met, evidence for mediation occurs when, in the latter regression equation, a previously significant relation between the predictor (attachment security) and the criterion variable (peer acceptance) is no longer significant.

Simple regression analyses showed that the second condition was met only for attachment to father (beta = .13, p < .05 at age 8 and age 11) and not for attachment to mother. Hence, the mediational model could be tested only for child–father attachment. Results from the series of regression analyses conducted for the attachment to father were as follows.

At age 8, evidence for a mediational effect of global self-worth was found. Global self-worth was predicted significantly by the perceived security of attachment with father (beta = .34, p < .0001; Condition 1), and when peer acceptance was regressed on both global self-worth (the proposed mediator) and perceived security with father, the effect of the mediator was significant (beta = .20, p < .01; Condition 3), whereas the effect of perceived security with father was reduced to zero (beta = .06, p = .36). The Sobel (1982) test indicated that the indirect effect of perceived security of attachment to father on peer acceptance via the child's self-worth was significant, z = 2.65, p < .01.

At age 11, no evidence for the proposed mediational effect was found. Conditions 1 and 2 were met, but when peer acceptance was regressed on both perceived security of attachment to father and global self-worth, the connection with the mediator (global self-worth) was not significant (beta = –.07, p = .31), whereas the connection with the predictor (perceived security of attachment to father) remained significant (beta = .16, p < .05).

In sum, the current study provides (partial) support for the attachment-theoretic assumption that linkages between children's attachment to parents and their acceptance by peers is mediated by their feelings of self-worth. Specifically, it shows that children with a more secure relationship with their fathers tend to be better accepted by their peers because of the effect of attachment security on their global feelings of self-worth. However, this mediating effect was found only when the children were in third grade. In grade 6, peer acceptance was still related to perceived security of attachment to father, but the mechanism through which attachment security was able to affect peer acceptance appeared to have changed. Other mediating mechanisms that have been suggested in the literature include social information processing, emotion regulation, communication skills, and social behavioral skills (Booth-LaForce et al., Chapter 8, this volume; Verschueren & Marcoen, 2002). Rather than speculate on the (increased) relevance of some of these intervening processes across middle childhood, it seems preferable to await the results of empirical investigations of these mediation models. Due to the lack of connection between attachment to mother and peer acceptance, the mediating effect of global self-worth could not be tested for attachment to mother.

GENERAL DISCUSSION AND CONCLUSION

In a longitudinal study across the middle-childhood years, we investigated the developmental changes in the perceived security of attachment to mother and father and their (changing) associations with self-perceptions and peer relationships at school.

Results revealed, first, that the Security Scale is a unidimensional and reliable measure of perceived security of attachment to one specific partner. This does not necessarily mean that this "perceived" security of attachment is an accurate reflection of the actual quality of parent–child interactions. As stated by Kerns and colleagues (Chapter 3, this volume), responses to self-report measures such as the Security Scale may be susceptible to different kinds of conscious or unconscious distortions. In particular, it may be too hurtful for children to openly admit not being able to use the attachment figure as a secure base or safe haven. Attachment research in childhood and adulthood has indeed shown that some people do not report negative experiences with attachment figures (at an abstract level), even though there is evidence for such experiences (based on observations or on reports of concrete experiences; e.g., Main & Goldwyn, 1984–1998). However, in our opinion, this does not a priori dismiss the significance of using self-report measures in future research on attachment. On the contrary, when examining connections with children's psychosocial functioning and quality of parenting, it may be important to include both self-report assessments of attachment quality and observational or representational assessments. Only that way can the predictive value of the perceived or self-reported versus observed or inferred quality of attachment be tested empirically.

With regard to the developmental changes, we found that, on average, perceptions of security with mother increased across the middle-childhood years. This increase was, however, only small. Perceptions of security with father remained the same over time, although there was a trend for decreasing perceptions of security in girls as opposed to stable perceptions of security in boys. When evaluating the stability of individual differences, our study showed that during middle childhood, children tended to retain their relative position among others with regard to their perceived attachment security. Finally, results from the Security Scale suggest that in middle childhood children generally differentiate between their perceptions of their relationships with mother and with father and show increasingly differentiated perceptions of these relationships over time.

With regard to the connections with self-worth and peer relationships at school, we found that acceptance in the peer group was predicted by the perceived quality of attachment to father, both at age 8 and at age

11. Only at age 8, however, could this relation be explained by the mediational role of children's global self-worth. Perceived security of attachment to mother was not related to children's peer acceptance. As stated before, and in line with suggestions from Schneider and colleagues (2001), this may be due to the fact that our study focused only on children's acceptance in the larger peer group. Felt security with mother may be more predictive of children's functioning in friendships or other more intimate relationships.

In general, results invite researchers to further investigate the attachment relationships that children form with both their mothers and their fathers and to be careful when assuming that patterns of connections between these attachment relationships and other variables (peer relations) are similar across different developmental periods.

REFERENCES

Ainsworth, M. D. S. (1990). Epilogue: Some considerations regarding theory and assessment relevant to attachments beyond infancy. In M. T. Greenberg, D. Cicchetti, & E. M. Cummings (Eds.), *Attachment in the preschool years* (pp. 463–488). Chicago: University of Chicago Press.

Baron, R. M., & Kenny, D. A. (1986). The moderator–mediator variable distinction in social psychological research: Conceptual, strategic, and statistical considerations. *Journal of Personality and Social Psychology, 51,* 1173–1182.

Belsky, J., & Cassidy, J. (1994). Attachment: Theory and evidence. In M. Rutter & D. F. Hay (Eds.), *Development through life: A handbook for clinicians* (pp. 373–402). Oxford, UK: Blackwell.

Bretherton, I. (1985). Attachment theory: Retrospect and prospect. In I. Bretherton & E. Waters (Eds.), Growing points in attachment theory and research. *Monographs of the Society for Research in Child Development, 50*(1–2, Serial No. 209), 211–227.

Cassidy, J. (1988). Child–mother attachment and the self in six-year-olds. *Child Development, 59,* 121–134.

Fields, L., & Prinz, R. J. (1997). Coping and adjustment during childhood and adolescence. *Clinical Psychology Review, 17,* 937–976.

Granot, D., & Mayseless, O. (2001). Attachment security and adjustment to school in middle childhood. *International Journal of Behavioral Development, 25,* 530–541.

Hamilton, C. E., & Howes, C. (1992). A comparison of young children's relationships with mother and teachers. In R.C. Pianta (Ed.), *Beyond the parent: The role of other adults in children's lives: Vol. 57. New directions of child development* (pp. 41–59). San Francisco: Jossey-Bass/Pfeiffer.

Harter, S. (1985). *Manual for the Self-Perception Profile for Children.* Denver, CO: University of Denver.

Harter, S. (1990). Developmental differences in the nature of self-representations: Implications for the understanding, assessment, and treatment of maladaptive behavior. *Cognitive Therapy and Research, 14,* 113–142.

Harter, S. (1998). The development of self-representations. In W. Damon (Series Ed.) & N. Eisenberg (Vol. Ed.), *Handbook of child psychology: Vol. 3. Social, emotional, and personality development* (5th ed., pp. 553–617). New York: Wiley.

Kerns, K. A., Klepac, L., & Cole, A. (1996). Peer relationships and preadolescents' perceptions of security in the child–mother relationship. *Developmental Psychology, 32,* 457–466.

Kerns, K. A., Tomich, P. L., Aspelmeier, J. E., & Contreras, J. M. (2000). Attachment-based assessments of parent–child relationships in middle childhood. *Developmental Psychology, 36,* 614–626.

Ladd, G. W. (1992). Themes and theories: Perspectives on processes in family–peer relationships. In R. D. Parke & G. W. Ladd (Eds.), *Family–peer relationships: Modes of linkage* (pp. 3–34). Hillsdale, NJ: Erlbaum.

Lieberman, M., Doyle, A., & Markiewicz, D. (1999). Developmental patterns in security of attachment to mother and father in late childhood and early adolescence: Associations with peer relations. *Child Development, 70,* 202–213.

Main, M., & Goldwyn, R. (1984–1998). *Adult attachment scoring and classification system.* Unpublished manuscript, University of California at Berkeley.

Papini, D. R., Roggman, L. A., & Anderson, J. (1991). Early adolescent perceptions of attachment to mother and father: A test of the emotional distancing and buffering hypotheses. *Journal of Early Adolescence, 11,* 258–275.

Rose-Krasnor, L., Rubin, K. H., Booth, C. L., & Coplan, R. (1996). The relation between maternal directiveness and child attachment security to social competence in preschoolers. *International Journal of Behavioral Development, 19,* 309–325.

Schneider, B. H., Atkinson, L., & Tardif, C. (2001). Child–parent attachment and children's peer relations: A quantitative review. *Developmental Psychology, 37,* 86–100.

Singleton, L., & Asher, S. (1977). Peer preferences and social interactions among third-grade children in an integrated school district. *Journal of Educational Psychology, 69,* 330–336.

Sobel, M. E. (1982). Asymptotic intervals for indirect effects in structural equation models. In S. Leinhart (Ed.), *Sociological methodology* (pp. 290–312). San Francisco: Jossey-Bass.

Stevenson-Hinde, J., & Verschueren, K. (2002). Attachment in childhood. In P. K. Smith & C. Hart (Eds.), *Handbook of childhood social development* (pp. 182–204). London: Blackwell.

Thompson, R. A. (1999). Early attachment and later development. In J. Cassidy & P. R. Shaver (Eds.), *Handbook of attachment: Theory, research, and clinical applications* (pp. 265–286). New York: Guilford Press.

Veerman, J. W., Straathof, M. A. E., Treffers, A., Van den Bergh, B. R. H., & ten Brink, L. T. (1997). *Handleiding Competentiebelevingsschaal voor kinderen CBSK.* Lisse, The Netherlands: Swets & Zeitlinger.

Verschueren, K., & Marcoen, A. (1999). Representation of self and socioemotional

competence in kindergartners: Differential and combined effects of attachment to mother and to father. *Child Development, 70,* 183–201.
Verschueren, K., & Marcoen, A. (2002). Perceptions of self and relationship with
parents in aggressive and nonaggressive rejected children. *Journal of School
Psychology, 40,* 501–522.
Verschueren, K., & Marcoen, A. (2003, April). Kindergartners' representations of
attachment to father and mother: Differential effects on socio-emotional
functioning in middle childhood. In K. Grossman & H. Kindler (Chairs), *Fathers in longitudinal studies of socio-emotional development: Steps towards a theory
of the child–father relationship.* Symposium conducted at the biennial meeting
of the Society for Research in Child Development, Tampa, FL.
Verschueren, K., Marcoen, A., & Schoefs, V. (1996). The internal working model
of the self, attachment and competence in five-year-olds. *Child Development,
67,* 2493–2511.

CHAPTER 11

◆ ◆ ◆

Examining Relationships
between Students and Teachers

A Potential Extension of Attachment Theory?

LAURA T. ZIONTS

This chapter describes teacher–student relationship quality as it contributes to positive school adjustment and how the relationship can serve as either a risk factor or a protective factor for elementary-age students who demonstrate externalizing disorders or disorganized (D) attachment relationships with their primary caregivers. The notion of the teacher–student relationship as a form of attachment relationship is discussed within a theoretical framework. The potential for a teacher to serve as a "secure base" from which an early-elementary-school child can navigate new, frightening, or intimidating school environments is described, particularly as it relates to children who have disorganized attachment relationships with their primary caregivers. Finally, the chapter presents considerations of culture and ethnic values that may influence the interpretation of observed attachment behaviors on the part of the teacher, student, or researcher.

DISORGANIZED ATTACHMENTS
AND EXTERNALIZING BEHAVIOR DISORDERS

Specifically, this chapter addresses the teacher–student relationship quality in relation to children who have disorganized attachments to their primary caregivers or who have or are at risk for developing externalizing behavior disorders (as defined by the two terms "oppositional defiant disorder" and "conduct disorder" in DSM-IV [American Psychiatric Association, 1994]). Researchers have found associations between many forms of dysfunctional behavior and disorganized attachment between infants and primary caregivers (Carlson, 1998; Lyons-Ruth, Alpern, & Repacholi, 1993; Speltz, Greenberg, & DeKlyen, 1990). For example, family risk factors play an important role in the development of D-type attachment relationships between child and primary caregiver: higher rates of cumulative adversity (as defined by more than one of the following factors: low socioeconomic status, un- or underemployment, residing in a high crime community, etc.); parental mental illness(es); domestic abuse or violence in the home; and drug or alcohol abuse by parents (Lyons-Ruth, 1996; Lyons-Ruth, Easterbrooks, & Cibelli, 1997). Kennedy and Kennedy (2002) assert that it is the *combination and interactions among multiple risk factors* (i.e., biological risks, family or community level factors, poor parenting, and/or insecure attachment) that leads to disorganized (D) attachment, which in turn leads to aggressive, hostile, cooperatively manipulative, and punitive behaviors by school age (see Lyons-Ruth, 1996; Main & Cassidy, 1988; Solomon, George, & DeJong, 1995). Many of the same risk factors influence the development of externalizing behavior disorders (Kauffman, 2001; Mash & Wolfe, 2002; Prinz & Miller, 1991).

Disorganized attachments and externalizing behaviors seem to have a direct impact on school adjustment and academic achievement. Relationships between disorganized attachments with the primary caregiver and global academic functioning in elementary school have been documented (Moss & St-Laurent, 2001; Solomon et al., 1995), as have decreased abilities in attention, engagement, and motivation for mastery of academic content, in children without compared with children with secure attachment relationships (Moss & St-Laurent, 2001). Lyons-Ruth and colleagues (1993) found that hostile behaviors in preschool children were six times more likely to be demonstrated by children who have disorganized attachment styles than by securely attached children. In fact, kindergarteners who demonstrated hostile behaviors in school were more likely to: (1) have established a D-type relationship during infancy and (2) have mothers with a form of mental illness, such as clinical depression or schizophrenia. As indicated by Lyons-Ruth and colleagues, disorganized attachments during infancy tend to redevelop themselves during preschool years as either controlling–caregiving or controlling–punitive behaviors toward the primary caregiver (Moss, St-Laurent, Dubois-Comtois, & Cyr, Chapter 9, this volume).

Externalizing behaviors such as conduct disorder and oppositional defiant disorder in early childhood years can be demonstrated in a mixed pattern of internalizing and externalizing responses to social stimuli that can be difficult to interpret (Lyons-Ruth, 1996; Stormshak, Bierman, & the Conduct Problems Prevention Research Group, 1998). For instance, comorbid aggressive and withdrawn behaviors have been documented in children who show higher levels of academic failure, distractibility, dependency, emotional dysregulation, and peer rejection (Hymel, Bowker, & Woody, 1993; Ledingham & Schwartzman, 1984; Milich & Landau, 1984). Main and Solomon (1990) described a variety of child responses to stress and unfamiliar situations in D-type children, such as helplessness, apprehension, depressed behavior, approach–avoidance toward attachment figure, emotional dysregulation, or pieces from the other three attachment behavior styles used in unpredictable ways. Ladd and Burgess (1999) described the aggressive–withdrawn child's tendency to use withdrawn behaviors (such as withdrawing from peer interactions, playing alone, isolating themselves) in order to "reduce the demands placed on them by peers and teachers, and limit obligations that stem from relationships (e.g., responsibilities to partners, reciprocation of resources)" (p. 926). Therefore, children who demonstrate early behavioral aggression and those who demonstrate D-type attachments share a comparable set of:

1. Behaviors (i.e., ambivalence, apprehension, approach–avoidance, aggressive behaviors, noncompliance, emotional dysregulation)
2. School adjustment characteristics (i.e., poor academic performance, weak peer and teacher relationships, limited classroom-related social abilities such as sharing of resources or cooperative learning behaviors)
3. Outcomes (stable trajectories for school performance; stable trajectories for aggressive behaviors; stable trajectories for poor-quality peer, teacher, and parent relationships).

The need to intervene with children who demonstrate D-type attachments and externalizing behaviors during early elementary grades is evident from the stability of their academic and social trajectories (Kelley, Loeber, Keenan, & DeLamatre, 1997; Ladd & Burgess, 1999; Prinz & Miller, 1991).

Within this chapter, the terms "disorganized attachment" and "externalizing disordered" will be referred to as "D/EBD." When only one of the terms is used, the research or point of discussion refers solely to the term indicated.

ATTACHMENT THEORY'S SECURE-BASE CONCEPT

A definition of attachment theory that lends itself to the present discussion was provided by Bowlby (1979): "a way of conceptualizing the propensity of human beings to make strong affectational bonds to particular others and of explaining the many forms of emotional distress and personality disturbance, including anxiety, anger, depression and emotional detachment, to which unwilling separation and loss give rise" (p. 127). Although most frequently associated with mother–child dyads (Ainsworth, 1969; Ainsworth et al., 1978; Bowlby, 1958, 1969/1982), attachment relationships have been documented between foster parent and child (Schofield, 2002), father and child (Grossman et al., 2002), peers during adolescence (West, Rose, Spreng, Sheldon-Keller, & Adam, 1998), and romantic partners among adults (Crowell & Treboux, 1995). One's ability to form attachment bonds with more than one significant person across the lifespan is referred to as "multiple attachment relationships." Bowlby pointed out in a lecture to the Royal College of Psychiatrists that the common association of attachment theory with mother–child dyads was arbitrary because of the preponderance of easily accessible subjects of study at that time. Furthermore, he clearly stated that the theory was intended to apply equally to adults and children and to *whomever* is acting for the individual as an attachment figure.

Owens and colleagues (1995) proposed that behaviors in attachment relationships apart from that with one's primary caregiver may differ from traditional attachment behaviors commonly between primary caregiver and child, but they may still maintain the purpose and experience of attachments in a more typical sense (i.e., to give and receive care, to provide a sense of security when a perception of threat or fear is present, to offer protection from various environmental factors). According to Bowlby's (1979) estimates, more than half the children in the United States and Britain grow up experiencing a secure attachment relationship with a primary caregiver, the result of which is development of a representational model of themselves as worthy of help when needed and as capable of self-help in many situations. The role of the attachment caregiver is defined as being available, responsive when wanted, and willing to judiciously intervene should a problem or threat to the child arise (Bowlby, 1979). Those children who do not experience a secure attachment relationship with a primary caregiver have a significantly increased risk for developmental maladjustment (Bowlby, 1979; Steele & Steele, 1994).

Some of the most thought-provoking theoretical commentary on the nature of attachment theory as a developmental (lifespan) process was presented by Waters and Cummings (2000). These researchers assert that the critical component of attachment theory is the notion of having a "secure base." They expand upon familiar infant–toddler attachment contexts and behaviors to propose differentiated caregiver supports and relationship contexts as a function of developmental period, from infancy through adulthood. Important to their thesis is the central role of cognitive development and its implications for understanding the changing topography of the "secure base" through the lifespan. Waters and Cummings argued that connections between cognitive development and secure-base representations fulfill an important role in understanding the organization of attachment working models. They introduced the phrase "secure-base figures of convenience" to indicate the somewhat fluid use of peers, teachers, friends, and others as attachment figures as childhood evolves into adolescence. This terminology has potential applications for teachers or other adults as alternative secure bases to one's primary caregiver.

The consideration of the early elementary grade teacher as a "secure-base figure of convenience" could play a pivotal role in the school adjustment trajectory of children who have a history of D/EBD. Research has validated the perspective that children who have a secure relationship with a parent or primary caregiver will experience more positive school adjustment in the early elementary school grades (Moss, Rousseau, Parent, St-Laurent, & Saintonge, 1998; Pianta & Harbors, 1996). Preliminary studies indicate that in the absence of a secure attachment to one's primary caregiver, a teacher can play a protective role in the early school years. For example, teachers can foster positive school adjustment among children who are disorganized in attachment style or externalizing and aggressive in psychoeducational evaluation (Hughes, Cavell, & Jackson, 1999; Hughes, Cavell, & Willson, 2001).

The possible application of attachment theory to the classroom scenario posits the teacher in a comparable role to that of an "attachment figure of convenience" for the child who demonstrates high risk of aggression, psychopathy, antisocial behavior, and/or other externalizing behavior disorders (such as attachment type D within the child's actual parent–child relationship). In light of the importance of preventative and ameliorative interventions for children early in their developmental trajectory, the teacher's role as a potential substitute "attachment figure" would seem a potentially viable option, given the significant findings by researchers studying the impact of teacher–student relationship quality on school adjustment and psychological functioning in early school experiences.

Arguably, a traditional view of attachment relationships has considered a true attachment figure to be someone with whom the individual maintains a long-term relationship, presumably over years. However, given the possible application of attachment theory to the classroom-intervention scenario, the duration of the relationship may be less than a year. Consequently, there are three considerations for situations in which an attachment may be limited in duration. First, the student–teacher relationship has begun being extended in several school reform models. For example, in the "Classroom Looping" model, teachers are assigned a group of students in kindergarten, and they remain the primary teachers for the same group of students for a set number of subsequent grade levels (frequently through two or three grade levels). In this type of reform model, a teacher and student would have the benefit of an extended period of time during which to develop a secure relationship.

A second point to consider regarding the length of time in which the person acts as a secure base may be illustrated through examples of other situations in which a caregiver may serve as a secure base for a limited time period, such as a parent or, in the case of the adult, a spouse, who has a fatal illness. Although these situations would be likely to have a negative affect on the person's overall well-being, it must be noted that as of yet, researchers have not attempted to study the impact of relationships with significant individuals in cases in which the relationship is intentionally time limited in duration. One might argue that in such a situation, the negative repercussions of the issues of abandonment may be lessened because both parties knew that the relationship would be of a limited duration.

A third and final consideration is that, although some relationships with a person who serves as a secure base may end (the relationship ceases), other relationships may simply be redefined, as in the case of the parent and the adolescent or adult child who must realign their goals and negotiate new meaning to their shared relationship as the youth develops a stronger sense of independence and self-identity (Bowlby, 1988). So may be the case with the teacher as an attachment figure substitute. Specifically, many people recall teachers who believed in their abilities and with whom they felt a particularly strong connection. In fact, some people continued relationships with those teachers long after they had left the teachers' classrooms, stopping back for visits or hugs when still within one school building, writing letters or making purposeful visits when in different locations. Again, this notion has yet to be pursued through research, but such behaviors may indicate that the goal of creating a safe haven or secure base to support growth and gradual independence of the child have been successful.

THE RATIONALE FOR TEACHERS
AS SECURE-BASE INTERVENTIONS: WHY TEACHERS?

This chapter proposes the "teacher-as-a-secure-base" as a potential source of intervention for children identified as at risk for development of externalizing behavior disorders and for children who have disorganized attachments (D/EBD) with their primary caregivers. In order to explain the rationale for identifying teachers as possible intervention mechanisms to promote the increased mental health and behavioral appropriateness of children who have evidenced signs of D/EBD, we need to consider the research on school adjustment trajectories for and teacher–student relationships with young "at-risk" children who have the aforementioned characteristics.

School Adjustment Trajectories

School adjustment has been defined by Spencer (1999) as "the degree of school acculturation required or adaptations necessitated for maximizing the educational fit between the student's qualities and the multidimensional character and requirements of learning environments" (p. 43). Children who have poor school adjustment are more likely to be retained or referred for special education, to fail course work, to have fewer friends, to be subject to more frequent disciplinary actions, to have higher absenteeism, and to fail to complete high school (Alexander, Entwistle, & Dauber, 1995; Robertson, Chamberlain, & Kasari, 2003). Current evidence points to the importance of the quality of the teacher–student relationship in mediating positive or negative school adjustment in elementary-school children (Hughes et al., 1999, 2001; Pianta, 1999).

Pianta (1999) reported that the early school years have a strong influence on the trajectories of children's later adjustment in school and in their relationships with adults and peers. Pianta and Walsh (1996) consider the early years to serve as a "sensitive period" in which developmental trajectories can be greatly influenced, a conclusion that was supported by Esposito's (1999) findings. Alexander and Entwistle (1988; Alexander, Entwistle, & Dauber, 1995) conducted a longitudinal study of a cohort of children from kindergarten throughout their school years and found that by the end of third grade the children's developmental pathways are reasonably stable. Children who have been identified as having emotional and behavioral problems often experience a history of conflict in their relationships with teachers and peers (Hughes et al., 1999, 2001; Pianta, Steinberg, & Rollins, 1995). Student relationships with peers and teachers interact with other risk factors to modify their developmental pathways (Berndt, 1999; Hughes et al., 1999, 2001; Pianta, 1999).

As indicated in a longitudinal study of the malleability of aggression from first grade through middle school, early elementary transition to first grade parallels the important transition to middle school in that both represent developmental challenges that draw upon existing social skills and strategies for adaptation to new demands, new natural raters (i.e., teachers), and more complex influences from peers (Kellam, Rebok, Ialongo, & Mayer, 1994). Kellam and his colleagues hypothesize that if this developmental trajectory has been disrupted at any earlier point (such as by parental abuse or neglect or by other family dysfunction), resulting in maladaptive skills or behaviors such as aggressive or withdrawn behaviors or relational aggression, the new challenges provided within these key childhood transitions will evidence further maladaptive responses from the child. However, protective interventions through the classroom teacher (such as reframing the relationship to better support and nurture the child, i.e., providing a secure base) can affect the quality of future school relationships with teachers and peers (Hughes et al., 2001; Ladd & Burgess, 2001; Pianta, Teitbohl, & Bennett, 1997), the future levels of aggression among males who exhibit early and high levels of aggression in first grade (Kellam et al., 1994), and future academic performance (Williams, Ayer, Abbot, Hawkins, & Catalano, 1999).

The Nature of Teacher–Student Relationships

Theoretical frameworks for teacher–student relationship analyses are based most frequently in Bronfenbrenner's (1979) human ecological theory in attachment theory (Bowlby, 1969/1982, 1973, 1980) and in general systems theory (Sameroff, 1983). Researchers have ascribed to many variations on these theories in their effort to explain variance in relationships between teachers, peers, and students and the impact of those relationships on individuals' developmental trajectories (Bergman & Magnusson, 1997; Cairns & Rodkin, 1997; Cairns, Cairns, Rodkin, & Xie, 1998; Magnusson, 1997). Despite the differences and variations in theoretical interpretation and research design, an undergirding philosophy of these theories is the common perception that perspectives on developmental risk and childhood psychopathology are significantly enhanced by the study of configurations of behaviors, relationships, and child and adult characteristics that predict negative or positive outcomes for children. Given that children who are identified as having a D/EBD are at higher risk for childhood maladjustment or psychopathology, it seems pertinent to examine teacher–student attachment relationships as a possible intervention mechanism.

Howes (Howes, Hamilton, & Matheson, 1994; Howes & Matheson, 1992; Howes, Matheson, & Hamilton, 1994) has examined the relationship parallels between child–teacher relationships and mother–child attachments. She concluded that mother–child relationship dynamics influence the quality and nature of teacher–child interactions and relationship quality. Although both have an impact on the child's interactions with peers, teachers have a stronger impact on the quality of peer interactions in the classroom than do mothers (Howes, Hamilton, & Matheson, 1994). Peers, through their rejection of a behaviorally disorganized student, have a statistically significant negative impact on a student's level of cooperation in the classroom (Ladd, 1997) and on increasing attention problems and decreasing school achievement (Ladd & Burgess, 2001).

Lynch and Cicchetti (1992) concluded from their research that children who have experienced neglectful or abusive relationships with their primary caregivers are prone to actively trying to engage their teachers in relational interactions that are patterned after their own maladjusted experiences. However, they continue to seek support from their teachers in order to validate their worth and ability. Several researchers have reasoned that close teacher–student relationships can provide students in the early years of schooling with the emotional security, guidance, and aid that will facilitate successful adaptation to the school environment (Birch & Ladd, 1996; Howes, Matheson, & Hamilton, 1994). In terms of attachment theory, this role could potentially be defined as a "secure base."

Teacher–child relationship dynamics are reported to have moderate levels of stability from kindergarten through second grade and to correlate with future teacher actions such as referral for special education evaluation, grade retention, and reports of school adjustment (Birch & Ladd, 1997; Pianta et al., 1995). However, a key finding by Pianta and his colleagues (1995) is that closeness to teachers appears to function as a protective factor against risk. In their study, "high risk" was defined as likelihood of special education referral or retention on the basis of emotional difficulties or behavioral aggression, both of which can be demonstrated by disorganized children. Children who were referred or retained experienced significantly greater levels of conflict with the teachers than those who were not retained or referred. Arranging classroom-based interventions for disorganized children and others who have emotional or behavioral disorders around a systematic attempt to increase secure-base behaviors may capitalize on the protective features of the close teacher–child relationship.

Student–Teacher Relationship Variables That May Moderate Secure-Base Use and Secure-Base Support

Teacher and student feelings about their relationship can influence continued or increased levels of conflict. Student behavior, attentiveness, and dependency are predictors of decreased teacher ratings of student–teacher relationship quality (Robertson, Chamberlain, & Kasari, 2003). Similarly, student interpretations of teacher affect toward the student can predict misbehavior, noncompliance, and decreased school performance (Birch & Ladd, 1998; Ladd & Burgess, 2001). Alternately, positive relationship qualities, such as caring, sharing of information, and the provision of emotional and academic support, can increase cooperation and compliance in classroom activities (Ladd & Burgess, 2001).

Children who have been identified as having behavioral problems often experience a history of conflict in their relationships with teachers and peers (Hughes et al., 1999, 2001; Pianta, Steinberg, & Rollins, 1995). This is a significant finding in that the teacher's or student's feelings and beliefs about their relationship can inform continued or increased conflict. Stormshak and colleagues (1998) describe the process whereby oppositional, impulsive/inattentive, and aggressive behaviors may increase the likelihood of a child becoming engaged in negative or coercive adult interactions, which in turn lead to the further development of such behaviors in a cyclical process. The predictability of decreased teacher–student relationship quality as a function of student behavior, attentiveness, and dependency is stable across children with and without disabilities (Robertson et al., 2003).

A final factor that may affect the likelihood of the teacher becoming a secure base for a given child (who has D/EBD) is the ability of the teacher to *serve as* a "secure base." Posada, Waters, Crowell, and Lay (1995) have found that it is easier for secure adults to serve as a secure base for others than it is for insecure adults because of their better caregiving and listening skills and responding patterns. There does not appear to be research available on the attachment status of teachers or how that may or may not be reflected in the quality of relationship they experience with externalizing (aggressive/oppositional) and D-type children. Nor is there research regarding the training of teachers to act as secure bases for students.

The Effects of Teacher–Student Relationship Quality on Peer Relations

Teachers and students who establish a strong supportive bond can positively influence the student's peer relationships. Teacher perceptions of the child–teacher relationship may also influence peer acceptance. A study of 229 children by Zionts, Anhalt, Devore and Davidson (2004) identified 96 children rated by their teachers as either "prosocial," "aggressive," or "both prosocial and aggressive" using the Teacher Report Form of the Achenbach Child Behavior Checklist (1991). Although students identified as "aggressive" in this analysis received above a .60 on the aggression subscale, sociometric measures completed by peers revealed that peers were significantly more likely to rate the aggressive child as "getting in trouble" than as "aggressive" or "mean." This indicates that children were more cognizant of teacher–student relationship dynamics than of the actual aggressive acts of the child. When a teacher has a negative perception of a child, which is more likely to occur when a child demonstrates relational or overt aggression, irritability, impulsivity, and academic difficulties, peers are likely to indicate lower levels of social acceptance of the student.

According to Hymel (1986; Hymel, Wagner, & Butler, 1990) peers may use information learned from interchanges between a student and a teacher to interpret future student interactions. In the situation in which teachers have developed a close, secure relationship with the child who exhibits disorganized behaviors or emotional disorders, the ameliorative effect of teacher acceptance may mediate the child's acceptance by peers. Taylor (1989) found that when teachers report liking a peer-rejected child and having a more positive relationship with the child, the child was less likely to be rejected by peers in subsequent years. These findings further substantiate the importance of the student-and-teacher relationship.

Ladd and Burgess (2001) studied 396 children during their first 2 years of school. They proposed an "additive risk" model that separated the risk associated with aggressive behaviors from relational risks with peers, parents, and other adults that typically result from aggression (such as peer rejection and teacher–child conflict). In their model, relational risks increased the probability that aggressive children would become dysfunctional or maladaptive in the school environment and would display increasing thought and attention problems. Relational risks were hypothesized to strengthen disobedience and decrease cooperation.

Risk factors were balanced in Ladd and Burgess's (2001) model by hypothesized protective factors, such as peer support, mutual friendships, and teacher–student caring. Protective factors predicted increases in school liking and scholastic engagement and decreases in misconduct. Among the many important findings was the fact that strength in teacher–student caring and lack of teacher–student conflict had a statistically significant impact on the overall school adjustment of aggressive children, regardless of initial level of aggression. Additionally, students who evidenced high, stable levels of aggression in kindergarten and first grade but who also experienced a caring teacher–student relationship and peer support demonstrated increased obedience during classroom activities and an increased level of school liking by the end of first grade (Ladd & Burgess, 2001). The results speak to the significance of promoting a strong attachment relationship between teacher and child for the child who does not have a strong relationship with a primary caregiver. A sense of belongingness in the class and peer acceptance had a significant impact on overall positive school adjustment for behaviorally aggressive children who display emotional maladjustment in early grades. Previous studies indicate that the teacher's support and caring, demonstrated through daily interactions, can affect peer acceptance (Hymel, 1986; Hymel et al., 1990).

Moreover, Ladd and Burgess (2001) found that these results were most significant when the child's exposure to relational risk factors was chronic (i.e., parental dysfunction, violence or abuse in the home, etc.) as opposed to situational (i.e., briefer exposure to risk factors). The D/EBD child is likely to live with chronic stressors; therefore, the findings indicate that using the teacher to provide security, safety, and support does seem to have a positive impact on school performance and on later intensified aggressive behavior. When aggressive children received sustained peer acceptance, they tended to demonstrate fewer attention problems in the classroom.

THE ISSUE OF CULTURAL DISCONTINUITY

The primary goal of a "secure attachment" relationship is to provide the child a safe haven from which the world can be explored for increasing periods of independence, with the security of knowing that protection and comfort will be available to him and her from the caregiver as needed (Bowlby, 1979). Healthy children experience gradual independence from their primary caregivers. This may affect their adult attachment relationships as they shift their primary attachments to peers and life partners throughout the lifespan (Carnelley, Pietromonaco, & Jaffe, 1994; Cooper, Shaver, & Collins, 1998; Owens et al., 1995; Weinfield, Sroufe, & Egeland, 2000).

Indeed, Bowlby (1979) argues that individuals will continue to demonstrate the characteristics of their attachment style, because whatever representational models of "attachment figures and of self the individual builds during his childhood and adolescence will tend to persist relatively unchanged into and throughout adult life" (p. 141). Still, the secure attachment theoretically provides the optimal condition for growth and development of independence, and "those who are most stable emotionally and making the most of their opportunities are [those who experience a secure attachment relationship with their parent]" (p. 12).

A final variable pertinent to the present discussion of attachment theory as it may relate to teacher–student relationship quality is that of cultural discontinuity. Although several studies have attempted to better understand the role of teacher–student ethnicities on the quality of the student-and-teacher relationship, none to date have examined this variable from the perspective of attachment theory. The relevance of ethnicity and culture to attachment theory as it may relate to student–teacher relationship quality is most evident in the interpretation of the relationship by each party and, importantly, also in the interpretation of the dyadic interactions by researchers. This section addresses both the general difficulty of behavioral interpretation of participants by observers and the ways in which culture-based behaviors and perspectives must be examined for their potential to affect the likelihood of using a teacher as a secure base.

The ethnic or cultural identity of an individual was considered by Bowlby (1988) a relevant source of variation in attachment behavior. He cited examples of studies by cultural anthropologists in which cultural patterns of caretaking and caregiving vary and are relative in their appropriateness and utility. A particular example was of a cultural group in the South Seas area who shared a custom during and after childbirth (Bowlby, 1988). The mother would be cared for by female relatives during the first month of the baby's life, so that she may in turn concentrate on caring for her baby. According to Bowlby's interpretation, the female relatives provided practical assistance and served as a "secure base" for the mother during a time of stress and uncertainty.

Still, Bowlby (1988) also recognized that within clinical circles attachment behaviors were at times misinterpreted or perceived inaccurately. An example he provides is that of the adolescent who manifests attachment behaviors that are interpreted by clinicians as "regressive" or inappropriate, whereas the adolescent him- or herself would have characterized those same behaviors as entirely appropriate, practical manifestations of attachment behavior as it occurs during adolescence. In much the same way, researchers from the majority culture who attempt to study ethnicity and culture within our broader society often seem as genuinely misled in their interpretations of observed behavior as the clinicians Bowlby previously described.

The notion of "role reversal" in attachment theory (Bowlby, 1973, 1980) is an example of a cultural interpretation that can seem clear at first and yet perhaps worthy of another view. Theoretically, role reversal indicates that interactions occur between child and caregiver in which the child takes on the role of the parent and the parent of the child. Bowlby (1979) argues that many children who suffer from school phobia and agoraphobia probably developed these phobias through exposure to an insecure attachment to a caregiver who pressured the child to act as the parent or adult in the dyadic interactions. In a typical role-reversal situation, a parent who has argued with her spouse is consoled by her child. However, it is possible that appropriate coding of observed attachment behaviors may not be thoroughly understood by a researcher from the primary (or majority) culture. An example may occur in a family in which the parent has intentionally chosen to raise her children to demonstrate interdependence rather than independence as a primary outcome for adulthood. Within an interdependent value, each member of the family learns to respect and care for the others, placing the needs of others in the family above their own. Independent self-care and responsibility are also strongly valued, following as a close second to caring for the family. Alternately, in a culture that chooses to emphasize independence, the value of self-responsibility and self-care are valued as primary outcomes, whereas caring for others is a second, though it also may be a valued, outcome. In a teacher–student relationship situation, the issue of independence versus interdependence may also be misunderstood due to differing cultural practices on the part of the teacher and the family.

According to a report from the National Educators Association (NEA, 2002), more than one third of students in today's public schools are children of color. By the year 2025, it is estimated that children of color will increase to at least 50%. Teachers of color, however, currently make up 13% of all teachers. Approximately 40% of U.S. schools do not have a school staff member who is a member of a cultural/ethnic minority group. The possible cross-cultural misinterpretations are evident.

To examine the school-based applications of cultural behaviors, take as an example the Mexican family whose credo is *"Todas para la familia"* (in English, "Everything for the family"). During a chaotic morning rush in which the elementary-age children must leave for school and both parents must leave for their respective jobs, the phone rings. A child answers the family phone. The morning continues at rapid-fire pace, as usual. Upon exiting the car when being dropped at school by the parent, the child says to the parent, "The doctor called. Your appointment today was cancelled. I wrote down her number and put it in your purse so you wouldn't forget it at home in the hurry of the morning." On the one hand, a majority-culture attachment researcher may code that exchange as "role reversal" because it could be interpreted that the child is taking care of the mother. On the other hand, the parent may be overwhelmed with satisfaction at a job well done—her child had independently demonstrated the exact skill the parent had been nurturing and modeling for years, interdependence (taking care of and responsibility for one another to accomplish a common goal, in this case getting the family to school or work on time in an orderly fashion).

Who is to say which interpretation is more accurate? Perhaps both. But if coded as role reversal, according to Bowlby (1988), an intervention might be recommended due to the negative outcomes that could be expected to result. If perceived from the perspective of the parent, this child is growing into the exact type of caring and dedicated family member she has tried so hard to raise. How does one determine which is the "correct" interpretation of the behavior that occurred? On what basis is the conclusion about the behavioral interpretation drawn? Is it incorrect to parent a child in ways that contradict the predominant culture (assuming that they do not cause physical injury nor include illegal or immoral activity)? Is it incorrect to determine that a parenting style is improper based on one's own values (when those values are shared by the majority of individuals around you)? At this point, these questions have only been raised, but no clear answers have been offered beyond the perspectives and opinions of individuals.

As a second example, consider the same family: The school principal has stopped the parent at the front desk of the school on a morning when he is dropping off a forgotten library book that was due that day. The principal is describing to the parent (again) that by bringing the child forgotten items, the parent is undermining the child's opportunity to develop responsibility and independence. It does the child an injustice, claims the principal. To this the parent calmly begins to explain (again) that in his family, the most important thing his children need to learn is that everyone looks out for one another. That value is what will assist them most as adults because no one lives their life independent of others. People are never successful only because of their own actions. Family support and a sense of shared responsibility will be what matters most when life becomes trying and stressful for his children, even when they become adults.

Again in this example, there is one set of events and behaviors and two very different interpretations of them. Clearly, the former (the principal's) perspective is the more traditional mainstream interpretation in our society. It reflects the belief system held within the predominant culture. Most of our researchers, direct-service providers, and teachers share membership within the majority culture. Therefore, it is often easy to find validation (interrater reliability) for one's observational coding and for interpretation of data collected, regardless of the relativity of the values being debated. This problem is compounded in importance by the recent federal regulations that funding agencies require inclusion of culturally diverse samples in all funded studies. Although the attempt to diversify our knowledge base and extend our generalizability is applauded, the obvious problem that remains is the interpretation of collected data (e.g., the actions and behaviors that reflect values and perspectives that are not obvious to researchers and easily misunderstood or misinterpreted). Some behavioral interpretations are not recognized as the value-laden judgments they truly are, even when specifically called to the attention of the researcher(s). The predominant culture is exactly that—predominant in thoughts, interpretations, and "scientific" theories and interventions.

There are no clear resolutions to situations in which interpretations must be made of the culture or values of another. Perhaps the best one can hope for is to be aware that the situations and challenges exist. Researchers are challenged to interpret behaviors that carry meaning and that may or may not fit well within a set theory. However, consider next the attempt to discern a goodness-of-fit between attachment theory and student–teacher relationships when the teacher and student do not share a common ethnic or cultural background.

Teacher–Student Relationship Issues of Cultural Discontinuity

When teachers and children do not share a common background, it is likely that misinterpretations of the others' behaviors, values, and intentions may arise. Current attachment research has not yet explored the intersection of ethnic/cultural values and behaviors with the demonstration of behaviors indicative of a secure-base relationship between student and teacher, nor has the potential for the use of teacher as intervention agent for children who demonstrate disorganized attachment to their primary caregiver been fully examined.

Specific correlates of relationship quality between teacher, child, and parent are needed in terms of how shared ethnicity/culture and differing cultures/ethnicities among the individuals may affect the validation, understanding, and shared teaching of "independent" behaviors and how "security" is conveyed to the child (both in terms of words and behaviors). Future studies need to interpret these nuances of attachment behaviors within U.S. culture by some measure of cultural identity for each participant. This will be difficult because children haven't yet reached a level of cognitive development to fully express such notions (Bracey, Bamaca, & Umana-Taylor, 2004; Prinz & Miller, 1991). It would also seem that differences in the findings (as in the examples provided in this chapter) would be much easier to overlook if all of the individuals shared a U.S. identity and separate cultural or ethnic group identifications (Mexican American and African American or white American), as opposed to comparing behavioral and value-based interpretations of Americans who live in America with Palestinians who live in Palestine.

How do the behavioral and value-laden interpretations of cultural and ethnic group relate to teacher–student relationships? In terms of home–school collaboration, there seems to be a link between the cultural/ethnic considerations and the provision of security and safety to any given child, as well as to the process of teaching independence in a way that is acceptable to both parents and teacher. If a teacher is to serve as a "secure-base figure of convenience" (Waters & Cummings, 2000) but his or her values of interdependence or dependence or methods for expressing comfort and security are not in agreement with the values or behavioral expectations of the family, then the relationship could feasibly create more chaos than comfort. Unresolved questions exist about the potential for secure-base relationships to form when the teacher-and-student dyad do not share the same cultural/ethnic identity (which is likely in U.S. public schools). Further research from an attachment orientation is needed to examine questions such as how easily (likely?) an attachment bond may be formed when the family and teacher do not share a common set of cultural behaviors or beliefs (i.e., the teacher is "into" independence and the parents are "into" interdependence or vice versa). How easily may a child form an attachment relationship with one or another adult (i.e., parent or teacher) when differences do exist? Do cultural values and practices matter to the child on any level, or does the child receive the message he or she needs of safety and security from either person, regardless of cultural nuances in which they are expressed?

Again, the option of teacher as attachment figure of convenience would seem appropriate only for the situation in which a dysfunctional attachment with the primary caregiver has already transpired. Research on the intended population would carry its own set of multivariate family-related factors (to include socioeconomic status, alcohol/drug abuse, and physical, sexual, or emotional abuse, each of which carries many of its own cultural behaviors and values). To be certain, better understanding the influence of authentic teacher and student ethnic/cultural contributions to the likelihood of a secure-base bond forming between teacher and child will be a difficult undertaking from a research perspective. However, it seems pertinent to the exploration of how plausible the teacher–student intervention may be.

CONCLUSIONS

Recently, Berryhill and Prinz (2003) argued that interventions to improve school adjustment, emotional functioning, and sense of school belongingness would be difficult to implement in schools in this era of teacher and student academic accountability. When testing is mandated, teachers and administrators must devote their attention first to interventions that improve student academic performance. However, they further argue, "it may be that environments that fit children well do not make all of them top students but nonetheless help them have more positive experiences that cause them to stay in school" (p. 82).

Clearly, research suggests that teachers can play a pivotal role in providing a "secure base" in academic settings and that the presence of a high-quality teacher–student relationship may ameliorate the effects of a lower quality relationship with one's primary caregiver. The children most at risk for developing externalizing behavior disorders share many overlapping causes, characteristics, and outcomes with children who have evidenced disorganized attachments to their primary caregiver. Evidence suggests that teachers who establish positive and caring relationships with such children can, over time, affect their current and future school adjustment and social and academic proficiency. Children who fail to attain a "secure base" as they adjust to the demands of school by middle childhood are at higher risk for academic failure, social exclusion, referral for special education, and grade retention; by high school they are at risk for a greater likelihood of dropping out prior to graduation, participating in risky behaviors, and finding social acceptance by other maladjusted youths. Through continued research into the dynamics of the teacher–child relationship, the nurturing of teacher–student relationships as a specific preventative intervention point may prove to become a viable option.

IMPLICATIONS FOR FUTURE RESEARCH

Many questions remain to be answered through systematic inquiry into teacher–student relationships. Despite the fact that existing research has suggested connections between and influences of teacher–child relationships and mother–child relationships, specific information has yet to be determined about what constitutes the quality of the teacher–student relationship and at what point along a relationship quality continuum school adjustment may be affected positively or negatively.

The notion of the "secure base of convenience" (Gao & Waters, 1998) must be further developed. What qualities of a secure-base relationship specifically align with a typical teacher's role in a classroom environment? What are the limitations to a teacher–student relationship in meeting the intended goals of independence and security? Are there modifications to the relationship that can make a secure relationship between an individually targeted child more plausible in an environment generally deprived of adequate time, attention to the individual, and resources? How would children most likely to fit the D-type category or the externalizing behavior category be identified for intervention? What are the impacts of the high-quality relationship or "secure base of convenience" outside of the classroom/school setting? How much time is needed to establish and maintain a high-quality relationship between a teacher and a behaviorally challenging or D-type student? How long does the relationship continue to support the child? What happens to the child's level of independence and security when the teacher with whom the child bonded is replaced? What amount of variance in the developmental trajectory of the child for whom this intervention may be considered is explained by such an intervention? Clearly there are numerous questions that remain before attachment theory can be proposed as a viable intervention option between teacher and child. These questions have not even broached the topic of culture discussed previously in the chapter.

Research into cultural variations on attachment theory within U.S. populations is a critical if one is to apply the concept of teacher–student attachment as a possible intervention approach for children at risk for poor school adjustment. Studies thus far have included teachers and students of varying races and ethnicities, but very specific questions about interpersonal relationship behaviors and attitudes, in addition to the possible cultural (mis)interpretations of social behaviors between students who do not share the same cultural group identity with their teachers, must be explored within the larger U.S. culture. Student–teacher dyads in which teacher–student ethnicity or culture are shared and those in which the student and teacher have different ethnicities or cultures must be studied with attention to the impact of cultural interpretation and expectations of the relationship. This research must also include other contextual factors, such as socioeconomic status, language, teacher training, and attachment issues of both primary-care provider and teacher.

Attachment theory shows promise in terms of its potential application for school-based settings. However, at this point in our theoretical and practical applications of the theory, there are more questions remaining than answers discernable through the existing research. This chapter has attempted to integrate attachment theory concepts with existing research and literature to provide the reader with a foundation from which to explore the plausibility of extending the theory to classroom-based intervention for children who have D-type attachments and/or externalizing behavior problems. Given the stability of academic and interpersonal outcomes for children who fit within these two categories, it seems necessary to find approaches to intervention that are based solidly in theory, that are effective and efficient to implement, and that have promising a longitudinal impact on children's developmental outcomes.

REFERENCES

Achenbach, T. M. (1991). *Manual for the Child Behavior Checklist/4–18 and 1991 profile*. Burlington: University of Vermont, Department of Psychiatry.

Ainsworth, M., Blehar, M., Waters, E., & Wall, S. (1978). *Patterns of attachment.* Hillsdale, NJ: Erlbaum.

Ainsworth, M. D. S. (1969). Object relations, dependency, and attachment: A theoretical review of the infant–mother relationship. *Child Development, 40,* 969–1025.

Alexander, K., & Entwistle, D. R. (1988). Achievement in the first two years of school: Patterns and processes. *Monographs of the Society for Research in Child Development, 53*(2, Serial No. 218).

Alexander, K., Entwistle, D. R., & Dauber, S. L. (1995). *On the success of failure.* New York: Cambridge University Press.

American Psychiatric Association. (1994). *Diagnostic and statistical manual of mental disorders* (4th ed.). Washington, DC: Author.

Bergman, L. R., & Magnusson, D. (1997). A person-oriented approach in research on developmental psychopathology. *Development and Psychopathology, 9*(2), 291–319.

Berndt, T. J. (1999). Friends' influence on adjustment to school. *Educational Psychologist, 34,* 15–28.

Berryhill, J. C., & Prinz, R. L. (2003). Environmental interventions to enhance student adjustment: Implications for prevention. *Prevention Science, 4*(2), 65–87.

Birch, S., & Ladd, G. (1996). Interpersonal relationships in the school environment and children's early school adjustment: The role of teachers and peers. In J. Juvonen & K. R. Wentzel (Eds.), *Social motivation: Understanding children's school adjustment* (pp. 199–225). New York: Cambridge University Press.

Birch, S., & Ladd, G. (1997). The teacher–child relationship and children's early school adjustment. *Journal of School Psychology, 35,* 61–79.

Birch, S. H., & Ladd, G. W. (1998). Children's interpersonal behaviors and the teacher–child relationship. *Developmental Psychology, 34,* 934–946.

Bowlby, J. (1958). The nature of the child's tie to its mother. *International Journal of Psycho-analysis, 39,* 350–373.

Bowlby, J. (1973). *Attachment and loss: Vol. 2. Separation, anxiety and anger.* New York: Basic Books.

Bowlby, J. (1979). The making and breaking of affectional bonds. In J. Bowlby (Ed.), *The making and breaking of affectional bonds* (pp. 126–160). London: Routledge.

Bowlby, J. (1980). *Attachment and loss: Vol. 3. Loss.* New York: Basic Books.

Bowlby, J. (1982). *Attachment and loss: Vol. 1 Attachment* (rev. ed.). London: Hogarth Press. (Original work published 1969)

Bowlby, J. (1988). *A secure base: Parent–child attachment and healthy human development.* New York: Basic Books.

Bracey, J. R., Bamaca, M. Y., & Umana-Taylor, A. J. (2004). Examining ethnic identity and self-esteem among biracial and monoracial adolescents. *Journal of Youth and Adolescence, 33,* 123–132.

Bronfenbrenner, U. (1979). *The ecology of human development: Experiments by nature and design.* Cambridge, MA: Harvard University Press.

Cairns, R. B., Cairns, B. D., Rodkin, P., & Xie, H. (1998). New directions in developmental research: Models and methods. In R. Jessor (Ed.), *New perspectives on adolescent risk behavior* (pp. 13–40). New York: Cambridge University Press.

Carlson, E. (1998). A prospective longitudinal study of attachment disorganization/disorientation. *Child Development, 69*, 1107–1128.

Carnelley, K. B., Pietromonaco, P. R., & Jaffe, K. (1994). Depression, working models of others, and relationship functioning. *Journal of Personality and Social Psychology, 66*(1), 127–140.

Cooper, D. H., & Speece, D. L. (1990). Ontogeny of school failure: Classification of first-grade children. *American Educational Research Journal, 27*(1), 119–140.

Cooper, M. L., Shaver, P. R., & Collins, N. L. (1998). Attachment styles, emotion regulation, and adjustment in adolescence. *Journal of Personality and Social Psychology, 74*(5), 1380.

Crowell, J., & Treboux, D. (1995). A review of adult attachment measures: Implications for theory and research. *Social Development, 4*, 294–327.

Esposito, C. (1999). Learning in the urban blight: School climate and its effect on the school performance of urban, minority, low-income children. *School Psychology Review, 28*, 365–377.

Gao, Y., & Waters, E. (1998, June). *Secure base behavior and attachment security in engaged couples.* Paper presented at the meeting of the International Society for the Study of Personal Relationships, Saratoga Springs, NY.

Grossman, K., Grossman, K. E., Fremmer-Bombik, E., Kindler, H., Scheuerer-Englisch, H., & Zimmerman, P. (2002). The uniqueness of the child–father attachment relationship and challenging play as a pivotal variable in a 16-year longitudinal study. *Social Development, 11*(3), 307–331.

Howes, C., Hamilton, C. E., Matheson, C. C. (1994). Children's relationships with peers: Differential associations with aspects of the teacher–child relationship. *Child Development, 65*(1), 253–263.

Howes, C., & Matheson, C. (1992). Contextual constraints on the concordance of mother–child and teacher–child relationships. In R. C. Pianta (Ed.), *New Directions in Child Development: Vol. 57. Relationships between children and nonparental adults* (pp. 25–90). San Francisco: Jossey-Bass.

Howes, C., & Matheson, C., & Hamilton, C. E. (1994). Maternal, teacher, and child care history correlates of children's relationships with peers. *Child Development, 65*, 264–273.

Hughes, J., Cavell, T., & Jackson, T. (1999). Influence of the teacher–student relationship on childhood conduct problems: A prospective study. *Journal of Clinical Child Psychology, 28*(2), 173–184.

Hughes, J. N., Cavell, T. A., & Willson, V. (2001). Further support for the developmental significance of the quality of the teacher–student relationship. *Journal of School Psychology, 39*(4), 289–301.

Hymel, S. (1986). Interpretation of peer behavior: Affective bias in childhood and adolescence. *Child Development, 57*(2), 431–445.

Hymel, S., Bowker, A., & Woody, W. (1993). Aggressive versus withdrawn unpopular children: Variations in peer- and self-perceptions in multiple domains. *Child Development, 64*, 879–896.

Hymel, S., Wagner, E., & Butler, L. J. D. (1990). *Peer rejection in childhood.* New York: Cambridge University Press.

Kauffman, J. M. (2001). *Characteristics of emotional and behavioral disorders of children and youth* (7th ed.). Upper Saddle River, NJ: Merrill Prentice-Hall.

Kellam, S. G., Rebok, G. W., Ialongo, N., & Mayer, L. S. (1994). The course and malleability of aggressive behavior from early first grade into middle school: Results of a developmental epidemiologically based preventive trial. *Journal of Child Psychology and Psychiatry, 35,* 359–382.

Kelley, B. T., Loeber, R., Keenan, K., & DeLamatre, M. (1997). *Developmental pathways in boys' disruptive and delinquent behavior.* Washington, DC: Office of Juvenile Justice and Delinquency Prevention.

Kennedy, J. H., & Kennedy, C. E. (2002, February). *Developmental trajectories of children classified as disorganized in attachment.* Poster presented at the annual meeting of the National Association of School Psychologists, Chicago.

Ladd, G. W. (1997). Classroom peer acceptance, friendship, and victimization: Distinct relational systems that contribute uniquely to children's school adjustment? *Child Development, 68*(6), 1181–1197.

Ladd, G. W., & Burgess, K. B. (1999). Charting the relationship trajectories of aggressive, withdrawn, and aggressive/withdrawn children during early grade school. *Child Development, 70*(4), 910–929.

Ladd, G. W., & Burgess, K. B. (2001). Do relational risks and protective factors moderate the linkages between childhood aggression and early psychological and school adjustment? *Child Development, 72*(5), 1579–1602.

Ledingham, J. E., & Schwartzman, A. E. (1984). A 3-year follow-up of aggressive and withdrawn behavior in childhood: Preliminary findings. *Journal of Abnormal Child Psychology, 16,* 539–552.

Lynch, M., & Cicchetti, D. (1992). Maltreated children's reports of relatedness to their teachers. *New Directions for Child Development, 37,* 81–108.

Lyons-Ruth, K. (1996). Attachment relationships among children with aggressive behavior problems: The role of disorganized early attachment patterns. *Journal of Counseling and Clinical Psychology, 64,* 64–73.

Lyons-Ruth, K., Alpern, L., & Repacholi, B. (1993). Disorganized infant attachment classification and maternal psychosocial problems as predictors of hostile aggressive behavior in the preschool classroom. *Child Development, 64,* 572–585.

Lyons-Ruth, K., Easterbrooks, M. A., & Cibelli, C. D. (1997). Infant attachment strategies, infant mental lag, and maternal depressive symptoms: Predictors of internalizing and externalizing behavior problems at age 7. *Developmental Psychology, 33,* 681–692.

Magnusson, D. (1997). The person in developmental research. *Report from the Department of Psychology, Stockholm University, 830,* 1–14.

Main, M., & Cassidy, J. (1988). Categories of response to reunion with the parent at age six: Predictable from infant attachment classifications and stable over a one-month period. *Developmental Psychology, 24,* 415–526.

Main, M., & Solomon, J. (1990). Procedures for identifying infants as disorganized/disoriented during the Ainsworth Strange Situation. In M. Greenberg, D. Chicette, & E. M. Cumings (Eds.), *Attachment in the preschool years: Theory, research and practice* (pp. 121–160). Chicago: University of Chicago Press.

Mash, E. J., & Wolfe, D. A. (2002). *Abnormal child psychology.* Belmont, CA: Wadsworth.

Milich, R., & Landau, S. (1984). A comparison of the social status and social behavior of aggressive and aggressive/withdrawn boys. *Journal of Abnormal Child Psychology, 12,* 277–288.

Moss, E., Rousseau, D., Parent, S., St-Laurent, D., & Saintonge, J. (1998). Correlates of attachment at school age: Maternal reported stress, mother–child interaction, and behavior problems. *Child Development, 69*(5), 390–405.

Moss, E., & St-Laurent, D. (2001). Attachment at school age and academic performance. *Developmental Psychology, 37,* 863–874.

National Educators Association. (2002). *2002 Tomorrow's Teachers: Help Wanted: Minority Teachers.* Washington, DC: National Educators Association.

Owens, G., Crowell, J. A., Pan, H., Treboux, D., O'Connor, C., & Waters, E. (1995). The prototype hypothesis and the origins of attachment working models: Adult relationships with parents and romantic partners. *Monographs of the Society for Research in Child Development, 60*(2–3), 216–233.

Pianta, R. C. (1999). *Enhancing relationships between children and teachers.* Washington, DC: American Psychological Association.

Pianta, R. C., & Harbors, K. (1996). Observing mother and child behavior in a problem-solving situation at school entry: Relations with academic achievement. *Journal of School Psychology, 34,* 307–322.

Pianta, R. C., Steinberg, M., & Rollins, K. (1995). The first two years of school: Teacher–child relationships and deflections in children's classroom adjustment. *Development and Psychopathology, 7,* 297–312.

Pianta, R. C., Tietbohl, P. J., & Bennett, E. M. (1997). Adult–child relationship processes and early schooling. *Early Education and Development, 8*(2), 137–152.

Pianta, R. C., & Walsh, D. (1996). *High-risk children in the schools: Creating sustaining relationships.* New York: Routledge.

Posada, G., Waters, E., Crowell, J., & Lay, K. L. (1995). Is it easier to use a secure mother as a secure base: Attachment Q-sort correlates of the Berkeley Adult Attachment Interview. *Monographs of the Society for Research in Child Development, 60*(2–3, Serial No. 244), 133–145.

Prinz, R. J., & Miller, G. E. (1991). Issues in understanding and treating childhood conduct problems in disadvantaged populations. *Journal of Clinical Child Psychology, 20*(4), 379–385.

Robertson, K., Chamberlain, B., & Kasari, C. (2003). General education teachers' relationships with included students with autism. *Journal of Autism and Developmental Disorders, 33*(2), 123–130.

Sameroff, A. J. (1983). Developmental systems: Context and evolution. In P. H. Mussen (Series Ed.) & W. Kessen (Vol. Ed.), *Handbook of child psychology: Vol. 1. History, theory, and methods* (pp. 237–294). New York: Wiley.

Schofield, G. (2002). The significance of a secure base: A psychosocial model of long-term foster care. *Child and Family Social Work, 7,* 259–272.

Solomon, J., George, C., & DeJong, A. (1995). Children classified as controlling at age six: Evidence of disorganized representational strategies and aggression at home and at school. *Development and Psychopathology, 7,* 447–463.

Speltz, M. L., Greenberg, M. T., & DeKlyen, M. (1990). Attachment in preschoolers with disruptive behavior: A comparison of clinic-referred and nonproblem children. *Development and Psychopathology, 2,* 31–46.

Spencer, M. B. (1999). Social and cultural influences on school adjustment: The application of an identity-focused cultural ecological perspective. *Educational Psychologist, 34,* 43–57.

Steele, H., & Steele, M. (1994). Intergenerational patterns of attachment. In D. Perlman & K. Bartholomew (Eds.), *Attachment processes in adulthood* (pp. 93–120). Bristol, PA: Jessica Kingsley.

Stormshak, E. A., Bierman, K., and the Conduct Problems Prevention Research Group. (1998). The implications of different developmental patterns of disruptive behavior problems for school adjustment. *Development and Psychology, 10,* 451–467.

Taylor, A. (1989). Predictors of peer rejection in early elementary grades: Roles of problem behavior, academic achievement, and teacher preference. *Journal of Clinical Child Psychology, 18,* 360–365.

Waters, E., & Cummings, E. M. (2000). A secure base from which to explore close relationships. *Child Development, 71*(1), 164–172.

Weinfield, N. S., Sroufe, L. A., & Egeland, B. (2000). Attachment from infancy to early adulthood in a high-risk sample: Continuity, discontinuity, and their correlates. *Child Development, 71*(3), 695–701.

West, M., Rose, S., Spreng, S., Sheldon-Keller, A., & Adam, K. (1998). Adolescent Attachment Questionnaire: A brief assessment of attachment in adolescence. *Journal of Youth and Adolescence, 27*(5), 661–673.

Williams, J. H., Ayer, C. D., Abbot, R. D., Hawkins, J. D., & Catalano, R. F. (1999). Racial differences in risk factors for delinquency and substance abuse among adolescents. *Social Work Research, 23,* 241–256.

Zionts, L., Anhalt, K., Devore, H., & Davidson, S. (2004, April). *Children's school adjustment: The impact of teacher and parent relationships.* Paper presented at the annual meeting of the National Association for School Psychologists, Dallas, TX.

CHAPTER 12

◆ ◆ ◆

Relationships Past, Present, and Future

Reflections on Attachment in Middle Childhood

H. ABIGAIL RAIKES
ROSS A. THOMPSON

It is no exaggeration to describe the contributors to this volume as pioneers at the frontiers of attachment research. Middle childhood is among the most important, and unexplored, developmental periods of attachment security. Chronologically situated between infancy and early childhood and adolescence and adulthood, middle childhood is the period in which the attachment behavioral system becomes a more fully representational system and attachment security begins to be characteristic of a person, not just of a specific relationship. In contrast to the well-established research literatures about other ages, however, less is known about attachment organization and functioning in middle childhood. This field is attracting new and experienced scientists who are interested in exploring influences on attachment and the implications of attachment security for personality and social development during this period.

It is not easy being a pioneer. In uncharted fields, it is often necessary to create makeshift tools and intuitive strategies when well-established procedures do not exist. This volume highlights the impressive creativity of researchers who have sought to shed new light on how to conceptualize and assess attachment security in older children. The contributors raise important issues concerning the hierarchy that may exist among attachment figures, the integration of representations of relationships into coherent, internal attachment patterns, and mediators of the relations between attachment security and its correlates. As one would expect, the chapters also reflect considerable diversity in measurement strategy: Observational, self-report, narrative, and other approaches are used. These contributions are essential to inaugurating new work in this area, but now the challenge in moving forward is to integrate this theoretical and methodological pluralism into a coherent view of attachment in later childhood. Perhaps this is why Solomon and George (1999) bemoaned the "frontier mentality" of contemporary attachment research. It is challenging to create new conceptions and measures of attachment functioning; it is even more difficult to systematically validate and integrate them.

We believe that the time is right to do so. Middle childhood is, for reasons we describe herein, a unique developmental period for the growth of attachment. As a consequence, it can be studied neither as a developmentally upward extension of the behavioral attachments of infancy nor as the downward extension of the representational sophistication of adulthood. Attachment in middle childhood must be understood in terms of its own developmental characteristics. In doing so, attachment researchers must address a number of conceptual and methodological problems that have the potential of contributing to the emergence of a genuine lifespan theory of attachment and to the implementation of lifespan theory in new assessment strategies. This is one reason that the study of attachment in middle childhood is so important.

In this commentary chapter, we draw on the provocative insights of the contributors to this volume to outline issues that are crucial to creating an integrative view of attachment in middle childhood. In the section that follows, we describe the core developmental achievements that make the later childhood years a unique period for parent–child relationships and for the internal working models that underlie attachment security. We then consider the implications of these developmental changes for how the security of attachment should be conceptualized in middle childhood. We argue that theory development is important for clarifying expectations of how attachment is organized and functions in later childhood and is essential as a guide to assessment strategies. This section poses some of the central questions for the growth of attachment theory in later childhood, drawing on the ideas of the contributors to this volume. In a third section, finally, we turn to methodological considerations in assessing attachment in middle childhood. We consider how the measurement of security should be validated and core validational criteria.

DEVELOPMENTS IN MIDDLE CHILDHOOD

In contrast to some traditional portrayals of middle childhood as a period of psychological latency, remarkable advances in conceptual skills and social competence take place during this period. The sophistication of thinking improves, influencing how children view themselves and others, and these changes provide a foundation for growth in social skills and social cognition. As noted throughout this volume, children's social worlds expand, and their relationships with peers and other adults become more intense and complex. Middle childhood is also marked by normative and non-normative events that influence children's socioemotional development. Most children enter puberty, which can begin as early as age 9. They spend increasing amounts of time in social contexts outside of the family, such as school, sports teams, and other social activities. In addition, many children experience the dissolution or reconstitution of their families during middle childhood. The host of cognitive and social changes experienced by children during this period makes the study of attachment in middle childhood important and challenging because such developments also provide the groundwork for new forms of attachment-related behaviors and representations.

Cognitive Development

Between the ages of 7 and 11, children's thinking becomes more internally consistent, logical, and objective as children move toward abstract reasoning (Flavell, Miller, & Miller, 2002). A generation of research inspired by Piagetian theory has shown that, whereas preschoolers are more intuitive and perception-bound thinkers, older children are capable of divorcing apparent phenomena from underlying (often invisible) causes and realities, and this makes them more insightful and systematic thinkers. They are also more flexible in their reasoning because of a developing capacity for recursive thought, enhanced ability to consider multiple perspectives or ideas simultaneously, and greater mental processing speed and efficiency. Memory retention increases in middle childhood, aided substantially by the use of mental strategies to organize and recall information. Some of these cognitive skills have particular significance for social interaction and emotional development, such as in older children's greater insight into the underlying mental, emotional, and motivational origins of people's actions and their greater capacities to reflect on themselves and their experiences.

One of the most significant cognitive advances in middle childhood is the ability to think about thinking, or metacognition (Flavell et al., 2002). Metacognitive skills arise during middle childhood as children gain the ability to reflect on their own cognitive processes. As a result, older children begin to use knowledge of their mental capacities to monitor internal reasoning processes, such as knowing when a spelling list has been mastered or realizing that the present strategy for learning words needs to be modified. Growth in metacognition emerges in the early elementary school years and continues to develop throughout middle childhood, and it is one reason that children are better learners at the end of elementary school than at the beginning.

Although metacognition supports children's academic competence in middle childhood, its influence on social and emotional development has been studied less extensively. However, in addition to providing strategies for organizing information mentally, the rise of metacognition means that children can also reflect on their own psychological processes—such as emotions, motives, and thoughts—and make them objects of conscious thought in ways that preschoolers cannot. In addition to changes in self-awareness, children also become more insightful interpreters of others' behavior, their concepts of relationships become more nuanced and sophisticated, and their capacities for self-regulation in general—and emotion regulation in particular—improve. We discuss these psychological advances in greater detail in the following sections.

Self-Concept and Self-Understanding

Self-concept develops substantially as older children become capable of thinking about themselves with greater psychological depth (Harter, 1999). Older children define themselves using psychological constructs, rather than exclusively in physical or behavioral terms. Although preschoolers can endorse psychological traits as self-descriptions (Eder, 1990), their spontaneous self-attributions tend to be defined by externally visible concepts (e.g., "I have brown hair"). By middle childhood, however, the self-concept becomes more inclusive of psychological criteria (e.g., "I am shy sometimes"), signaling a more nuanced and self-reflective view of the self. Consistent with this, the self-concept also becomes more multifaceted in middle childhood and taps many different dimensions of functioning, in contrast to the more global, unrealistic, and positive self-descriptions that generally characterize the preschool years. Older children begin to perceive themselves as having different constellations of strengths and weaknesses with respect to academic skills, athletic competence, relationships with friends, and other areas. Thus self-understanding becomes more sophisticated and differentiated (Harter, 1999).

Self-awareness also becomes more integrated in middle childhood. Children are forming overall impressions of themselves that are incorporated into representations of "global self-worth," or one's skills and deficiencies across a number of areas (Harter, 1999). The creation of global self-worth hinges on interactions with others, as children incorporate the messages they receive from significant others and the social world at large into models comparing who they should be with who they really are (Higgins, 1991). Global self-worth is especially influenced by how children perceive their strengths and weaknesses in areas that matter to them: Being poor athletically may have little influence on self-worth if athletic prowess is unimportant, but self-perceived interpersonal strengths are an asset to self-worth if getting along with others is important to the child. In this respect, therefore, self-worth incorporates social evaluations within the context of personal priorities. In addition, children's self-definitions in middle childhood more extensively incorporate comparisons of themselves with other people. Consequently, self-esteem tends to decline in middle childhood as children begin to notice areas of strengths and weaknesses in themselves in relation to those of others (Powers & Wagner, 1984).

In middle childhood, children become better reporters of their own emotional states, and they can describe feelings and their causes with greater depth and insight than can younger children (Saarni, Mumme, & Campos, 1998). However, they still tend to report more positive reactions to emotional situations than they might actually experience. An older child might report, for example, that he would not be sad at losing an important soccer game, but that other children would be. Despite this tendency, children are also more aware of the multifaceted emotions they feel in social situations. For example, a child of 10 might report, "I was excited to go to the amusement park, but scared to ride on the roller coaster," whereas preschool-age children will report that it is impossible to feel conflicting emotions at the same time (Flavell et al., 2002). Toward the end of middle childhood, children can also acknowledge ambivalence in important relationships. They will report complexities such as loving a parent but being angry at him or her in the moment (Harter & Whitesell, 1989).

These conclusions about the growth of self-concept and self-understanding have potentially important implications for understanding the nature of attachment security and the internal working models arising from relational experience in middle childhood. The greater psychological insight of children of this age makes them more open to the diverse and, at times, inconsistent facets of themselves and of their experiences that younger children may have more difficulty acknowledging, and it suggests that working models of the self are growing significantly in scope and complexity. Social evaluations and social comparisons are also increasingly important influences on how older children regard themselves at this age. Although little work has addressed the potential significance

of these developments for children's understanding of attachment relationships, the ability to consciously recognize the existence of positive and
negative emotions toward important people may alter both how children
comprehend and internalize feelings about attachment figures and their
ability to verbalize ambivalent or conflicting relational experiences in assessment procedures. For children of this age, perceiving problems in relationships or in other partners is not inconsistent with having strong
emotional attachments.

Social Understanding

Building on advances in theory of mind and emotion understanding in
the preschool years, children continue to refine their understanding of
other people's intentions, motives, and feelings in middle childhood, mir-
roring advances in self-understanding. During this period, children grasp
the concept of mixed emotions in other people as well as in themselves
(Harter, 1999), become more adept at deciphering social cues (Rubin,
Bukowski & Parker, 1998), and refine their skills in monitoring others'
emotion displays and communicating their emotions. They acquire more
capable social problem-solving skills, based on information-processing
strategies that entail more nuanced interpretation of others' social cues
and an awareness of alternative strategies for accomplishing social goals
and evaluating their outcomes (Crick & Dodge, 1994). Enhanced social
understanding improves children's insight into the behaviors of others
and gives children more control over the messages they send in interpersonal interaction.

Enhanced social understanding arises, in part, because children
increasingly perceive others as psychologically complex individuals
(Cillessen & Bellmore, 2002). Consistent with transitions in self-concept
development, by the end of the elementary school years, children tend to
see others' psychological characteristics as their most salient features and
to create descriptions of other people that are primarily psychological in
nature. The emphasis on psychological characteristics reflects children's
greater facility in tracing the psychological roots of behaviors, which
makes it easier to understand others. Children become better at predicting future behavior and actions because they begin to focus on the motivational and affective origins of behavior. This conceptual advance also
means that children perceive other people as differentiated and consistent
individuals, because they consciously comprehend others' behaviors as reflecting relatively stable and predictable psychological characteristics,
rather than seeing behavior as primarily a response to external conditions. Children's definition of friendship also matures; instead of seeing
friends as primarily partners in shared activity, friendships are now seen

as mutually selective and enduring, based on psychological compatibility. Older children are motivated to maintain relationships even during times of conflict with friends—which are frequent (Rubin et al., 1998).

It is probable that children's understanding of their parents changes in similar ways, such as increasingly focusing on psychological attributes, perceiving each parent as a differentiated personality with unique underlying qualities, and understanding better the connections between behavior and emotions, motivations, and thoughts. If so, it suggests that the "goal-corrected partnership" that Bowlby (1969/1982, 1973) highlighted as the fourth stage of attachment development, emerging in the early preschool years, becomes increasingly sophisticated in middle childhood, with older children far more sensitive to the complex psychological origins of parental conduct. To date, however, there has been little research describing developmental transitions in children's understanding of their relationships with parents, which is a significant gap in the research literature.

Children also have greater knowledge and competence in using emotional display rules in middle childhood, owing partly to conceptual advances that cause children to realize how internal, psychological experiences can be withheld or dissembled. Saarni and colleagues (1998) report that as children grow older, they are more likely to mask emotions in order to maintain cohesion within a relationship. However, children's decisions to display or hide emotions are also related to their perceptions of available emotional support, as children are more likely to display negative feelings if they perceive that parents are nearby to provide comfort. On the other hand, children's growth in social understanding also improves their ability to deceive others (Feldman, Tomasian, & Coats, 1999) and to engage in emotional manipulation such as bullying (Sutton, Smith, & Swettenham, 1999). Social understanding can be used for negative, as well as positive, ends. Also apparent by middle childhood are gender differences in emotional displays, with boys showing negative emotions such as sadness less frequently than girls. Children's ability to engage in strategic thinking regarding their emotional displays demonstrates the tightening links between conscious emotional thought and behavior in middle childhood (Saarni, 1999).

Emotion Regulation

In contrast to infancy and toddlerhood, children are increasingly managing their own emotional states in middle childhood. This shift in regulation from parent to child depends on the metacognitive skills mentioned previously: Children use their knowledge of themselves and their feelings to predict their emotional responses to challenging situations, increasing their ability to manage both emotional experience and expression (Thompson, 1994). Children are aware, for example, that emotional intensity decreases over time, especially if one does not think about an emotional event; that emotions can be altered by changing one's mental focus; and that reinterpreting the situation can also change emotional arousal (see Harris, 1989, for a general discussion). These and other cognitive controls may reflect some conscious understanding of defensive processing in older children. The growth in emotion self-regulation and cognitive self-control means that parents become decreasingly involved in children's moment-to-moment emotional states; but their role remains important, as children continue to turn to parents for emotional support and guidance throughout middle childhood (and well into adolescence).

The growth of emotion regulation—as part of the development of broader skills in self-regulation—has potentially significant implications for the organization and assessment of attachment security. Just as the manifestation of secure-base behavior shifts from an emphasis on physical proximity in infancy to the need for physical accessibility in early childhood, another change may occur in middle childhood as youths seek support that is psychological in nature and that harmonizes with the child's own self-regulatory efforts. Older children seek personal understanding in a way that preschoolers do not, understanding that adolescents will require even more. Moreover, anticipating the dynamic tension between autonomy and support in adolescence, secure-base behavior in middle childhood is likely to incorporate self-regulation with support-seeking activities, and sensitive parents will respect these dual needs. In addition, different varieties of insecurity may emerge as children of this age develop more elaborate and psychologically based styles of emotional self-regulation and, possibly, defensive processes (although there is little research into developmental changes in psychological defenses during this period; see, however, Ammaniti, van IJzendoorn, Speranza, & Tambelli, 2000, who found greater defensive processing at age 14 than at age 10). Taken together, therefore, growing capacities for self-management in middle childhood potentially change what is needed from the parent when difficult times arise, and this shift may alter the manifestations of secure-base behavior and other reflections of attachment security.

Although the social and cognitive changes described herein are normative, substantial individual differences exist in the content of self-representations and in the degree to which children are able to successfully maintain friendships, regulate emotions, and demonstrate knowledge of skills such as using emotion display rules. Many of the influences leading to these differences, such as troubled family relationships, temperamental vulnerability, and the availability or lack of social support, are also likely to influence the growth of attachment security in middle childhood. Consequently, understanding these contextual influences on psychological growth in older children may provide insights into developmental processes related to attachment.

Contextual and Physical Changes in Middle Childhood

Changes in Social Context

Along with the growing capacity of children to process and respond to social information in middle childhood, the number and types of relationships expands. Children develop meaningful relationships with teachers, coaches, peers, and others, and most of these relationships arise independently of parents; nearly 30% of all social interactions children experience are with peers in middle childhood, for example, compared with only 10% in early childhood (Rubin et al., 1998). Moreover, there is greater diversity in the types of social settings children experience, each of which calls for different kinds of social skills: school classrooms, peers' homes, practice fields, shopping malls, and other environments that children can often access independently of parental supervision. The host of relationships widens the circle of influences on children's ideas of relationships and stretches children's skills in relationship development and maintenance. These new relationships also give children opportunities to form significant bonds with people other than parents, although the associations they develop are not the same as the parent–child relationship and do not assume the same functions for the child.

Changing Family Dynamics

As many as 40% of children living in the United States experience the dissolution or reconstitution of their families during middle childhood (U.S. Bureau of the Census, 1998). This means that a large portion of children will spend at least some time growing up in a single-parent home, and many children will experience a period of renegotiation of familiar family relationships that, for younger children, is often associated with changes in attachment security (Thompson, 1998). As aptly described by Richardson (Chapter 2, this volume), the amount of parental monitoring, exposure to conflict within the family, and expectations for children's involvement in family life vary according to family structure. In turn, children may also have differing expectations for the level of emotional support provided by parents and peers, depending on experiences of significant changes or disruptions in family life. At the least, these patterns of change in family life suggest that, as older children are developing a more sophisticated and nuanced understanding of family relationships, many also encounter significant challenges to their sense of security and stability of the family.

Puberty

From a child's perspective, puberty is perhaps the most dramatic of all developmental changes in middle childhood. For most, it begins between the ages of 9 and 12 (Malina, 1990). More traditionally viewed as a rite of passage for children in early adolescence, children in the United States are beginning puberty at earlier ages than in the past. Richardson (Chapter 2, this volume) describes the many psychological and physical changes that take place during puberty and reviews the implications of these changes for relationships with parents and peers. Of particular note is her observation that the onset of puberty is highly individualized and may begin as early as the fourth grade. Puberty and the timing of puberty alter parent–child relationships and change how children view parents and themselves. In short, the biological transition of puberty has important social and emotional dimensions that alter close relationships and may influence attachment security.

Limitations

Although the social cognitive gains of middle childhood are impressive, it is also important to recognize cognitive limitations. Although older children are capable of greater psychological insight than younger children, they nevertheless lack the abstract representational skills and self-reflection of adolescents. The metacognitive skills that enable children to reflect on their own psychological states continue to develop throughout middle childhood and are inconsistently applied (Kuhn, 2001). Although children possess the ability to think more objectively about themselves and others, there is evidence that the sophistication of their problem-solving capabilities is inconsistently enlisted when children are experiencing emotionally challenging events (Ganzel, 1999). These findings are important to research on attachment in middle childhood because many of the relational experiences affecting the growth and maintenance of attachment security are likely to be emotionally charged, and the extent to which the conceptual capabilities of older children are enlisted in their assessment of relational experience remains to be explored.

One of the most notable changes from middle childhood to adolescence is the transition from concrete to abstract thinking. The transitional status of middle childhood has particular implications for the measurement of attachment security, especially for the use of measures that enlist metacognitive skills in reflecting on past relational experience, such as the Adult Attachment Interview (AAI). As described by Ammaniti,

Speranza, and Fidele (Chapter 6, this volume), measures such as the AAI assess security or insecurity based on the quality of discourse used to describe attachment relationships. Yet discourse styles vary by age. For example, Ammaniti and his colleagues (2000) noted that children in middle childhood more frequently engaged in the types of discourse that are taken to indicate insecurity among adolescents and adults, such as movement between past and present tenses and difficulty reaching an abstract level of description. Although Ammaniti and his colleagues adjusted the scoring of their interviews with younger children to account for these age-related differences, age differences in discourse raise broader questions about the suitability of measures for middle childhood that entail sophisticated metacognitive capabilities. More broadly, understanding the conceptual capabilities of children of different ages is a foundation for conceptualizing attachment security at each developmental period and the design of appropriate measures, discussed in greater detail subsequently.

Further, the term "middle childhood" encompasses a heterogeneous population. Individual differences in cognitive accomplishments and social skills highlight the considerable variation that exists between children of the same age, and children of different ages within this developmental period are likely to show significant differences in representational skills and social understanding. The challenge this presents to attachment theory and research is how to conceptualize attachment security in middle childhood, how attachment is related to attachment processes at earlier (and later) ages, and the implications for assessing attachment.

IMPLICATIONS FOR ATTACHMENT THEORY

What do these conceptual and contextual changes mean for theory and research on attachment in middle childhood? In concert with the chapters of this volume, the foregoing review poses several significant questions for attachment theorists to consider.

How Does the Goal-Corrected Partnership with Attachment Figures Change in Middle Childhood?

The distinctive feature of a goal-corrected partnership, in Bowlby's theory, is the mutual understanding of each partner's intentions and needs in the service of the attachment system. As earlier noted, middle childhood witnesses many advances in psychological and relational understanding that are likely to alter this partnership. Children are far more capable than they were in early childhood of understanding the complex influences on a parent's behavior—that a mother's abrupt or distracted demeanor may arise from the feelings elicited by a prior spousal argument, for example, or that each parent's personality can explain why they are sources of support in different circumstances. Although these capabilities are inconsistently enlisted in their understanding of actual relational experience, children also understand relationships to be based on psychological sharing between partners and to endure despite conflict, and they begin considering relational processes (e.g., friendship formation; ingroup and outgroup relations) for the first time. Each of these conceptual achievements means that the parent–child partnership is more mutual, with shared psychological understanding between partners and psychological inferences, attributions (and misattributions), and expectations shaping relational security. Conceptual advances also have important implications for the internal working models that arise from attachment relationships because they guide the conceptual skills by which children interpret new relational experience and, perhaps, reinterpret past relationships. One important task of attachment theorists is to elucidate further what these implications are.

As the contributors to this volume note, relational intimacy is also forged in more diverse interactive contexts in middle childhood. Moss, St-Laurent, Dubois-Comtois, and Cyr (Chapter 9, this volume) comment, for example, that the emotional sharing of parent–child communication is an important influence on attachment security for older children and on the stability of attachment from earlier ages (see also Thompson, 2000; Thompson, Laible, & Ontai, 2003). This may occur, as Richardson (Chapter 2, this volume) reminds us, because children's daily experience is more independent of the family, and thus conversations about school, peers, clubs, and other activities become more important forums for disclosing and discussing significant events. As Mayseless (Chapter 1, this volume) notes, different attachment figures may also assume different attachment functions for older children because of the distinctive relationships that children develop with different partners. For these reasons, it is unsurprising that Ammaniti, Moss, Steele, their colleagues, and other contributors to this volume note that attachment security in middle childhood is a product both of developmental history and of current experience in the relationship. This view, which was shared by Bowlby, emphasizes that, as their partnership evolves with the psychological growth of the child, the continuing quality of parent–child interaction maintains a crucial influence on the security of attachment.

How Do the Developmental Changes of Middle Childhood Alter Attachment Functioning?

In light of this, and because of the psychological growth of the child, it is reasonable to expect that the attachment system changes in middle childhood. In Chapter 1 (this volume), Ofra Mayseless identifies some of the most important functional changes. Rather than seeking physical proximity to their caregivers, older children desire their accessibility and, we have argued, psychological support. The activating and terminating conditions for the attachment system also change to reflect older children's greater ease with being separated from partners, the greater psychological complexity of the threatening conditions activating the attachment systems, children's greater responsibility for monitoring and maintaining access to attachment figures, and their capacities to interact with their partners symbolically (such as through notes) or through distal means (such as phone calls or "instant messaging"). Mayseless also underscores the decreased intensity of attachment behavior, at least with respect to manifestations of distress at the absence of the attachment figure. She proposes that middle childhood is a phase of "preparation for refocusing (reorienting) attachment investment" from parents to other partners.

The view that parent–child attachments become psychologically less intense in middle childhood and that peer attachments become relatively more important during this time is consistent with widespread views of the relational transitions of adolescence. But it is also valuable to keep in mind the continuing unique role of parents as attachment figures throughout much of life. As Kerns, Schlegelmilch, Morgan, and Abraham comment (Chapter 3, this volume), older children may prefer peers for companionship, but parents remain critical for fulfilling core attachment needs. This is consistent with the research on adolescence that shows that, although peers gain influence over many teenage decisions about style, appearance, and taste, adolescents still prefer parents for guidance on core moral values, political and religious beliefs, and planning and achieving life goals (Coleman & Hendry, 1990). The central issue for attachment theory is thus whether the decreased intensity of the expression of attachment to parents in middle childhood signals a transfer of attachment functions to peers (such as romantic partners) or instead reflects a change in the functioning and expression of the parent–child attachment system in the context of its continuing importance to the child. Addressing such a question requires a better understanding of the course of parent–child attachment throughout the adolescent and adult years and the evolving functions of this relationship with psychological maturity.

Who Are Attachment Figures in Later Childhood?

In view of the increasing diversity of the social worlds of older children and the growing importance of peers, it is common to conclude that middle childhood witnesses a growing number of attachment figures. Such a view looks ahead to young adulthood, when peer relationships are central to social experience and relationships with romantic partners assume attachment-like functions. In Chapter 1 of this volume, Mayseless describes the growing number of attachment figures as one of the hallmarks of middle childhood. In Chapter 4, Kobak, Rosenthal, and Serwick explore whether children create reliable hierarchies among their attachment figures and the implications of hierarchy violations for children's psychological well-being.

How do we know whether an individual has become an attachment figure to a child? Attachment partners are believed to be distinct from other affiliative partners because they provide a psychological safe haven, especially when children are stressed or threatened, and constitute a psychological secure base that promotes confident exploration and mastery and that contributes to emotional self-regulation. The behaviors that reflect attachment to a partner (such as a stepparent) in middle childhood might include seeking that person out when distressed, desiring psychological access to that person (especially when it is precluded), sharing events of significance, seeking help with problems, and perhaps even making efforts to maintain the esteem of the attachment partner and competing for that person's exclusive attention. It is not apparent when, or if, peers or teachers begin to assume these attachment-related functions in middle childhood or later. To be sure, older children certainly develop close friendships characterized by support, intimacy, and exclusivity. Whether these constitute attachments—and how they compare with parent–child attachments—remains one of the central questions about which attachment theorists disagree. Using a behavioral systems analysis, for example, Ainsworth (1989) distinguished even close romantic relationships from attachments because of the different systems relevant to each, even though others (e.g., Hazan & Shaver, 1994) consider adult pair bonds as a kind of attachment. Thus, defining the nature of attachment and its generality beyond the parent–child relationship constitutes a critical theoretical concern.

An equally critical question about which less is known is: How do we know when a partner fails to remain an attachment figure? The demographics of marital divorce and separation indicate that many children are living in single-parent homes or with stepparents by middle childhood. The research on divorce and custody suggests that, even as children are progressively losing contact with their noncustodial fathers, they remain emotionally committed to their relationships with their absent dads (Thompson & Laible, 1999). How long can attachments—or, more broadly, representations of a close relationship with a parent—endure in the context of limited continuing contact with that person? Attachment research could yield important insights into this issue that would serve both theory development and social policy.

Do New Forms of Security and/or Insecurity Emerge with Psychological Growth?

In light of the changes in parent–child relationships and attachment functioning described previously, it would be unsurprising to discover that new forms of security or insecurity emerge in middle childhood. Such a view has been proposed by Crittenden (2000), who has argued that psychological growth in childhood and adolescence yields organizational changes in attachment. In her dynamic–maturational approach, new attachment patterns are expected to emerge from the fourfold Strange Situation classifications of infancy as children and youth develop more differentiated forms of security and insecurity in relationships and a broader array of behavioral strategies for expressing them.

Yet Crittenden's view is contrary to most contemporary research, in which attachment studies of childhood, adolescence, and adulthood maintain close fidelity to the fourfold classifications identified in infancy. The approach of most researchers is to follow the example of the AAI, which was developed to predict the attachment classifications of offspring based on parental interviews, and consequently adult classifications closely parallel the fourfold infancy classifications developed from the Strange Situation (Hesse, 1999). Many attachment researchers focus even more exclusively on the differences between securely and insecurely attached children, ignoring variations within each group. The contributors to this volume reflect these trends in contemporary scholarship. Some (such as Kerns and her colleagues, Chapter 3; Verschueren & Marcoen, Chapter 10; and Booth-LaForce, Rubin, Rose-Krasnor, & Burgess, Chapter 8), focus exclusively on the security–insecurity distinction, but others (such as Moss et al., Chapter 9; Ammaniti et al., Chapter 6; and Yunger, Corby, and Perry, Chapter 5) emphasize the importance of exploring variations among insecure attachment groups as well. Yet with the exception of some D classification subgroups that emerge in early childhood (see Moss et al., Chapter 9, this volume), none of the authors of this volume has proposed that middle childhood witnesses the emergence of qualitatively new forms of attachment security or insecurity that are not anticipated in infancy Strange Situation classifications, nor have other researchers in this field (see the review by Kerns et al. in Chapter 3, this volume).

Assessing attachment organization in ways that maintain consistency with the original fourfold classification system of the Strange Situation is ideal for identifying consistency in attachment status over time, which has been a major concern of attachment researchers. But when measures are designed in this way, it begs the question of whether new forms of attachment organization emerge with psychological growth in childhood, adolescence, or adulthood. The question it raises is not only methodological but also theoretical. What are the implications of the developmental changes in psychological understanding and of parent–child relationships for the organization of attachment after infancy? If the organization of attachment security is believed to remain unchanging from infancy to adulthood, why? Are the psychological changes from infancy to adolescence irrelevant to how attachment security is organized? And if the organization of attachment security changes, why is it not reflected in more diverse classifications?

How Do Internal Working Models Develop in Middle Childhood?

Crucial to addressing these questions is understanding the nature of the internal working models that are believed to arise from secure or insecure attachments. Beginning in infancy, these representations of relational experience are thought to be related to broader representations of the attachment figure and the self and to contribute to implicit decision rules about how to relate to others that cause new relationships to be influenced by one's relational history (Bretherton & Munholland, 1999). But beyond these heuristically powerful ideas, there is considerable confusion about what internal working models are, how they develop, and how they relate to other mental constructs of interest to developmental psychologists (Thompson & Raikes, 2003). In some views, internal working models are conceptualized in a manner resembling the dynamic unconscious, shaped by relational experience that is interpreted through the perceptual–affective schemas of infancy, and thus largely inaccessible to conscious influences. From this perspective, the initial organization of attachment security is likely to persist throughout the life course because it endures as an affective core beneath the conscious changes that occur with relational experience. In other views, internal working models are portrayed as functioning more like scripts or schemas, and they become associated over time with other conscious mental constructs such as event representations and autobiographical memory. From this perspective, one would expect working models to change developmentally with conceptual growth and further relational experience. Few attachment theorists argue that internal working models do not change at all over time. But without greater theoretical clarity and specificity concerning the nature of internal working models, it is difficult to address central questions concerning developmental changes in attachment and its internal representations. It is also difficult to offer clear predictions concerning the relations between attachment security and broader features of sociopersonality development, because these predictions are usually based on the internal working models concept.

Perhaps the most important change in attachment representations in middle childhood is the progressive integration of relationship-specific internal working models into attachment representations that are characteristic of the person, not just of specific relationships. In infancy and early childhood, we typically think of children as secure with respect to a specific caregiver; in adolescence and adulthood, we commonly think of secure or insecure persons. But this volume presents somewhat inconsistent evidence as to whether attachment security is more characteristic of a relationship, or of the person, in middle childhood. Whereas Amminiti and his colleagues (Chapter 6, this volume) enlisted data from the Attachment Interview for Childhood and Adolescence (AICA; patterned on the AAI) to describe children's overall attachment security, and Kerns and her colleagues (Chapter 3, this volume) reported high concordance between mother–child and father–child security, Verschueren and Marcoen (Chapter 10, this volume) found that the correlates of attachment security in middle childhood were relationship specific, not necessarily generalized across partners. Their findings suggest that attachments perhaps influence children's development in a domain-specific fashion. This is a very different conceptualization from the model of an attachment hierarchy proposed by Kobak and colleagues (Chapter 4, this volume), which compares specific relationships according to consistent attachment-related criteria. Each view highlights, however, that the identity of the partner is crucial to the security children experience.

These conclusions suggest that the question of whether and how attachment-related representations become integrated in middle childhood must remain open. Further research is needed to empirically clarify the extent to which children's internal working models at this age are generalized across relationships or are relationship specific. In doing so, attachment researchers exploring middle childhood will again be breaking new ground. Measures of attachment security for older individuals have incorporated the assumption that attachment styles or states of mind are characteristic of the person, and researchers have rarely examined whether adolescents or adults also maintain relationship-specific representations. Is it possible that both exist within the hierarchically organized representational systems that internal working models are believed to be (Bretherton & Munholland, 1999)? If internal working models exist as *both* relationship-specific representations and as more generalized states of mind, it might help to clarify how attachment security can be both a personality construct and a relationship-specific construct at many periods of development.

How Is Attachment in Middle Childhood Associated with the Development of Competence?

A final question is one of the classic challenges for attachment theory: How is security of attachment related to competence in middle childhood? The contributors to this volume explore this question in relation to a range of developmental outcomes, including emotion understanding (Steele & Steele, Chapter 7), peer relations (Verschueren & Marcoen, Chapter 10; Booth-LaForce et al., Chapter 8), coping and adjustment (Yunger et al., Chapter 5; Moss et al., Chapter 9; Booth-LaForce et al., Chapter 8), and even academic achievement (Moss et al., Chapter 9). Importantly, they not only examine the direct relations between attachment and developmental outcomes but also explore the role of mediating variables. These mediators include self-worth, social support and social skills, parent–child communication, and relational stability and consistency in care. Attachment theorists have long acknowledged the necessity of examining mediators of the association between attachment and its sequelae, but studies are not often designed to elucidate them (and samples are often underpowered to reliably identify them). The research in this volume is a model, therefore, for future research efforts to explore the relations between attachment and developmental outcomes in a manner that recognizes that these outcomes are complex and multidetermined.

IMPLICATIONS FOR ATTACHMENT ASSESSMENT

The myriad of developmental transitions outlined herein means that assessing attachment in middle childhood is necessarily complex. The wide variety of measures used to index attachment in middle childhood reflects the ingenuity of attachment researchers but has also required researchers to examine what attachment means in older children. In this section, we consider a variety of methodological questions related to the study of attachment in middle childhood that arise from the preceding discussion of developmental and theoretical issues.

Should Attachment Representations in Middle Childhood Be Linked to Relational Interaction?

The Strange Situation has been the empirical anchor for attachment research because of the careful validational work of Ainsworth and her colleagues (Ainsworth, Blehar, Waters, & Wall, 1978). By linking detailed longitudinal observations of secure-base behavior at home with patterns of attachment in the Strange Situation, Ainsworth demonstrated that a 20-minute lab procedure could capture important dimensions of relational security in infancy. As Strange Situation observations were subsequently found to be associated with later features of socioemotional and personality functioning, attachment theorists began to understand Strange Situation behavior as reflecting underlying representations—or "working models"—of the caregiver's behavior that in certain circumstances maintained continuity over time (see Thompson, 1998, 1999). In the Strange Situation, behavioral manifestations of attachment security were closely linked to representations of the caregiver. Indeed, working models were inferred from behavior.

A key question for the study of attachment in middle childhood is whether researchers should similarly expect that the content of internal working models will be manifested in children's interactions with attachment partners (and, perhaps, other relational partners such as peers). If the preschool years witness the transition to more fully representational models of attachment, the reliance on semiprojective measures, self-report interviews and questionnaires, and narrative assessment approaches underscores how important are representations in defining attachment security in middle childhood (see Kerns et al., Chapter 3, this volume). Behavioral manifestations of attachment are complex and difficult to operationalize in middle childhood; the social and cognitive skills of older children make it easier to achieve felt security without requiring physical contact with caregivers or other manifestations of secure-base behavior that are apparent at younger ages. For both theoretical and methodological reasons, therefore, attachment researchers have used representational assessments in postinfancy research far more often than behavioral measures of attachment security, and they have rarely sought to validate self-report or narrative measures in relation to observations of parent–child interaction at home, as Ainsworth did in validating the Strange Situation. It is arguable, in fact, that representations are important regardless of their associations with actual relational interaction because they constitute the locus of consistency in attachment functioning.

However, an alternative view is suggested by lifespan research on attachment and, in particular, studies that link representations yielded by the AAI with adult caregiving behavior. Adult attachment classifications in the AAI reliably predict the sensitivity of parental care (see van IJzendoorn, 1995, for a review), suggesting that attachment representations at all stages of life should be reliably associated with attachment-relevant behavior in developmentally appropriate ways. Indeed, the connection between attachment behavior and attachment representations in adulthood is striking given the representational complexity and sophistication of adults and the importance of this connection for validating the AAI, which was designed to predict attachment in offspring through the quality of parental care.

If attachment representations and relational interaction are expected to meaningfully converge in middle childhood, this leaves unaddressed the question of how to design age-appropriate behavioral assessments of attachment. One approach is offered by Waters and Cummings (2000), who describe attachment in middle childhood as a "supervision partnership." Inherent in this concept is that children cooperate with parents to achieve goals of both exploration and security. Accordingly, attachment behaviors in middle childhood could be conceptualized as promoting security within parent–child relationships while maintaining cohesion and balance as the child strives for greater self-regulation and independence. Behaviors associated with attachment in middle childhood could include seeking a parent's assistance when stressed or upset, sharing affection with parents, disclosing information about important events in their lives, and seeking help with school or social problems. Other behaviors could include the child's cooperation with a parent's supervision of his or her activities, using the home as an important venue of activity, and participating in family activities (Waters & Cummings, 2000). Research indicating that children decide whether to reveal feelings of sadness and vulnerability based on the perceived availability of parental support (Saarni et al., 1998) suggests that self-disclosure about sensitive or difficult emotional issues may also reflect the extent to which children experience security in relationships with parents. The identification of age-appropriate attachment behaviors, coupled with investigations of how such behaviors change as children mature psychologically, could significantly enhance understanding of the relation between behavioral patterns and internal working models beyond infancy and early childhood. Central to such an effort is determining whether relationship-specific representations are in better concordance with children's behavior with specific partners or whether more global attachment representations (integrated across multiple partners) are better correlates of relational interaction. In addition, identifying behaviors related to security in middle childhood may also provide new insights into the types of behaviors that are associated with the correlates of security, such as peer acceptance, friendship quality, and social competence.

As this important work proceeds, there still remain significant challenges for conceptualizing the expected relations between attachment representations and behavior. The multidetermination of relational behavior and the complexity of relational representations together suggest that a tight linkage between the two is unlikely to occur and unreasonable to expect in middle childhood and beyond. For example, children's relational dispositions are likely to be shaped by experience in several close relationships, and representations of relationships likewise influenced by relational experience, discourse about relationships, and self-reflection. Denoting connections between relational representations and relational behavior is a conceptual challenge for middle childhood. Yet where assessment of attachment security is concerned, how valid are representations of relationships that are not manifested in relational interaction?

How Much Continuity Should We Expect from Infancy to Assessments in Later Childhood?

For many years, later-age attachment assessments have been validated by showing their concordance with infant attachment classifications in the Strange Situation. If children received the same security classifications at later ages as they did in infancy, the later assessments were believed to be valid. Yet the significant developmental changes from infancy to later childhood raise important questions about whether this is a reasonable expectation for at least two reasons. First, representational advances may themselves trigger a substantial reorganization of earlier representations because of the new understandings of self, others, and relationships that they are likely to foster (Stern, 1985). As older children become capable of new understanding of the workability and success of attachment strategies in the relationships and social contexts that characterize middle childhood, attachment security (or insecurity) may be prone to change because of the representational advances of this period. This may be why Bowlby (1973) portrayed attachment-related working models as slowly constructed throughout childhood and adolescence, becoming consolidated only at the end of this long period of gestation. Second, the years from infancy to middle childhood may also witness changes in close relationships and in the sensitivity of parents to children's developmental needs. Thus changes in attachment security may arise also because of changes in relationships themselves. This is consistent with Bowlby's view, shared by the contributors to this volume, that attachment security arises from both developmental history and current experience. A secure attachment history does not inoculate a child against later threats to security arising from marital discord, parental insensitivity, or family difficulty, nor does an insecure attachment history make the development of more secure parent–child relationships impossible.

These considerations are consistent with the empirical evidence: Short-term, as well as long-term, consistency in attachment classifications is extremely variable, with some children exhibiting consistency in security over a period of years, but with many showing instability in the security of attachment over several months (Thompson, 1998, 2000). There is also suggestive evidence that when attachment security changes, it is associated with changes in other features of the child's life related to their experience of close relationships. Although the stability evidence is inconsistent with expectations that attachment security should endure over time, it is consistent with our understanding of the developmental dynamics of relationships in childhood and of representational changes in children's understanding of relational experience, as well as with Bowlby's (1973) views of the long consolidation of attachment security and the working models with which it is associated.

This conclusion suggests, however, that in addition to considering the possibility that new forms of attachment organization emerge after infancy, continuity in security from infancy to later childhood may not be a satisfactory criterion for the validity of later-age attachment assessments. Because attachment strategies could experience substantial modification as children mature (Crittenden, 2000; Moss et al., Chapter 9, this volume), and because relational security may change as relationships evolve with the child's psychological maturing, the structure of internal working models should not necessarily be expected to remain consistent over time.

How Should Attachment Assessments in Middle Childhood Be Validated?

The research described in this volume offers abundant evidence that efforts to assess attachment security in middle childhood and to relate security to important developmental outcomes (such as emotional understanding, global self-worth, and friendship quality) are important and valuable. With these pioneering efforts having proven their worth, it is now important to address the validity of attachment assessments to ensure the enduring contribution of this work. If consistency with infancy Strange Situation classifications is not the validity standard, and if face validity is only one criterion, how else should researchers seek to validate their assessments of attachment in middle childhood?

Convergent Validity

Aptly elaborated by Kerns and colleagues (Chapter 3, this volume), there are many definitions of attachment security in middle childhood that encompass such potentially distinct features as the willingness to rely on parents for emotional support and children's openness and coherence in discussing emotional issues. Moreover, attachment itself is operationalized in various ways (e.g., security as relationship specific vs. integrated representations; hierarchy of attachment figures; insecurity as unidimensional vs. multidimensional; peers and teachers as potential attachment figures). Do these alternative conceptions assess a consistent underlying attachment construct? We concur with Kerns and her colleagues that more work is needed to reconcile differences between measures of security and that convergent validity is important, while acknowledging that the conceptual sophistication and complex relationships of older children make this challenging. Existing evidence is limited, but it suggests moderate concordance between measures of attachment in middle childhood (see Kerns et al., Chapter 3, this volume), which is consistent with the mixed convergence between different measures of attachment at younger ages also (Solomon & George, 1999).

Failure to find convergence between middle-childhood attachment measures does not necessarily raise validity concerns. Instead, lack of convergence may indicate that different attachment measures assess different dimensions of security in close relationships. A child's sense of security with parents as indexed by self-report, for instance, may be sensitive to current relational experience and influenced by the changes in interactional dynamics that accompany psychological growth in middle childhood. Responses to semiprojective narrative assessments, by contrast, may capture affective dimensions of the parent–child relationship that are more enduring but may also be affected by other, nonconscious influences less directly related to attachment security. If observations of attachment behaviors are used, they may reveal even more complexity in attachment functioning, because children's secure-base behaviors may be sensitive to *both* immediate relational experience and nonconscious processing. Thus lack of concordance between attachment measures may be further testament to the multifaceted nature of attachment security in middle childhood and the various functions of attachment relationships at this age. These constitute only working hypotheses, however, and more research is needed to evaluate assessments and how they are affected by relational processes and other influences (e.g., narrative processes, social desirability biases, culture and ethnicity) that may not be directly related to attachment security. The differentiation of attachment measures and their underlying cognitive and affective components may be particularly critical when addressing discriminant validity.

Discriminant Validity

Another important question concerns the extent to which measures of attachment security in middle childhood reliably predict outcomes and interactional styles theoretically related to security, while showing little association with outcomes not theoretically linked to security. Discriminant validity is critically important to ensuring that measures of attachment security are not simply assessments of good psychosocial functioning. But evaluating discriminant validity requires clear theoretical predictions concerning the outcomes that attachment should—and should not—predict (Thompson & Raikes, 2003). Although Kerns, Tomich, Aspelmeier, and Contreras (2000) made substantial progress in this area by demonstrating that children's reports on the Security Scale were relatively consistent over time and related to parents' reports of parenting styles and to children's reports of coping styles with parents, for example, there was still some indication that "all good things go together" with the finding that children with higher security scores also had higher scores on various measures of scholastic adjustment (Kerns, Klepac & Cole, 1996; Granot & Mayseless, 2001). Clarifying whether the latter finding is consistent with theoretical expectations (e.g., secure children should be more academically competent), arises from the influence of third variables (e.g., supportive parenting is related both to security and to academic achievement), or is inconsistent with attachment theory is crucial to clarifying issues of convergent and discriminant validity. At present, the lack of clarity and consistency in theoretical predictions makes discriminant validity more difficult to demonstrate, and increases the risk that attachment theory will be tested against predictions that it should not be evaluated against because they are inappropriate extensions of the theory (Thompson & Raikes, 2003).

Moreover, consistent with the idea that different measures of security in middle childhood may address distinct components of security, we may find that some measures of security are better predictors of some outcomes than others. For instance, Granot and Mayseless (2001) found that responses to the Doll Story Completion Task were more predictive of sociometric ratings than responses to the Security Scale but were also more strongly related to grade point averages. In addition to helping establish the validity of assessments of attachment in middle childhood, therefore, tests of discriminant validity may provide valuable insight into the types of functioning tapped by various measures of security in middle childhood.

In sum, considering the methodological questions associated with measuring attachment in middle childhood may provide new ideas about the nature of secure-base behavior and internal working models for children in this developmental stage. In addition, understanding how measures of attachment differentially predict children's outcomes may provide important insights into the various components of security among children in middle childhood. Perhaps most important, attachment assessments in middle childhood should be driven by theoretically based hypotheses regarding the nature of attachment during this period.

CONCLUSION

Attachment theory became prominent when infancy researchers established reliable empirical associations between secure-base functioning at home, Strange Situation behavior, and children's later developmental outcomes. At that time, researchers were guided by clear and straightforward (albeit provocative) hypotheses concerning developmental continuity, and the Strange Situation was the exclusive assessment of attachment security. Indeed, security of attachment was so readily indexed in the Strange Situation that some critics worried that the construct and index had become confounded, making it difficult to know whether influences on Strange Situation behavior were also influences on attachment security.

Contemporary attachment research is messier and more interesting. A wide variety of attachment assessments unconfound index and construct but raise new questions about the nature of the attachment construct they measure. The greater psychological sophistication of the older child makes it more challenging to conceptualize internal working models, attachment organization, and the nature of parent–child relationships in developmentally appropriate ways. And a quarter century of attachment research provides a framework within which research on middle childhood is conceived and interpreted. We believe that the contributors to this volume have broken new ground in theory and measurement and, equally important, have brought the field to the vanguard of new advances. These advances are ensured if attachment scholars take up the challenge of perceiving attachment in middle childhood as the product of a unique developmental period for close relationships, forged by the conceptual advances and relational challenges of the school-age years, and at the nexus of the behavioral and representational processes that shape attachment security throughout life.

REFERENCES

Ainsworth, M. D. S. (1989). Attachments beyond infancy. *American Psychologist, 44,* 709–716.

Ainsworth, M. D. S., Blehar, M. C., Waters, E., & Wall, S. (1978). *Patterns of attachment.* Hillsdale, NJ: Erlbaum.

Ammaniti, M., van IJzendoorn, M., Speranza, A.M., & Tambelli, R. (2000). Internal working models of late childhood and early adolescence: An exploration of stability and change. *Attachment and Human Development, 2,* 328–346.

Bowlby, J. (1973). *Attachment and loss: Vol. 2. Separation: Anxiety and anger.* New York: Basic Books.

Bowlby, J. (1982). *Attachment and loss: Vol. 1. Attachment* (2nd ed.). New York: Basic Books. (Original work published 1969).

Bretherton, I., & Munholland, K. A. (1999). Internal working models in attachment relationships: A construct revisited. In J. Cassidy & P. R. Shaver (Eds.), *Handbook of attachment: Theory, research, and clinical applications* (pp. 89–111). New York: Guilford Press.

Cillessen, A. H. N., & Bellmore, A. D. (2002). Social skills and interpersonal perception in early and middle childhood. In P. K. Smith & C. H. Hart (Eds.),

Blackwell handbook of childhood social development (pp. 355–374). Oxford, UK: Blackwell.

Coleman, J. C., & Hendry, L. (1990). *The nature of adolescence* (2nd ed.). London: Routledge.

Crick, N. R., & Dodge, K. A. (1994). A review and reformulation of social information processing mechanisms in children's social adjustment. *Psychological Bulletin, 115,* 74–101.

Crittenden, P. M. (2000). A dynamic–maturational exploration of the meaning of security and adaptation: Empirical, cultural, and theoretical considerations. In P. M. Crittenden & A. H. Claussen (Eds.), *The organization of attachment relationships: Maturation, culture, and context* (pp. 358–383). New York: Cambridge University Press.

Eder, R. A. (1990). Uncovering young children's psychological selves: Individual and developmental differences. *Child Development, 61,* 849–863.

Feldman, R. A., Tomasian, J. C., & Coats, E. J. (1999). Nonverbal deception abilities and adolescents' social competence: Adolescents with higher social skills are better liars. *Journal of Nonverbal Behavior, 23,* 237–249.

Flavell, J. H., Miller, P. H., & Miller, S. A. (2002). *Cognitive development* (4th ed.). Upper Saddle River, NJ: Prentice Hall.

Ganzel, A. K. (1999). Adolescent decision-making: The influence of mood, age, and gender on the consideration of information. *Journal of Adolescent Research, 14,* 289–318.

Granot, D., & Mayseless, O. (2001). Attachment security and adjustment to school in middle childhood. *International Journal of Behavioral Development, 25,* 530–541.

Harris, P. (1989). *Children and emotion: The development of psychological understanding.* Oxford, UK: Blackwell.

Harter, S. (1999). *The construction of the self: A developmental perspective.* New York: Guilford Press.

Harter, S., & Whitesell, N. R. (1989). Developmental changes in children's understanding of single, multiple, and blended emotion concepts. In C. Saarni & P. Harris (Eds.), *Children's understanding of emotion* (pp. 81–116). Cambridge, UK: Cambridge University Press.

Hazan, C., & Shaver, P. R. (1994). Attachment as an organizational framework for research on close relationships. *Psychological Inquiry, 5,* 1–22.

Hesse, E. (1999). The Adult Attachment Interview: Historical and current perspectives. In J. Cassidy & P. R. Shaver (Eds.), *Handbook of attachment: Theory, research, and clinical applications* (pp. 395–433). New York: Guilford Press.

Higgins, E. T. (1991). Development of self-regulatory and self-evaluative processes: Costs, benefits and tradeoffs. In M. R. Gunnar & L. A. Sroufe (Eds.), *Self processes and development: The Minnesota Symposia on Child Development* (Vol. 23, pp. 125–166). Hillsdale, NJ: Erlbaum.

Kerns, K. A., Klepac, L., & Cole, A. (1996). Peer relationships and preadolescents' perceptions of security in the child–mother relationship. *Developmental Psychology, 33,* 703–710.

Kerns, K. A., Tomich, P. L., Aspelmeier, J. E., & Contreras, J. M. (2000).

Attachment-based assessments of parent–child relationships in middle childhood. *Developmental Psychology, 36,* 614–626.

Kuhn, D. (2001). Why development does (and doesn't) occur: Evidence from the domain of inductive reasoning. In J. McClelland & R. Siegler (Eds.), *Mechanisms of cognitive development: Behavioral and neural perspectives* (pp. 221–249). Mahwah, NJ: Erlbaum.

Malina, R. M. (1990). Physical growth and performance during the transitional years (9–16). In R. Montemayor, G. R. Adams, & T. P. Gullotta (Eds.), *From childhood to adolescence: A transitional period?* (pp. 41–62). Newbury Park, CA: Sage.

Powers, S., & Wagner, M. J. (1984). Attributions for school achievement of middle school students. *Journal of Early Adolescence, 4,* 215–222.

Rubin, K., Bukowski, W., & Parker, J. (1998). Peer interactions, relationships and groups. In W. Damon (Series Ed.) & N. Eisenberg (Vol. Ed.), *Handbook of child psychology: Vol. 3. Social and personality development* (pp. 621–700). New York: Wiley.

Saarni, C. (1999). *The development of emotional competence.* New York: Guilford Press.

Saarni, C., Mumme, D., & Campos, J. (1998). Emotional development: Action, communication, and understanding. In W. Damon (Series Ed.) & N. Eisenberg (Vol. Ed.), *Handbook of child psychology: Social and personality development* (Volume 3, pp. 238–309). New York: Wiley.

Solomon, J., & George, C. (1999). The measurement of attachment security in infancy and childhood. In J. Cassidy & P. R. Shaver (Eds.), *Handbook of attachment: Theory, research, and clinical applications* (pp. 287–316). New York: Guilford Press.

Stern, D. N. (1985). *The interpersonal world of the infant.* New York: Basic.

Sutton, J., Smith, P. K., & Swettenham, J. (1999). Social cognition and bullying: Social inadequacy or skilled manipulation? *British Journal of Developmental Psychology, 17,* 435–450.

Thompson, R. A. (1994). Emotion regulation: A theme in search of definition. In N. A. Fox (Ed.), The development of emotion regulation and dysregulation: Biological and behavioral aspects. *Monographs of the Society for Research in Child Development, 59*(2–3, Serial No. 240), 25–52.

Thompson, R. A. (1998). Early sociopersonality development. In W. Damon (Series Ed.) & N. Eisenberg (Vol. Ed.), *Handbook of child psychology: Vol. 3. Social and personality development* (pp. 25–104). New York: Wiley.

Thompson, R. A. (1999). Early attachment and later development. In J. Cassidy & P. Shaver (Eds.), *Handbook of attachment: Theory, research, and applications* (pp. 265–286). New York: Guilford Press.

Thompson, R. A. (2000). The legacy of early attachments. *Child Development, 71*(1), 145–152.

Thompson, R. A., & Laible, D. J. (1999). Noncustodial parents. In M. E. Lamb (Ed.), *Parenting and child development in "nontraditional" families* (pp. 103–123). Hillsdale, NJ: Erlbaum.

Thompson, R. A., Laible, D. J., & Ontai, L. L. (2003). Early understanding of emotion, morality, and the self: Developing a working model. In R. V. Kail (Ed.), *Advances in child development and behavior* (Vol. 31, pp.137–171). San Diego, CA: Academic.

Thompson, R. A., & Raikes, H. A. (2003). Toward the next quarter-century: Conceptual and methodological challenges for attachment theory. *Development and Psychopathology, 15,* 691–718.

U.S. Bureau of the Census. (1998). Marital status and living arrangements. *Current population reports* (Series No. P20–514). Washington, DC: U.S. Government Printing Office.

van IJzendoorn, M. H. (1995). Adult attachment representations, parental responsiveness, and infant attachment: A meta-analysis on the predictive validity of the Adult Attachment Interview. *Psychological Bulletin, 117,* 387–403.

Waters, E., & Cummings, E. M. (2000). A secure base from which to explore close relationships. *Child Development, 71,* 164–172.

Index

283